Positive Airway Pressure Therapy

Guest Editor

RICHARD B. BERRY, MD

SLEEP MEDICINE CLINICS

www.sleep.theclinics.com

September 2010 • Volume 5 • Number 3

SAUNDERS an imprint of ELSEVIER, Inc.

W.B. SAUNDERS COMPANY
A Division of Elsevier Inc.

1600 John F. Kennedy Boulevard • Suite 1800 • Philadelphia, PA 19103-2899

http://www.sleep.theclinics.com

SLEEP MEDICINE CLINICS Volume 5, Number 3
September 2010, ISSN 1556-407X, ISBN-13: 978-1-4377-2495-0

Editor: Sarah E. Barth
Developmental Editor: Donald Mumford

Sleep Medicine Clinics (ISSN 1556-407X) is published quarterly by Elsevier Inc., 360 Park Avenue South, New York, NY 10010-1710. Months of issue are March, June, September and December. Business and Editorial Offices: 1600 John F. Kennedy Blvd., Ste. 1800, Philadelphia, PA 19103-2899. Customer Service Office: 3251 Riverport Lane, Maryland Heights, MO 63043. Periodicals postage paid at New York, NY and additional mailing offices. Subscription prices are $150.00 per year (US individuals), $76.00 (US residents), $346.00 (US institutions), $185.00 (foreign individuals), $106.00 (foreign residents), and $381.00 (foreign institutions). Foreign air speed delivery is included in all *Clinics* subscription prices. All prices are subject to change without notice. **POSTMASTER:** Send change of address to *Sleep Medicine Clinics*, Elsevier Health Sciences Division, Subscription Customer Service, 3251 Riverport Lane, Maryland Heights, MO 63043 Customer Service, (orders, claims, online, change of address): **Elsevier Health Sciences Division, Subscription Customer Service, 3251 Riverport Lane, Maryland Heights, MO 63043. Tel: 1-800-654-2452 (U.S. and Canada); 314-447-8871 (outside U.S. and Canada). Fax: 314-447-8029. E-mail: journals customerservice-usa@elsevier.com (for print support); journalsonlinesupport-usa@elsevier.com (for online support).**

Reprints. For copies of 100 or more of articles in this publication, please contact the Commercial Reprints Department, Elsevier Inc., 360 Park Avenue South, New York, NY 10010-1710. Tel.: 212-633-3812; Fax: 212-462-1935; E-mail: reprints@elsevier.com.

Printed and bound in the United Kingdom
Transferred to Digital Print 2011

Sleep Medicine Clinics

THE CLINICS ARE NOW AVAILABLE ONLINE!

Access your subscription at:
www.theclinics.com

Contributors

CONSULTING EDITOR

TEOFILO LEE-CHIONG Jr, MD
Professor of Medicine and Chief, Division of Sleep
Medicine, National Jewish Health; Associate
Professor of Medicine, University of Colorado
Denver School of Medicine, Denver, Colorado

GUEST EDITOR

RICHARD B. BERRY, MD
Professor of Medicine, Medical Director,
UF & Shands Sleep Disorders Center; Division
of Pulmonary, Critical Care, and Sleep Medicine,
University of Florida, Gainesville, Florida

AUTHORS

OMER AHMED, MD
Fellow, Pulmonary and Critical Care Medicine,
Department of Medicine, University of Arizona,
Tucson, Arizona

W. MCDOWELL ANDERSON, MD
Professor of Medicine, University of South Florida;
Chief of Pulmonary, Critical Care and Sleep
Medicine, James A. Haley Veterans Affairs
Hospital; Medical Director, Sleep Disorder Center,
Tampa General Hospital, Tampa, Florida

RAMI ARFOOSH, MD
Staff Physician, Pulmonary Service, John D.
Dingell Veterans Affairs Medical Center;
Division of Pulmonary, Critical Care and Sleep
Medicine, Department of Internal Medicine,
Wayne State University School of Medicine,
Detroit, Michigan

KENDRA A. BECKER, MD, MPH
Sleep Medicine Fellow, Pulmonary, Critical Care
and Sleep Medicine, Veterans Affairs Greater
Los Angeles Healthcare System (VA GLA),
Sepulveda, California

PHILIP J. BERGER, PhD
Ritchie Centre for Baby Health Research, Clayton,
Victoria, Australia

RICHARD B. BERRY, MD
Professor of Medicine, Medical Director,
UF & Shands Sleep Disorders Center; Division
of Pulmonary, Critical Care, and Sleep Medicine,
University of Florida, Gainesville, Florida

NITIN Y. BHATT, MD
Assistant Professor of Medicine, Division
of Pulmonary, Allergy, Critical Care, and Sleep
Medicine, The Ohio State University,
Columbus, Ohio

**LEE K. BROWN, MD, BS (Electrical
Engineering)**
Professor of Internal Medicine and Pediatrics;
Vice Chair, Clinical Affairs, Department of Internal
Medicine, University of New Mexico School
of Medicine; Executive Director, Program in
Sleep Medicine, University of New Mexico Health
Sciences Center, Albuquerque, New Mexico

SANGEETA CHAKRAVORTY, MD
Assistant Professor of Pediatrics; Director,
Pediatric Sleep Laboratory, Children's Hospital
of Pittsburgh of University of Pittsburgh Medical
Center, University of Pittsburgh School of
Medicine, Pittsburgh, Pennsylvania

TAPAN DESAI, MD
Sleep Medicine Fellow, Division of Pulmonary, Allergy, Critical Care, and Sleep Medicine, The Ohio State University, Columbus, Ohio

BRADLEY A. EDWARDS, PhD
Ritchie Centre for Baby Health Research, Clayton, Victoria, Australia; Brigham and Women's Hospital, Division of Sleep Medicine, Sleep Disorders Program and Harvard Medical School, Boston, Massachusetts

JONATHAN D. FINDER, MD
Professor of Pediatrics; Clinical Director, Pediatric Pulmonology, Children's Hospital of Pittsburgh of University of Pittsburgh Medical Center, University of Pittsburgh School of Medicine, Pittsburgh, Pennsylvania

S. JAVAHERI, MD
Emeritus Professor of Medicine, College of Medicine, University of Cincinnati; Medical Director, Sleepcare Diagnostics, Cincinnati, Ohio

KIRK KEE, MBBS
Department of Allergy, Immunology and Respiratory Medicine, Alfred Hospital, Melbourne, Australia

THOMAS G. KEENS, MD
Attending Pulmonologist, Childrens Hospital Los Angeles; Professor of Pediatrics, Physiology, and Biophysics, Keck School of Medicine at the University of Southern California, Los Angeles, California

MEENA KHAN, MD
Assistant Professor of Medicine, Division of Pulmonary, Allergy, Critical Care, and Sleep Medicine, The Ohio State University, Columbus, Ohio

CLETE A. KUSHIDA, MD, PhD
Stanford University Center of Excellence for Sleep Disorders, Stanford, California

MICHAEL R. LITTNER, MD
Pulmonary, Critical Care and Sleep Medicine, Veterans Affairs Greater Los Angeles Healthcare System (VA GLA), Sepulveda; Professor, Department of Medicine, David Geffen School of Medicine at University of California Los Angeles, Los Angeles, California

ATUL MALHOTRA, MD
Associate Professor of Medicine, Sleep Division, Brigham and Women's Hospital, Boston, Massachusetts

SHERWIN M. MINA, MS, MD
Sleep Medicine Fellow, University of South Florida, Tampa, Florida

MATTHEW T. NAUGHTON, MD
Professor, Department of Allergy, Immunology and Respiratory Medicine, Alfred Hospital, Melbourne; Faculty of Medicine, Monash University, Clayton, Victoria, Australia

SAIRAM PARTHASARATHY, MD
Chief of Research, Southern Arizona Veterans Administration Healthcare System; Associate Professor of Medicine, Department of Medicine, University of Arizona, Tucson, Arizona

IRIS A. PEREZ, MD
Attending Pulmonologist, Childrens Hospital Los Angeles; Assistant Professor of Pediatrics Keck School of Medicine at the University of Southern California, Los Angeles, California

CHARLES A. POON, MD
Sleep Medicine Fellow, Pulmonary, Critical Care and Sleep Medicine, Veterans Affairs Greater Los Angeles Healthcare System (VA GLA), Sepulveda, California

SHILPA RAHANGDALE, MD
Instructor in Medicine, Sleep Division, Brigham and Women's Hospital, Boston, Massachusetts

KANNAN RAMAR, MD
Division of Pulmonary, Center for Sleep Medicine, Sleep and Critical Care Medicine, Mayo Clinic, Rochester, Minnesota

JAMES A. ROWLEY, MD
Professor of Medicine, Division of Pulmonary, Critical Care and Sleep Medicine, Department of Internal Medicine, Wayne State University School of Medicine, Detroit, Michigan

SCOTT A. SANDS, BSc, BE
Ritchie Centre for Baby Health Research, Clayton, Victoria, Australia

ADRIAN VELASQUEZ, MD
Medical Resident, Department of Internal
Medicine, Caritas Carney Hospital, Tufts
University School of Medicine, Dorchester,
Massachusetts

SALLY L. DAVIDSON WARD, MD
Associate Professor of Pediatrics, Keck School
of Medicine at the University of Southern
California; Attending Pulmonologist, Head,
Division of Pediatric Pulmonology, Childrens
Hospital Los Angeles, Los Angeles, California

Contents

> Optimal adherence to nasal positive airway pressure as therapy for obstructive sleep apnea is a major problem faced by practicing sleep physicians. This article discusses the scope of the problem with adherence, predictors of adherence, including both demographic and psychological factors, and recent research on interventions to improve adherence, including behavioral therapy, interfaces, positive airway pressure modality, and treatment of adverse effects.

> The optimal pressure to treat sleep-related breathing disorders (SRBDs) using positive airway pressure (PAP) devices is usually obtained through performing an overnight attended polysomnography. Titration protocols to identify the optimal pressure vary widely from among sleep centers. Standardizing titration protocols brings uniformity to the whole titration process and improves reliability of treatment and overall quality of care. To help standardize the current practice, the American Academy of Sleep Medicine recently published clinical guidelines for the manual titration of PAP in patients with obstructive sleep apnea (OSA) but not for other SRBDs. This article describes the continuous PAP (CPAP) and bilevel PAP (BPAP) titration protocols for SRBDs (for not only OSA but also other SRBDs) in adults.

> Obstructive sleep apnea (OSA) is a condition characterized by intermittent upper airway closure during sleep that results in fragmented sleep and hypoxemia. Positive airway pressure (PAP) is the main form of treatment, with the most common mode of delivery being continuous positive airway pressure (CPAP). Despite its effectiveness in treating OSA, compliance with CPAP has been a long-standing problem. Issues with CPAP compliance include mask discomfort, pressure intolerance, nasal congestion, claustrophobia, and dryness. Many modifications have been developed to improve adherence, but with varying success. This article addresses the different forms of PAP therapy used to treat OSA. The authors also discuss the factors that have been shown to affect adherence and the innovations developed to improve compliance.

Omer Ahmed and Sairam Parthasarathy

> Positive airway pressure therapy (PAP) is a commonly prescribed treatment for obstructive sleep apnea (OSA). Traditionally, a sleep technician determined the optimal pressure for treatment of sleep-disordered breathing (SDB) through manual titration of the device during polysomnography. However, alternative methods for determination of optimal PAP, such as autotitrating PAP (APAP), have seen tremendous growth over the past decade. The purpose of this article is to improve understanding of the currently available alternative methods for titration of PAP in patients with SDB with special emphasis on OSA. Recent prospective randomized studies of alternative methods of titration suggest that pressure determinations made by these devices are comparable to traditional manual titrations made in the sleep laboratory. Obstacles to the adoption of these alternative modes of titration into daily practice may be attributable to issues surrounding appropriate patient selection, differences between devices, reimbursement policies of third-party payors, consensus among sleep experts, and individual physicians' practice patterns and volumes. Although newer generations and types of APAP devices are entering the sleep field constantly, providers' knowledge and time availability remain limiting factors. Tremendous growth is occurring in technology and scientific evidence supporting alternative modes of PAP titration for SDB, but barriers to implementation remain.

W. McDowell Anderson and Sherwin M. Mina

> Continuous positive airway pressure (CPAP) therapy has many adjunctive measures for controlling obstructive sleep apnea (OSA). Sedatives and hypnotics may have a role in improving adherence to CPAP use, but long-term studies of the effectiveness of these medications are pending. Although evidence showing that heated humidification improves adherence is conflicting, it does have a role in improving nasal symptoms related to CPAP use. Oxygen clearly has a role in improving oxygen saturation nadir in patients with sleep-disordered breathing. It can also be helpful as a supplement to CPAP or bilevel devices for patients experiencing hypoventilation. Here authors propose a simple algorithm for evaluating patients with a clinical impression of OSA. In the end, the goal of health care providers is to improve the quality of life in patients with OSA and prevent the adverse consequences of untreated disease. For patients who agree to CPAP therapy, health care providers must work together with individual patients to tailor their care to improve adherence and, consequently, treatment of OSA.

Adrian Velasquez, Shilpa Rahangdale, and Atul Malhotra

> In recent years, a continuous influx of theories and data suggest that obstructive sleep apnea (OSA) has a negative effect on cardiovascular health. OSA is likely an independent cardiovascular risk factor. Treatment of OSA with continuous positive airway pressure (CPAP) has been associated with significant improvement of certain cardiovascular diseases. CPAP use can improve hypertension in patients with OSA. In OSA patients with coronary artery disease, CPAP resulted in decreased numbers and severity of cardiovascular events. OSA patients with arrhythmias had decreased recurrence of atrial fibrillation with CPAP therapy. There is some evidence that CPAP use may also be beneficial in reducing visceral adiposity, although further investigation is needed to better characterize that effect. CPAP use in patients with OSA may

lead to improvement in vascular inflammation, endothelial function, and platelet function. Given the positive effect of CPAP on certain cardiovascular risk factors, long-term outcomes in patients with OSA and cardiovascular comorbidities may be improved with early recognition and appropriate treatment of OSA.

Positive Airway Pressure in Congestive Heart Failure   393

Kirk Kee, Scott A. Sands, Bradley A. Edwards, Philip J. Berger, and Matthew T. Naughton

Congestive heart failure (CHF) is a common disabling and costly condition, which is responsible for most hospital admissions and has a mortality rate on par with many malignancies. In recent years, positive airway pressure (PAP) has emerged as a novel therapeutic tool for pneumatically splinting open the sleep-related upper airway collapse; increasing lung volume, thereby increasing oxygen storage; and reducing the pressure gradient across the left ventricular wall, thereby reducing afterload. Strong evidence exists of physiologic efficacy and improved survival with PAP in acute pulmonary edema. Good evidence exists of physiologic improvement with PAP in chronic CHF associated with obstructive or central sleep apnea; however, good quality survival data are lacking.

Positive Airway Pressure Treatment of Central Sleep Apnea with Emphasis on Heart Failure, Opioids, and Complex Sleep Apnea   407

S. Javaheri

Central sleep apnea is due to temporary failure in the pontomedullary inspiratory pacemaker generating breathing rhythm. There are many causes of central sleep apnea. The focus of this article is on three disorders: systolic heart failure, opioid-induced sleep apnea, and complex sleep apnea.

Adaptive Servo-Ventilation for Sleep Apnea: Technology, Titration Protocols, and Treatment Efficacy   419

Lee K. Brown

In the United States, two manufacturers currently market adaptive servo-ventilators for the noninvasive treatment of sleep-disordered breathing including obstructive sleep apnea, central sleep apnea/Cheyne-Stokes ventilation, and complex sleep apnea syndromes. Each manufacturer uses substantially different technology; this technology is not always completely described and often uses algorithms that are not intuitive, with the result that behavior in any particular clinical situation cannot always be predicted. Moreover, relatively few published studies explore the intricacies of these devices. Consequently, it is recommended that the clinician ascertain the efficacy of a particular adaptive servo-ventilation device in each patient to be treated before prescribing such for home use.

Positive Airway Pressure Therapy in Children   439

Sangeeta Chakravorty and Jonathan D. Finder

This article addresses basic pathophysiology of childhood sleep-disordered breathing (SDB) in general, and obstructive sleep apnea in particular. It explains the rationale behind the use of positive airway pressure treatment and its role in the long-term management of children with SDB. Clinical practice guidelines and laboratory techniques for titration are also included, and an overview of current concepts and treatment strategies in children with SDB is given.

Foreword
Positive Airway Pressure Therapy Revisited

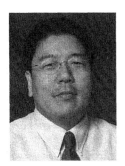

Teofilo Lee-Chiong Jr, MD
Consulting Editor

The year was 1981. The average price of a gallon of gasoline was $1.31, just having tripled over the previous 8 years. People were reading Jane Fonda's workout book, watching Cats on Broadway, and singing with MTV on cable. The first space shuttle, Columbia, took off successfully from Cape Canaveral, Florida, ushering in a new age of space exploration using reusable vehicles.

The year was 1981. In a brief 4-page article published in the journal *Lancet*, Drs Colin Sullivan, Michael Berthon-Jones, Faiq Issa, and Lorraine Eves from the University of Sydney in New South Wales first described the reversal of obstructive sleep apnea (OSA) by continuous positive airway pressure (CPAP) therapy applied through the nares using a mask.[1] OSA is a common disorder resulting from occlusion of the oropharyngeal airway during sleep; this, in turn, leads to multiple apneic episodes during the sleep period, sleep fragmentation, and excessive daytime sleepiness. Before this report, a tracheostomy, which is left open at night, was the only effective treatment available for the disorder. The effect of weight loss in obese persons with OSA was inconsistent and unreliable.

This study determined whether CPAP applied through the nares prevents upper airway occlusion by acting as a pneumatic splint. Two soft plastic tubes were strapped to the patient's face, with one end shaped to fit in each nares and the other end connected to a wide-bore tube. A comfortable seal over the nose was achieved using medical-grade silicone rubber. One end of the wide-bore tube was connected to a vacuum-cleaner blower

motor to produce continuous positive pressure, and the other end was narrowed with mechanical resistance. High airflow of 20 to 40 L/min was provided. Pressure and airway CO_2 were monitored continuously using catheters inserted in the nasal tubes. Five patients with severe OSA, all of whom had a history of snoring and excessive daytime sleepiness, were treated using this setup. At baseline, the mean apnea index was 62 and 64 episodes per hour during non–rapid eye movement and rapid eye movement sleep, respectively. In each of the 5 patients, CPAP at levels of 10.0, 4.5, 6.0, 7.0, and 4.5 cm H_2O completely prevented upper airway occlusion. Sleep quality improved, and each patient awoke spontaneously and remained alert and awake for the rest of the day.

Further advances in positive airway pressure (PAP) technology rapidly followed. Bilevel PAP was introduced in 1990,[2] automatic PAP in 1996,[3] and adaptive servoventilation in 2001.[4] Clinicians now can choose among a wide variety of PAP devices to manage cases of sleep-disordered breathing.

Now, if only we can convince our patients with OSA to use them! There have been numerous investigations on how to enhance adherence to PAP therapy, but despite these attempts, its use remains suboptimal for many patients. This realization along with the rising costs of providing PAP devices has prompted a reassessment of policies relating to their use. The Centers for Medicare and Medicaid Services have recently developed guidelines on the payment for PAP devices

Sleep Med Clin 5 (2010) xiii–xv
doi:10.1016/j.jsmc.2010.06.001

for OSA. This includes face-to-face clinical reevaluation and documentation of benefit from PAP therapy as well as objective evidence of adherence to use of the PAP device, anytime from days 31 to 91 after initiating therapy, to meet requirements for continued coverage of a PAP device beyond the first 3 months of therapy. Adherence to therapy is defined as the use of PAP for at least 4 hours per night on 70% of nights during a consecutive 30-day period anytime during the first 3 months of initial usage.

While it can be argued that this will result in substantial cost savings and eliminate any misuse of scarce resources (after all, why should insurers continue to pay for interventions that are not being used), it is equally important to consider some of the potential adverse ramifications. Firstly, in no other chronic serious medical disorder is continued reimbursement for therapy predicated on patient adherence to the prescribed intervention (eg, medications or oxygen therapy). Furthermore, it is only with OSA that objective monitoring of adherence is necessary. Needless to say, these two requirements place undue burden on the patient and health providers. There are no data to support that this approach is superior to simply asking patients to return their PAP device if they are not satisfied with this form of therapy. Although it may be true that patterns of future PAP use can be discerned during the first few days to weeks of initiating therapy, this does not address cases in which adjustments are still being made (and that might extend for several weeks and months) on both the PAP setting or mask interfaces to enhance patient comfort. The current guidelines appear to suggest that PAP use cannot, and does not, change after 3 months; this suggestion, however, is not supported by current literature.[5]

It is generally accepted that greater duration of use of PAP therapy is accompanied by greater improvements in several measured cardiovascular and neurocognitive parameters, and, therefore, is advisable. Nonetheless, it has yet to be proved that PAP use of less than 4 hours daily, or intermittent use, is entirely without benefits. This replaces clinical judgment by both the patient and physician of PAP-related improvements in sleep quality, mood, or quality of life by an arbitrarily defined "acceptable" PAP use. Furthermore, an optimal PAP pressure that reverses obstructive apnea-hypopneas in all sleep positions, in all sleep stages, and every night of use may not be easily determined for many patients with OSA. There is significant internight variability in PAP pressure requirements because of varying use of alcohol, sleep positions, and, possibly, degree of nasal congestion. No published data have distinguished between the benefits of using optimal or suboptimal prescribed PAP settings among adherent and nonadherent patients. Unanswered still is whether a fully compliant patient using suboptimal PAP settings obtains more benefit than a partially compliant individual using optimal pressures.

Most importantly, there is no evidence that patient acceptance or adherence of any therapy improves with punitive penalties (eg, termination of coverage) for not complying with prescribed therapies. Although every physician would agree that a patient can choose to ignore recommended therapies against medical advice, removing the ability to use, or possibility of reinitiating, treatment poses, for some, a major ethical dilemma. If documentation of adherence to PAP use is required during the initial 3 months of prescription, why is continued monitoring and documentation of PAP adherence not necessary after this period? Because the benefits from therapy continue to accrue long-term, would not these subsequent data be more meaningful to patient care?

Other more effective and efficient cost-saving measures related to PAP therapy should be considered. We should instruct patients on proper care of their equipment and supplies, including identifying signs of wear that indicate the need for replacement, rather than simply allowing Durable Medical Equipment companies to continue dispensing replacement supplies for PAP equipment based on Medicare guidelines (eg, replacement mask every 3 months or a headgear every 6 months) whether or not they are needed, and even if not requested by the patient. We should also encourage the use of PAP initiation and management sessions conducted by qualified personnel because patient education has been demonstrated to enhance PAP acceptance and use. Finally, more research funding should be allocated to help address the many unanswered concerns related to this subject.

Teofilo Lee-Chiong Jr, MD
Division of Sleep Medicine
National Jewish Health
University of Colorado Denver School of Medicine
1400 Jackson Street, Room J221
Denver, CO 60206, USA

E-mail address:
Lee-ChiongT@NJC.ORG

REFERENCES

1. Sullivan CE, Berthon-Jones M, Issa FG, et al. Reversal of obstructive sleep apnea by continuous positive airway pressure applied through the nares. Lancet 1981;1(8225):862–5.

2. Sanders MH, Kern N. Obstructive sleep apnea treated by independently adjusted inspiratory and expiratory positive airway pressures via nasal mask. Physiologic and clinical implications. Chest 1990;98(2):317–24.

3. Meurice JC, Marc I, Series F. Efficacy of auto-CPAP in the treatment of obstructive sleep apnea/hypopnea syndrome. Am J Respir Crit Care Med 1996;153(2): 794–8.

4. Teschler H, Döhring J, Wang YM, et al. Adaptive pressure support servo-ventilation: a novel treatment for Cheyne-Stokes respiration in heart failure. Am J Respir Crit Care Med 2001;164(4):614–9.

5. Aloia MS, Goodwin MS, Velicer WF, et al. Time series analysis of treatment adherence patterns in individuals with obstructive sleep apnea. Ann Behav Med 2008;36(1):44–53.

Preface

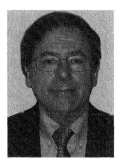

Richard B. Berry, MD
Guest Editor

This issue of *Sleep Medicine Clinics* provides a current review of the many facets of positive airway pressure (PAP) treatment for sleep apnea and chronic hypoventilation disorders in adults and children. It has been almost 30 years since Sullivan and colleagues[1] described continuous positive airway pressure (CPAP) as a treatment for obstructive sleep apnea (OSA). Since that time, the information about PAP treatment has truly exploded. Although there have been several technological advances in PAP devices as well as improved methods to monitor adherence, directing the delivery of effective PAP treatment remains challenging for the clinician.

Inadequate patient acceptance and adherence to PAP treatment remains the biggest challenge that sleep clinicians face. The devices are not effective if stored in the closet. Drs Arfoosh and Rowley have authored an article discussing methods to monitor and improve PAP adherence. It has been said that PAP titration remains an art as well as a science. Although most sleep centers have titration protocols, there has been no widely accepted standard. The American Academy of Sleep Medicine (AASM) formed a task force to create guidelines based on a review of the literature and consensus voting. The Clinical Guidelines for the Manual Titration of Positive Airway Pressure in Patients with Obstructive Sleep Apnea was published in 2008.[2] Dr Kushida was the chair of that task force and we are fortunate that he and Dr Ramar have authored an article on PAP titration based on those guidelines and the Stanford experience. Drs Desai, Khan, and Bhatt have given us a useful overview of PAP treatment in adults, including suggestions for the effective delivery of

long-term treatment to patients and interventions for commonly encountered problems. The development of auto-titrating and auto-adjusting positive airway pressure (APAP) devices has provided another treatment alternative for patients with OSA. The devices can be used to determine an effective single pressure level for CPAP treatment or as long-term treatment without the need for a PAP titration. Understanding the use and limitations of APAP devices is essential for sleep clinicians. Therefore, we are fortunate to have Drs Ahmed and Parthasarathy share their research and clinical experience using the APAP device. There are circumstances where adjunctive measures will improve the efficacy of PAP treatment. The addition of supplemental oxygen may be required in some patients who have continued arterial oxygen desaturation after airway patency has been restored. Many recent publications have examined the utility of hypnotics and humidification for improving the use of CPAP. Drs Mina and Anderson discuss the pros and cons of these adjunctive measures for use with PAP treatment.

There is a large volume of literature concerning the utility of PAP treatment in patients with sleep apnea who have cardiovascular disease or congestive heart failure. Drs Velasquez, Rahangdale, and Malhotra have authored an interesting article discussing the benefits of PAP treatment for hypertension, arrhythmias, and vascular endothelial function. Drs Kee, Sands, Edwards, Berger, and Naughton have written an informative article on the use of PAP in patients with sleep apnea and congestive heart failure.

The best treatment for patients with central apnea and Cheyne-Stokes breathing or central

Sleep Med Clin 5 (2010) xvii–xix
doi:10.1016/j.jsmc.2010.05.014
1556-407X/10/$ – see front matter © 2010 Elsevier Inc. All rights reserved.

apnea due to narcotics remains somewhat controversial. Other OSA patients without these conditions also manifest central apneas either at baseline or during the initial PAP titration (treatment emergent or persistent central sleep apnea) and are said to have complex sleep apnea. Adaptive servo-ventilation (ASV) is a new form of PAP developed for treating these patients who have an instability in ventilatory control. Should ASV be used to treat all patients with central apnea associated with Cheyne-Stokes breathing, narcotics, or complex sleep apnea? Dr Javaheri provides us with a practical approach to the treatment of central apnea associated with systolic heart failure, narcotics, and complex sleep apnea based on his extensive clinical experience and research. Dr Brown gives us insights into the technology of different ASV devices as well as some tips on ASV titration.

Delivery of PAP treatment to children has a unique set of challenges. Certainly with the obesity epidemic, more children with OSA will likely require PAP treatment in the future. Drs Chakravorty and Finder have provided a useful and interesting discussion on the use of PAP in children. As there are a limited number of pediatric sleep specialists, many sleep physicians who treat mainly adult patients may be called on to help deliver care to children with OSA.

Bilevel PAP is a form of PAP treatment increasingly used to provide noninvasive ventilation via mask interface to both adults and children with chronic hypoventilation syndromes. Drs Poon, Becker, and Littner have provided us with an overview of use of PAP in patients with chronic hypercapnia from a wide variety of medical disorders. Drs Perez, Keens, and Davidson Ward present a useful discussion of the PAP treatment of hypoventilation in children. Finally, I have written an article outlining methods for noninvasive positive pressure ventilation (NPPV) treatment initiation with or without attended titration. The AASM created a task force to develop guidelines for NPPV titration in the sleep center. These guidelines are yet to be finalized. I have presented some preliminary suggestions for NPPV initiation and titration based on the deliberations of the task force and protocols from industry and institutions experienced with NPPV treatment.

I was introduced to sleep medicine in 1983 during my pulmonary fellowship, when Dr A. Jay Block, a pioneer in sleep medicine, suggested I try to construct a CPAP device. There were no commercial CPAP devices available and I put together an odd assortment of parts used on ventilators, fashioned a nasal mask from a pediatric anesthesia mask, and used the medical grade air supply in the hospital (**Fig. 1**).[3] The first night I treated a patient with severe sleep apnea in the research laboratory, I was astonished when the nearly continuous apneas and snorting suddenly ceased as an effective pressure was reached. I was hooked on sleep medicine. Even though PAP devices have come a long way since then, treating patients with sleep apnea is still rewarding. I hope the reader of this issue of *Sleep Medicine Clinics* will share my enthusiasm for PAP treatment of sleep apnea. I thank all the authors for the hard work and dedication required to write their articles.

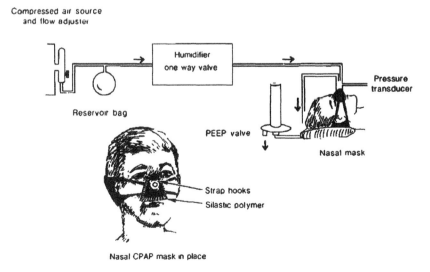

Fig. 1. Nasal CPAP apparatus and nasal mask. (*From* Berry RB, Block AJ. Positive nasal airway pressure eliminates snoring as well as obstructive sleep apnea. Chest 1984;85:16; with permission.)

I hope the information provided will be useful to the clinician taking care of patients with a wide variety of sleep-related breathing disorders.

Richard B. Berry, MD
Division of Pulmonary
Critical Care, and Sleep Medicine
University of Florida
Box 100225 HSC
Gainesville, FL 32610-0225, USA

E-mail address:
Sleep_doc@msn.com

REFERENCES

1. Sullivan CE, Berthon-Jones M, Issa FG. Remission of severe obesity-hypoventilation syndrome after short-term treatment during sleep with nasal continuous positive airway pressure. Am Rev Respir Dis 1983;128:177–81.
2. Kushida CA, Chediak A, Berry RB, et al. Clinical guidelines for the manual titration of positive airway pressure in patients with obstructive sleep apnea. J Clin Sleep Med 2008;4:157–71.
3. Berry RB, Block AJ. Positive nasal airway pressure eliminates snoring as well as obstructive sleep apnea. Chest 1984;85:15–20.

Adherence to Positive Airway Pressure Therapy

Rami Arfoosh, MD[a,b], James A. Rowley, MD[b,*]

KEYWORDS

- Positive airway pressure
- Obstructive sleep apnea–hypopnea syndrome • Adherence

Obstructive sleep apnea-hypopnea syndrome (OSAHS) is a common medical disorder[1] characterized by recurrent episodes of either complete (apnea) or partial (hypopnea) upper airway collapse and obstruction during sleep. These episodes of obstruction are associated with recurrent oxyhemoglobin desaturations and arousals from sleep. Recent literature clearly shows that OSAHS is associated with significant clinical sequelae including excessive daytime sleepiness,[2] decreased quality of life,[3] metabolic abnormalities[4,5] and cardiovascular morbidity and mortality.[6,7] Positive airway pressure (PAP) therapy is the mainstay of therapy for moderate-to-severe OSAHS. PAP therapy works primarily by mechanically splinting the upper airway, preventing the soft tissues from collapsing. By this mechanism, PAP effectively eliminates apneas and hypopneas, decreases recurrent arousals, and normalizes oxygen saturation. Evolving evidence suggests that PAP treatment leads to improvement in the sequelae of OSAHS.[6,8–10] Nevertheless adherence to the prescribed treatment has been less than ideal and is a major challenge for sleep specialists and primary providers.

Currently, PAP devices commonly used for OSAHS come in three modalities: continuous PAP (CPAP), bilevel PAP (BPAP), and automatic self-adjusting PAP (APAP). CPAP devices generate a fixed continuous pressure during inspiration and expiration. In BPAP, the pressure alternates between a fixed inspiratory and lower expiratory level during the respiratory cycle. In APAP, the pressure changes throughout the night in response to changes in airflow, respiratory events, and snoring.

This article will discuss the scope of the problem with compliance to PAP therapy and highlight recent research on the interventions to improve adherence with PAP. The words adherence and compliance will be used interchangeably in this article.

DEFINITION OF COMPLIANCE

The most frequently used definition of adequate compliance was first proposed in 1993 in one of the earliest studies with objective measurement of CPAP use.[11] In this study, the authors defined a minimal use criteria (>4 hours per night) and an optimal use criteria (>7 hours per night) and found that CPAP use met minimal criteria on about 50% of nights and optimal criteria on about 20% of nights. By consensus of the authors, regular users were those who used CPAP at least 4 hours per day on at least 70% of nights; 46% of patients met this criteria. Thus, the most frequently used definition of compliance is use for a minimum of 4 hours per night, 5 to 7 nights per week. This definition recently has been adopted by the Centers for Medicare and Medicaid Services as the minimal objective compliance a patient must demonstrate for continued reimbursement for PAP therapy.

[a] Pulmonary Service, John D. Dingell Veterans Affairs Medical Center, 4646 John R, Detroit, MI 48201, USA
[b] Division of Pulmonary, Critical Care and Sleep Medicine, Department of Internal Medicine, Wayne State University School of Medicine, 3990 John R, Detroit, MI 48201, USA
* Corresponding author. Pulmonary Critical Care, Harper University Hospital, Wayne State University School of Medicine, 3 Hudson, 3990 John R, Detroit, MI 48201.
E-mail address: jrowley@med.wayne.edu

Sleep Med Clin 5 (2010) 321–334
doi:10.1016/j.jsmc.2010.05.012
1556-407X/10/$ – see front matter © 2010 Elsevier Inc. All rights reserved.

Many studies have shown improvement with various symptoms and cognitive and cardiovascular parameters, with an average of 4 to 5 hours of sleep per night. Recent studies, however, have questioned whether the standard definition is an adequate measure of optimal CPAP use.[8,12,13] Weaver and colleagues[8] examined the nightly duration of use that was required to normalize daytime functioning as assessed by three common measures: the Epworth Sleepiness Scale, the Multiple Sleep Latency Test, and the Functional Outcomes of Sleep Questionnaire. The threshold of use above which further improvements were less likely was identified as 4 hours for the Epworth Sleepiness Scale, 6 hours for the Multiple Sleep Latency Test, and 7.5 hours for the Functional Outcomes of Sleep Questionnaire. A linear dose–response relationship between increased use and achieving normal levels was shown for objective and subjective measures of daytime sleepiness, but only up to 7 hours of use for functional status. This study illustrates that patients who are considered to have good adherence by accepted definitions may, in fact, be undertreated and that patients should be encouraged to use PAP for at least 7 hours per night.

In addition, cardiovascular morbidity and mortality may be influenced by the degree of regular PAP use. Campos-Rodriguez and colleagues[12] followed a historical cohort of 871 patients with OSAHS for a mean of 48 months. Five-year cumulative survival was highest in the group of patients who used PAP therapy more than 6 hours per night on average (96.4% survival) compared with patients who used PAP 1 to 6 hours per night (91.3% survival) and patients who used PAP less than 1 hour per night (85.5%). The same group conducted a prospective cohort study of 55 patients with hypertension.[13] In this group, a significant decrease in 24-hour mean arterial blood pressure after 24 months of therapy was primarily observed in patients with greater than 5.3 hours per night use of PAP therapy, and there was an overall correlation between hours of PAP therapy and change in blood pressure. These studies indicate that greater cardiovascular benefit would be achieved with regular use of PAP therapy more than 5 hours per night, rather than the 4 hours that are considered sufficient to be labeled compliant.

MONITORING OF COMPLIANCE

Early studies measuring objective compliance showed that patient self-reported use was found to be inaccurate, since patients with poor adherence overestimated their use of CPAP.[11,14] Therefore, objective monitoring is now a standard recommendation of the American Academy of Sleep Medicine (AASM), found in both a practice parameter on PAP therapy[15] and a clinical guideline on the long-term treatment of OSAHS.[16] Most modern PAP machines measure both machine-on and mask-on times, with the mask-on time used to measure adherence. Adherence data are stored on electronic chips from which compliance reports can be downloaded during follow-up appointments. Generally, these reports provide data such as number of days used, number of days used greater than 4 hours, and mean hours of use. Newer models of PAP machines also allow measurement of mask leak and apnea–hypopnea index. These reports provide physicians with real-time data on adherence, allowing them to immediately address problems in patients with marginal or poor adherence (**Fig. 1**).

PREDICTORS OF ADHERENCE

Acceptance and adherence with PAP therapies are major problems faced by sleep physicians in managing their patients with OSAHS. It has been hypothesized that acceptance of and adherence to PAP therapy are for the patient a balance between costs and benefits, similar to treatments of other diseases and syndromes.[17] Costs include not just financial costs but also lifestyle restrictions, adverse effects, aesthetics, discomfort, and ongoing commitment. Benefits include symptom and functional improvements.

Acceptance generally is defined as a patient's willingness to undergo a PAP titration study and accept a PAP device in his or her home. There is evidence that many patients do not accept CPAP and therefore do not initiate therapy, with a previous review of the literature finding that nonacceptance rates vary from 5% to 50%, with an average of approximately 20%.[17] There are few studies that have investigated which factors influence a patient's acceptance of PAP therapy. A study from Scotland found that patients who refused CPAP were more likely to be female, current smokers, and to have been referred by a specialist, rather than a primary care physician. Additionally, they were less likely to have witnessed apneas and had lower weekly alcohol consumption.[18] In a recent study from Israel, 162 consecutive patients with OSAHS were offered a PAP titration study and a 2-week trial period of PAP therapy.[19] All patients received an educational program on OSAHS and the benefits of PAP therapy. In this cohort, 30 patients declined the titration study; 27 declined PAP after the titration study, and 40 patients declined therapy after the 2-week trial period; in other words, only 40% (n = 65) of patients accepted PAP therapy. Predictors of acceptance included increased income level, increasing age, increasing apnea–hypopnea index of at least 35 per hour, and a family member or friend with a positive experience with CPAP.

A related problem in managing patients with PAP therapy is adherence with follow-up visits. In a study from the authors' sleep center, approximately 25% of patients did not present for regular follow-up with their sleep physician; of these, 75% were noncompliant.[20] Therefore, there is need for more research into the predictors PAP therapy acceptance and interventions that can taken to increase PAP acceptance.

Adherence or compliance is defined as the extent to which a person's behavior coincides with the medical or health advice. Previous reviews have found that 12% to 15% of patients who accept PAP therapy discontinue treatment within 3 years,[17] although more recent studies indicate that by 3 to 6 months, 25% to 50% patients will be either noncompliant or intermittent users,[21,22] and at 1 year, 10% to 35% will have discontinued their therapy.[23,24] In the largest study of long-term adherence with nasal CPAP, only 68% of patients were still using CPAP at 5 years.[18] This degree of adherence is comparable to that of oral medications used for chronic disorders, with studies indicating that at least 40% of patients take prescribed medications incorrectly or not at all.[25] Similarly, in a study on adherence to inhaler therapy with asthma, 50% of study participants took less than 70% of the expected dose of medication over the study period.[26] It is unclear if reasons for nonadherence to PAP therapy are similar to those for oral medication therapy. For instance, it has been hypothesized that patients who are nonadherent to PAP therapy would be nonadherent to medical therapies also. In a recent study, however, Villar and colleagues[27] found that the rates of adherence for oral medications for cardiovascular diseases were the same for patients' adherent to nasal CPAP and those nonadherent to nasal CPAP.

There is a large body of research investigating the determinants of adherence with CPAP in hopes that identification of risk factors for poor adherence will allow sleep physicians to intervene on individual patients.[11,17,18,21,22,24,28–37] Results from these studies are not uniformly consistent, likely because of study differences in patient characteristics (including baseline severity of disease and symptoms), degree of education and support provided to patients, length of follow-up, and which factors were analyzed for relationship to compliance. Despite the inconsistencies, several factors appear to be related to good compliance: increased apnea–hypopnea index, increased daytime sleepiness, and greater perception of benefit from regular use. Factors related to poor compliance include lower body mass index, lower apnea–hypopnea index (AHI), lack of perceived benefit, lack of daytime sleepiness, and nasal symptoms and other adverse effects. Most studies have not found a relationship between the pressure settings and compliance, with one study indicating poor compliance with a CPAP set greater than or equal to 12 cm H_2O.[24] Similarly, age and gender have not been consistently correlated with compliance.

Studies also have shown that long-term compliance is determined early in the course of treatment, with recent studies showing that perceptions of PAP and long-term adherence are established during the first 1 to 2 weeks of treatment.[21,23,38] For instance, in a study of 32 patients followed for 9 weeks, the nightly duration of use differed between compliant and noncompliant patients by the fourth night of use.[38] Several studies have shown that 6-month to 12-month compliance is determined by the pattern of use during the first 2 weeks.[21,23,34] In these studies, patients demonstrating long-term compliance had used the PAP device more than 2 hours more per night during the first 2 weeks compared with noncompliant patients. In addition, problems with PAP therapy during the first 2 weeks therapy, including problems even on the first night of therapy, are predictive of noncompliance.[33,34]

Given that PAP adherence appears to be determined early in the course of therapy and is not reliably predicted by demographic and physiologic factors, investigators have hypothesized that psychological and social factors may play a role in determining adherence to PAP therapy. Pretreatment anxiety and depression scores have not been found to correlate with adherence.[33,39] On the other hand, patients with the ability to apply active coping strategies to new situations were found to be more compliant with therapy,[39] while those with recent life events were found to be less likely to be compliant with therapy.[33] There is little evidence supporting a role for a spouse or bed partner in determining compliance.[32] Living alone was found to be predictive of poor compliance in one study.[33] In another study, however, if the evaluation for OSAHS was the idea of the spouse or bed partner, PAP compliance was actually lower.[40]

Several investigators have applied psychological models of adherence that have been derived from other domains and disease syndromes.[32,34,36,41] For instance, social cognitive

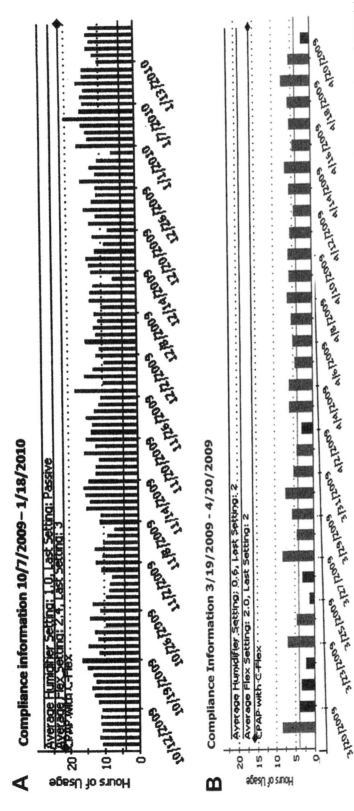

Fig. 1. Patterns of positive airway pressure (PAP) therapy adherence. (A) 62-year-old woman with moderate obstructive sleep apnea-hypopnea syndrome (OSAHS) (AHI =18 per hour) on CPAP 15 cm H_2O with pressure relief of 2 cm H_2O. Compliance reports showed that patient used CPAP 100% of nights with mean nightly use of 12 hours 10 min. Compliance by standard definition was 100%. The patient was still sleepy (Epworth sleepiness scale = 23). As she had gained weight since previous titration, a repeat CPAP titration was ordered. (B) 47-year-old man with severe OSAHS (AHI = 51 per hour) on CPAP 15 cm H_2O with pressure relief of 2 cm H_2O. Compliance report shows that patient used CPAP 100% of nights with mean nightly use of 5 hours 8 min. Compliance by standard definition was 79%. Patient subjectively improved. Patient encouraged to continue regular CPAP use. (C) 76-year-old man with severe OSAHS (AHI = 31 per hour) on CPAP 13 cm H_2O with pressure relief of 3 cm H_2O. Compliance reports show that patient used CPAP 97% of nights with a mean nightly use of 3 hours 51 min. Despite near nightly use, the patient was not considered compliant, as his compliance by standard definition was only 47%. Patient complained of mask leak and dry mouth, so his mask was changed, and the humidifier setting was increased. On a subsequent visit, the patient continued regular use but with insufficient hours to meet minimal criteria for adherence. At that visit, the patient admitted to often only being in bed 4 to 5 hours per night; therefore, increased hours of sleep were recommended. (D) 70-year-old woman with severe OSAHS (AHI = 38 per hour) on CPAP 13 cm H_2O. Compliance reports show that the patient used CPAP only 26% of nights with a mean nightly use of 1 hour 7 min. Compliance by standard definition was 0%. Patient complained of the high pressure preventing regular use. Review of the titration study indicated that CPAP setting could be lowered to 10 cm H_2O. At a subsequent visit, patient had continued complaints of high pressure, and compliance had only improved to 1.4%. A trial of auto-PAP was recommended.

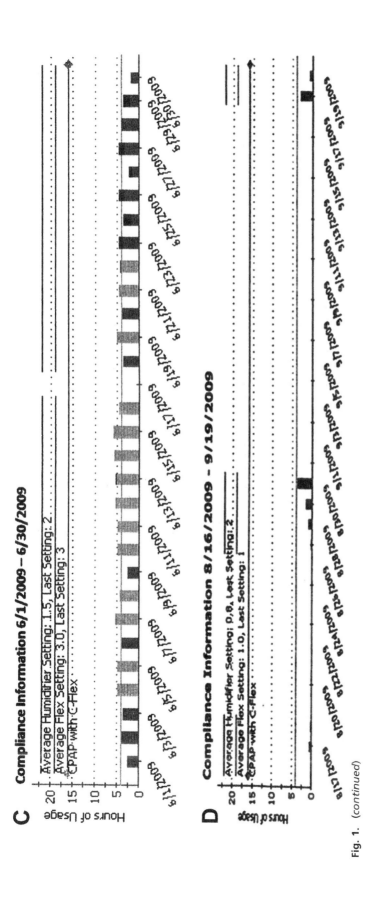

Fig. 1. (continued)

theory posits that a patient's expectations for good or bad outcomes and his or her belief in their ability to engage in the necessary behaviors to affect change are predictive of adherence.[31] Using this model, Stepnowsky and colleagues[36] found that OSAHS-specific scales of self-efficacy, outcomes expectations, social support, knowledge, and decisional balance (balance between the pros and cons of therapy) contributed significantly to a logistic regression model predicting adherence to therapy. Using the same theoretic model, Aloia and colleagues found that regular users of PAP therapy were more ready and confident to continue use with a positive decisional balance at 1 week of therapy, which subsequently predicted 3- and 6-month compliance. Interestingly, measures of self-efficacy and outcomes expectations pretreatment were not predictive of compliance.[34] Wild and colleagues[32] used a slightly different theoretic model that investigated the psychological constructs of health value (importance individual places on maintaining good health), internality (extent to which an individual believes he or she is responsible for his or her own health), powerful others (extent to which an individual believes that others, usually sleep health care workers, are responsible for their health), and self-efficacy (individual's belief in his or her own capacity to organize and carry out activities to deal with a new situation). Applying this model in a cohort of 119 patients, CPAP adherence at 3 months was associated with stronger internal locus of control, greater health value, and less belief in powerful others. These results indicate that patients who have a greater sense that their health is under their control (and not under the control of others) have increased ability for self-management (a hallmark of a greater internal locus of control), internalization of physician advise, and therefore, greater adherence.

In summary, there is clear evidence that psychologic factors, particularly patient knowledge, positive outcomes expectations, perceived benefit from treatment, active ooping strategies, and increased sense of control over health decisions are important determinants of CPAP adherence. To date, however, there are no large studies applying these results to create interventions that will modify these factors in such a way as to improve compliance.

COMPLIANCE IN THE ELDERLY

There also have been several studies looking at compliance in the elderly. Parish and colleagues[42] compared compliance in an elderly cohort (age older than 65 years) with that in a nonelderly cohort

(younger than 65 years). Compliance at 3 months, measured by percentage of patients using CPAP and mean hours of nightly use, was not different between the two groups. In a study of 33 elderly veterans, 20 were found to be compliant (regular use >5 hours per night).[43] Compliant patients were more likely to have had initial resolution of symptoms. Predictors of poor compliance included cigarette smoking, nocturia, and benign prostatic hypertrophy.

Two studies address the issue of long-term compliance in the elderly. In a cohort study of 163 patients, Pelletier-Fleury and colleagues[24] found that elderly patients (age older than 60 years) were significantly less compliant at 3 years (56% vs 74%). However, when compliance of the whole cohort was analyzed using Cox proportional hazards analysis, age was not a predictor of compliance. In contrast, a recent long-term prospective follow-up study on the impact of PAP therapy on mortality in elderly (mean age approximately 70 years) patients with ischemic stroke, 45% of patients offered PAP therapy withdrew from therapy within 6 months.[44] Only 29% were compliant (using the standard definition of good compliance) at the end of the 5-year follow-up period, which is significantly lower percentage of compliant patients when compared with another 5-year follow-up study in which 68% of patients (median age approximately 50 years) were still compliant at the end of the study.[18]

Further studies need to be performed to better determine long-term compliance and predictors of compliance in the elderly. In the meantime, data suggest that long-term compliance may be poorer in the elderly, indicating that special care must be taken when managing these patients.

INTERVENTIONS TO IMPROVE COMPLIANCE
Patient Education, Behavioral Therapy, and Intensive Monitoring

In a retrospective review, attendance in a group clinic designed to encourage patient adherence with CPAP therapy provided a simple and effective means of improving treatment on average 1 hour per night, with 29% of patients demonstrating an increase in use of 2 hours or more.[45] Similarly, group cognitive–behavioral therapy seems to be a promising modality to improve adherence. In a randomized study, two 1-hour sessions that included an educational talk and video of real CPAP users were compared with usual treatment. The group undergoing cognitive–behavioral therapy had a higher proportion of patients initiate therapy and a mean increase in nightly use of 2.9 hours.[46] Written literature and weekly phone calls during the first month of use also have been shown to improve adherence,[47] as has use of an instructional video.[48] Finally, motivational techniques and a self-management approach to therapy also have been described in the literature.[49,50]

An interesting pilot project using telemonitoring of patient compliance has recently been published.[51] In this study, 45 patients with severe OSAHS being treated with PAP therapy were randomized to receive either daily monitoring of their PAP therapy using telemonitoring or usual care. Patients assigned to the telemonitoring group had their compliance reviewed on a regular basis, daily if indicated, during the first 2 months of treatment; based upon the compliance information, clinical pathways were followed, and in partnership with the patient, interventions were taken to improve PAP use. In this study, average daily use in the telemonitoring group was 1.3 hours longer than the usual care group, and the telemonitoring group used their CPAP on more nights (78% vs 60%). Although these results are encouraging, it is unclear if a similar program could be replicated by most sleep centers, given the intensive nature of a daily monitoring program.

A recent Cochrane review evaluated the evidence about educational, supportive, and behavioral interventions to improve usage of CPAP machines for adults with OSA.[52] The review concluded that there is some evidence that a supportive intervention that encourages people to continue to use their CPAP machines leads to greater levels of CPAP machine usage than control, although the variation across the studies introduces some uncertainty over how consistent is the effect. The review could not find evidence that a short-term educational intervention led to improvements in usage. Cognitive–behavioral therapy led to the largest increases in average machine usage, partly because more participants were prepared to try out the treatment.

Patient education is a long-term process that starts on the initial visit and continues afterward. The practice parameters from the American Academy of Sleep Medicine stated that the addition of a systematic educational program is indicated to improve PAP use should be a standard of care.[15] Patient education should optimally be delivered as part of a multidisciplinary chronic disease management team including the sleep physician, the referring provider, and allied health care providers. In addition, videotapes, handouts, Web sites, and brochures can be employed. A recent Adult Obstructive Sleep Apnea Task Force of the American Academy of Sleep Medicine has identified essential components of patient education program.[16] These components are listed in

Box 1. The authors recommend that the educational points be reviewed on a regular basis, particularly in patients who show poor compliance with therapy.

Heated Humidification and Inhaled Steroids

Nasal dryness and mouth dryness are frequent adverse effects of PAP therapy. Nasal congestion and rhinorrhea are also frequent complaints of PAP users (Table 1). Several studies have examined the use of humidification to improve dryness and improve compliance.[53–56] Two prospective cohorts[53,54] and one randomized cross-over study[56] support the use of heated humidification to decrease nasal symptoms and improve compliance, although it should be noted that the increase in the number of hours used per night was small and generally less than 1 hour. A more recent, randomized study of 98 patients, however, did not show a difference in compliance between a control group and the group using heated humidification despite a lower incidence of dry nose and mouth in the humidification group.[55]

A recent study was the largest study to date to address the role of humidification and nasal steroids.[57] In this study, 125 patients were divided into three groups: dry air, heated humidified air, and heated humidified air with nasal steroids. Although nasal symptoms decreased with the

---

Box 1
Recommended components of patient education programs

Findings of study, severity of disease

Pathophysiology of obstructive sleep apnea

Explanation of natural course of disease and associated disorders

Risk factor identification, explanation of exacerbating factors, and risk factor modification

Treatment options

Expectations from treatment

Discuss the patient's role in treatment, address his or her concerns, and set goals

Consequences of untreated disease

Drowsy driving/sleepiness counseling

Patient quality assessment and other feedback regarding evaluation

Adapted from Epstein LJ, Kristo D, Strollo PJ, et al. Clinical guideline for the evaluation, management, and long-term care of obstructive sleep apnea in adults. J Clin Sleep Med 2009;5:263–76; with permission.

Table 1
Common problems with continuous positive airway pressure and recommended solutions

Problem	Possible Cause	Solution
Dry nose or throat epistaxis	Dry air	Intranasal saline before sleep Heated humidification
Nasal congestion	Dry air, vasodilatation	Intranasal saline before sleep Heated humidification Intranasal corticosteroid
Rhinorrhea	Dry air, vasodilatation	Intranasal anticholinergic Nonsedating antihistamine
Dry mouth	Sleeping with mouth open Air leak through the mouth Dry air	Chin strap Full face mask Heated humidification
Sore, dry, irritated eyes	Mask leaks	Readjust headgear/straps Repositioning of mask on face Change interface if necessary
Mask leak Skin irritation Pressure sores/blisters	Improper strap adjustment Incorrect mask size Worn-out mask	Readjust headgear/straps Mask fitting with respiratory therapist or sleep technologist Replacement mask
General discomfort with mask Mask comes off during night	Improper strap adjustment Incorrect mask size Wrong mask for patient	Readjust headgear/straps Mask fitting with respiratory therapist or sleep technologist with change in mask Replacement mask
Pressure too high	Unadjusted patient Overtitration	Use of ramp function Consider pressure relief mode Consider retitration

use of heated humidification, compliance was the same between the three groups (approximately 5 hours), as was the improvement in daytime sleepiness and quality of life. This study was specifically powered to find a 1-hour difference in compliance, which may be one reason that a significant difference was not found between the groups.

Based upon the available evidence and the AASM practice parameters on PAP therapy of OSAHS, the addition of heated humidification is indicated to improve CPAP use with a recommendation level of standard.[15] In addition, the AASM practice parameters on the medical therapy of OSAHS reported that topical nasal corticosteroids may improve the AHI in patients with OSA and concurrent rhinitis, and thus may be a useful adjunct to primary therapies for OSA with a recommendation level of guideline (a patient-care strategy, which reflects a moderate degree of clinical certainty).[58] Further studies, however, need to be performed, specifically on the role of nasal steroids in improving nasal symptoms and compliance. Despite these limitations, the authors have found that it is important to ask all patients about nasal symptoms and treat patients who report significant congestion with nasal congestions.

Change of the Interface

There are many different CPAP interfaces now available for the treatment of OSA. The type of CPAP delivery interface is likely to influence a patient's acceptance of CPAP therapy and long-term compliance. Patients who have mask-related complaints such as mask leaks (often manifested as irritated eyes), skin irritation, or pressure sores should be evaluated by a respiratory therapist for improper mask size or fit, with an order for a new mask interface provided if needed. Patients with dry mouths may be mouth breathing; for these patients, either a chin strap or change in mask to a full-face mask (the authors' preference) is indicated. Unfortunately, there are few studies directly comparing mask interfaces and their effect on patient compliance. A recent review evaluated the role of mask interface in compliance and concluded that more studies need to be performed.[59] The reviewers, however, suggested that nasal pillows may be a useful alternative when a patient is unable to tolerate conventional nasal masks and that a full-face mask should be considered if nasal obstruction or dryness limits the use of a nasal mask.

Change of PAP Modality

Pressure relief CPAP

Pressure-relief CPAP, which is a system that lowers the pressure at the onset of expiration, is hypothesized to improve adherence by reducing the uncomfortable sensation of breathing against high pressure while maintaining a patent upper airway. Three studies have been performed evaluating the effect of pressure-relief CPAP on compliance.[60–62] These studies varied in size (n = 19 to 184 patients), type of study (cross-over vs parallel), and length of follow-up (4 weeks to 6 months). All were uniform, however, in showing that pressure-relief CPAP did not improve compliance compared with fixed CPAP. A recent Cochrane database review, which also included several studies reported only in abstract form, concluded that pressure-relief CPAP did not improve compliance.[63] Despite these findings, in the authors' center, pressure-relief CPAP frequently is prescribed for all patients who require a setting of 10 cm H_2O.

There has been one study evaluating whether pressure-relief BPAP improved compliance. In this prospective study, 104 persistently noncompliant patients (patients had failed simple interventions to improve compliance) were randomized to CPAP or flexible or pressure relief BPAP.[64] In this study, compliance was defined as mean average use of greater than 4 hours per day. After 3 months, the proportion of patients who were compliant with PAP therapy was higher in the flexible BPAP group (49%) than in the CPAP group (28%). Further studies will need to be performed on this modality to determine if flexible BPAP consistently improves compliance.

BPAP

In BPAP, the pressure alternates between a fixed inspiratory and lower expiratory level during the respiratory cycle. The lower expiratory pressure originally was theorized to be more comfortable for patients (less resistance of exhalation) and thus was hypothesized to lead to improved adherence. However, two studies have not shown any difference in adherence or changes in AHI or daytime sleepiness when the CPAP and BPAP were directly compared with each other.[65,66] A recent Cochrane review that also included several studies published in abstract format only concluded that BPAP does not result in improved adherence compared with fixed CPAP.[63]

The most recent AASM guidelines recommend BPAP as an optional therapy in some cases when high pressure is needed and the patient experiences difficulty exhaling against a fixed pressure or coexisting central hypoventilation is present. BPAP also is optional in treating some forms of restrictive lung disease or hypoventilation syndromes associated with daytime hypercapnia.[15]

APAP

The rationale for autotitrating devices is that the pressure required to treat OSAHS may vary over the course of the night and between different nights, sleep stages, and body positions, and these variations are not captured by a 1-night titration study. In theory, the mean pressure delivered by APAP devices is lower than that with fixed CPAP. APAP devices were designed to continuously measure airflow, airway resistance, respiratory events, and snoring, and, using an integrated algorithm, deliver the minimal PAP required to eliminate obstructive apnea and hypopnea events. Each manufacturer's device uses different sensors and algorithms to achieve the changes in pressure.

A recent Cochrane database review evaluated the overall evidence for the effect of APAP devices on patient adherence to PAP therapy.[63] The authors included 30 studies that included fully published articles and abstracts presented at conferences. There were 10 studies that directly compared APAP with fixed CPAP in a parallel design. Only one of these 10 studies showed a significant improvement in compliance with APAP,[67] and the overall analysis showed a nonsignificant increase in numbers of hours used, 0.22 hours per night, favoring APAP. There were 18 studies that compared APAP with fixed CPAP in a crossover design (patients wore both APAP and fixed CPAP). Of these 18 studies, two studies showed improved compliance with APAP; however, only one of these has been published in a peer-reviewed journal.[68] For the 18 studies as a whole, there was a statistically significant increase in numbers of hours used of 0.21 hours per night, favoring APAP. In summary, the review found that improvement in average machine use of auto-CPAP was superior in studies with a crossover design; the point estimate in parallel group trials was similar, but did not reach statistical significance. The authors concluded that APAP does not increase machine usage by a meaningful amount in unselected patients with OSAHS. In addition, it is uncertain how use of machines in study settings relates to real-world use, especially given that the average increased use per night was only 12 minutes. It should be noted, however, that when preference was measured, participants routinely preferred auto-CPAP to fixed-pressure CPAP.

The precise role of autotitrating CPAP systems in the treatment of OSAH is unclear, in part because while several studies have shown that outcomes measures are similar between APAP and regular CPAP devices, adherence has not been consistently shown to be improved with APAP, as originally theorized. It should be noted that recent practice parameters from the AASM do not recommend APAP devices as a PAP modality to improve adherence to therapy.[69] Although the authors have switched an occasional noncompliant patient to an APAP device in hopes to improve compliance, it is not a routine practice in their center.

Use of Sedatives During Titration or for the Short Term Upon Starting PAP

It has been suggested that the quality of the titration may influence compliance. Specifically, in a cohort study of 71 patients with severe OSAHS, short-term (1 to 2 months) compliance was highest in patients who had a significant improvement in their sleep efficiency during the titration study compared with the diagnostic study.[70] In other words, patients whose sleep improved the most during the titration study were more likely to be compliant with PAP therapy. This finding led one group of investigators to hypothesize that improving sleep quality during the titration study would improve compliance.[71,72] In these studies, patients with OSAHS undergoing a PAP titration study were randomized to either eszopiclone or placebo. Patients medicated with eszopiclone had greater sleep efficiency during the titration studies. In addition, the titration studies with eszopiclone had fewer residual events and were less likely to be incomplete.[72] Patients then were followed for 4 to 6 weeks and had their compliance objectively measured. Patients in the eszopiclone group used their CPAP on a higher percentage of nights (76% vs 60%) and for more hours per night (4.8 hours vs 3.9 hours on average).

Many patients have difficulty initiating therapy because of discomfort with CPAP. Intolerance may establish poor compliance patterns or may cause patients to abandon therapy. Conversely, as discussed previously, patients who have positive initial experiences with CPAP may show greater use. Compliance patterns, as stated earlier, may be established very early in the course of treatment, and initial exposure to CPAP, therefore, may have a tremendous impact on subsequent use. It has been hypothesized that use of a sedative–hypnotic during the initial treatment period may result in improved sleep during the initiation phase of PAP therapy in the home, thus improving compliance.

This hypothesis has been studied by two groups. Bradshaw and colleagues[73] conducted a randomized trial with 72 patients with severe OSAHS comparing the effect of two weeks of zolpidem or placebo with standard treatment (no zolpidem or placebo) on compliance. The group found no difference in compliance whether measured by number of days used, number of hours used, or percentage of patients considered regular users. Lettieri and colleagues[74] studied 160 adults with severe OSAHS, comparing 2 weeks of eszopiclone with placebo. In contrast to the previous study, patients in the eszopiclone group used CPAP more nights (64.4% vs 45.2%) and more hours per night (4.05 hours vs 3.02 hours) on nights used. Time to discontinuing regular CPAP use was longer in the eszopiclone group (19.7 vs 17.2 weeks), with fewer patients discontinuing therapy (42.1% vs 57.7%). The eszopiclone group had a larger decrease in the Epworth score compared with placebo, with no difference in the Functional Outcomes of Sleep Questionnaire. The contrasting conclusions of these two studies likely arise from differences in study design (including time at which compliance was measured) and different sedative–hypnotic used (eszopiclone is a longer-acting medication than zolpidem, which could influence the results). Thus, further studies will need to be performed before the routine use of a sedative–hypnotic as an adjunctive therapy for PAP therapy can be recommended.

TREATMENT OF ADVERSE EFFECTS

PAP therapy for OSAHS is safe, and its adverse effects are mainly minor and reversible. The major adverse effects of PAP are either pressure-related or interface-related. The pressure-related complications include dry mouth, rhinitis, nasal and sinus congestion, and rhinorrhea. The nasal and sinus congestion can be particularly severe in patients with pre-existing sinus disease. These adverse effects are generally effectively treated with humidification and the addition of either an intranasal corticosteroid or antihistamine at bedtime. Rhinorrhea usually responds to treatment with either an intranasal corticosteroid or anticholinergic spray. Occasionally, eye irritation secondary to air leak may warrant changing the mask.

Interface-related effects include allergic reactions to the mask and abrasions at the ridge of the nose. These are treated with either a change in the mask type or by refitting the mask to prevent it from being too tight on the face.

Other uncommon adverse effects include claustrophobia, gastric and bowel distention, and recurrent ear and sinus infections. Rare instances of cerebrospinal fluid leakage, both spontaneous and associated with prior skull trauma, have been reported.

THE AUTHORS' EXPERIENCE

Using PAP therapy is likely a life-long process. Therefore, it is essential to establish a good rapport with patients who require PAP therapy. Early in the course of treatment, close follow-up is indicated to establish effective patterns of use and to remediate problems, if needed. The importance of early intervention for adverse effects and other concerns cannot be overestimated. Follow-up is especially important during the first few weeks of therapy given that long-term adherence is established in this period. The authors' overall approach is shown in the algorithm (**Fig. 2**).

The authors have established a PAP compliance clinic. They schedule all patients for follow-up within the first 4 weeks of starting therapy. Those with poor adherence are subsequently evaluated every 2 to 3 months until problems are addressed and adherence improves. Patients with good adherence can be seen less frequently. Objective compliance is reviewed on every visit. Patient education should be provided on each visit. The education team usually includes a sleep physician, a respiratory therapist, and a nurse.

To determine reasons for poor adherence, a systematic approach should be taken. Poorly adherent patients should be asked about mask fit, mask leak, sinus/nasal congestion, mouth breathing, and general sleep habits to determine reasons for nonadherence. Patients should be encouraged to contact the sleep center if they encounter a problem, rather than waiting for the follow-up appointment to address it.

Patients also need to be asked about other reasons for poor adherence, including bed partner intolerance, poor sleep habits (such as sleeping on the couch instead of in bed), frequent awakenings with nocturia, inability to fall asleep with the device, and general inability to tolerate the device. These complaints need to be addressed on an individualized basis and may require education of bed partners, use of the ramp function, and sleep hygiene education. Regular reinforcement of the negative consequences of OSAHS and the benefits of CPAP should be part of every visit for nonadherent patients.

Repeated polysomnography and PAP titration should be considered if the patient demonstrates poor compliance,[15] has significant complaints

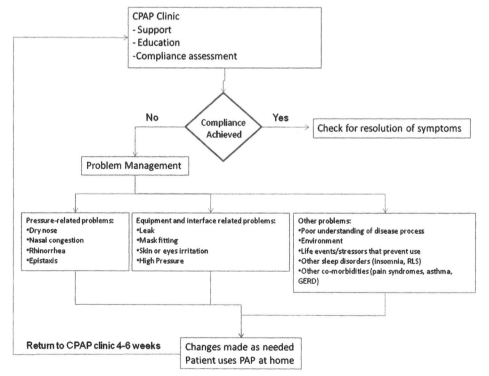

Fig. 2. Algorithm used by the authors to monitor and improve adherence to positive airway pressure therapy.

about the level of pressure, demonstrates change in weight, or if his/her symptoms do not improve or worsen after initial improvement.

REFERENCES

1. Young T, Palta M, Dempsey J, et al. The occurrence of sleep-disordered breathing among middle-aged adults. N Engl J Med 1993;328(17):1230–5.
2. Jenkinson C, Davies RJ, Mullins R, et al. Comparison of therapeutic and subtherapeutic nasal continuous positive airway pressure for obstructive sleep apnoea: a randomised prospective parallel trial. Lancet 1999;353(9170):2100–5.
3. Weaver TE, Laizner AM, Evans LK, et al. An instrument to measure functional status outcomes for disorders of excessive sleepiness. Sleep 1997; 20(10):835–43.
4. McArdle N, Hillman D, Beilin L, et al. Metabolic risk factors for vascular disease in obstructive sleep apnea: a matched controlled study. Am J Respir Crit Care Med 2007;175(2):190–5.
5. Punjabi NM, Shahar E, Redline S, et al. Sleep-disordered breathing, glucose intolerance, and insulin resistance: the Sleep Heart Health Study. Am J Epidemiol 2004;160(6):521–30.
6. Marin JM, Carrizo SJ, Vicente E, et al. Long-term cardiovascular outcomes in men with obstructive sleep apnoea–hypopnoea with or without treatment with continuous positive airway pressure: an observational study. Lancet 2005;365(9464):1046–53.
7. Punjabi NM, Caffo BS, Goodwin JL, et al. Sleep-disordered breathing and mortality: a prospective cohort study. PLoS Med 2009;6(8):e1000132.
8. Weaver TE, Maislin G, Dinges DF, et al. Relationship between hours of CPAP use and achieving normal levels of sleepiness and daily functioning. Sleep 2007;30(6):711–9.
9. Kohler M, Pepperell JC, Casadei B, et al. CPAP and measures of cardiovascular risk in males with OSAS. Eur Respir J 2008;32(6):1488–96.
10. Pepperell JC, Ramdassingh-Dow S, Crosthwaite N, et al. Ambulatory blood pressure after therapeutic and subtherapeutic nasal continuous positive airway pressure for obstructive sleep apnoea: a randomised parallel trial. Lancet 2002;359(9302):204–10.
11. Kribbs NB, Pack AI, Kline LR, et al. Objective measurement of patterns of nasal CPAP use by patients with obstructive sleep apnea. Am Rev Respir Dis 1993;147(4):887–95.
12. Campos-Rodriguez F, Pena-Grinan N, Reyes-Nunez N, et al. Mortality in obstructive sleep apnea–hypopnea patients treated with positive airway pressure. Chest 2005;128(2):624–33.
13. Campos-Rodriguez F, Perez-Ronchel J, Grilo-Reina A, et al. Long-term effect of continuous positive airway pressure on BP in patients with hypertension and sleep apnea. Chest 2007; 132(6):1847–52.
14. Reeves-Hoche MK, Meck R, Zwillich CW. Nasal CPAP: an objective evaluation of patient compliance. Am J Respir Crit Care Med 1994;149(1):149–54.
15. Kushida CA, Littner MR, Hirshkowitz M, et al. Practice parameters for the use of continuous and bilevel positive airway pressure devices to treat adult patients with sleep-related breathing disorders. Sleep 2006;29(3):375–80.
16. Epstein LJ, Kristo D, Strollo PJ Jr, et al. Clinical guideline for the evaluation, management, and long-term care of obstructive sleep apnea in adults. J Clin Sleep Med 2009;5(3):263–76.
17. Engleman HM, Wild MR. Improving CPAP use by patients with the sleep apnoea/hypopnoea syndrome (SAHS). Sleep Med Rev 2003;7(1):81–99.
18. McArdle N, Devereux G, Heidarnejad H, et al. Long-term use of CPAP therapy for sleep apnea/hypopnea syndrome. Am J Respir Crit Care Med 1999; 159:1108–14.
19. Simon-Tuval T, Reuveni H, Greenberg-Dotan S, et al. Low socioeconomic status is a risk factor for CPAP acceptance among adult OSAS patients requiring treatment. Sleep 2009;32(4):545–52.
20. Lin HS, Zuliani G, Amjad EH, et al. Treatment compliance in patients lost to follow-up after polysomnography. Otolaryngol Head Neck Surg 2007;136(2): 236–40.
21. Aloia MS, Arnedt JT, Stanchina M, et al. How early in treatment is PAP adherence established? Revisiting night-to-night variability. Behav Sleep Med 2007; 5(3):229–40.
22. Hui DS, Choy DK, Li TS, et al. Determinants of continuous positive airway pressure compliance in a group of Chinese patients with obstructive sleep apnea. Chest 2001;120(1):170–6.
23. Popescu G, Latham M, Allgar V, et al. Continuous positive airway pressure for sleep apnoea/hypopnoea syndrome: usefulness of a 2 week trial to identify factors associated with long-term use. Thorax 2001;56(9):727–33.
24. Pelletier-Fleury N, Rakotonanahary D, Fleury B. The age and other factors in the evaluation of compliance with nasal continuous positive airway pressure for obstructive sleep apnea syndrome. A Cox's proportional hazard analysis. Sleep Med 2001;2(3):225–32.
25. DiMatteo MR, Giordani PJ, Lepper HS, et al. Patient adherence and medical treatment outcomes: a meta-analysis. Med Care 2002;40(9):794–811.
26. Bosley CM, Fosbury JA, Cochrane GM. The psychological factors associated with poor compliance with treatment in asthma. Eur Respir J 1995;8(6): 899–904.
27. Villar I, Izuel M, Carrizo S, et al. Medication adherence and persistence in severe obstructive sleep apnea. Sleep 2009;32(5):623–8.

28. Pepin JL, Krieger J, Rodenstein D, et al. Effective compliance during the first 3 months of continuous positive airway pressure. A European prospective study of 121 patients. Am J Respir Crit Care Med 1999;160(4):1124–9.

29. Sin DD, Mayers I, Man GC, et al. Long-term compliance rates to continuous positive airway pressure in obstructive sleep apnea: a population-based study. Chest 2002;121(2):430–5.

30. Janson C, Noges E, Svedberg-Randt S, et al. What characterizes patients who are unable to tolerate continuous positive airway pressure (CPAP) treatment? Respir Med 2000;94(2):145–9.

31. Olsen S, Smith S, Oei TP. Adherence to continuous positive airway pressure therapy in obstructive sleep apnoea sufferers: a theoretical approach to treatment adherence and intervention. Clin Psychol Rev 2008;28(8):1355–71.

32. Wild MR, Engleman HM, Douglas NJ, et al. Can psychological factors help us to determine adherence to CPAP? A prospective study. Eur Respir J 2004;24(3):461–5.

33. Lewis KE, Seale L, Bartle IE, et al. Early predictors of CPAP use for the treatment of obstructive sleep apnea. Sleep 2004;27(1):134–8.

34. Aloia MS, Arnedt JT, Stepnowsky C, et al. Predicting treatment adherence in obstructive sleep apnea using principles of behavior change. J Clin Sleep Med 2005;1(4):346–53.

35. Stepnowsky CJ, Dimsdale JE. Dose–response relationship between CPAP compliance and measures of sleep apnea severity. Sleep Med 2002;3(4):329–34.

36. Stepnowsky CJ Jr, Marler MR, ncoli-Israel S. Determinants of nasal CPAP compliance. Sleep Med 2002;3(3):239–47.

37. Yetkin O, Kunter E, Gunen H. CPAP compliance in patients with obstructive sleep apnea syndrome. Sleep Breath 2008;12(4):365–7.

38. Weaver TE, Kribbs NB, Pack AI, et al. Night-to-night variability in CPAP use over the first three months of treatment. Sleep 1997;20(4):278–83.

39. Stepnowsky CJ Jr, Bardwell WA, Moore PJ, et al. Psychologic correlates of compliance with continuous positive airway pressure. Sleep 2002;25(7):758–62.

40. Hoy CJ, Vennelle M, Kingshott RN, et al. Can intensive support improve continuous positive airway pressure use in patients with the sleep apnea/hypopnea syndrome? Am J Respir Crit Care Med 1999;159:1096–100.

41. Olsen S, Smith S, Oei T, et al. Health belief model predicts adherence to CPAP before experience with CPAP. Eur Respir J 2008;32(3):710–7.

42. Parish JM, Lyng PJ, Wisbey J. Compliance with CPAP in elderly patients with OSA. Sleep Med 2000;1(3):209–14.

43. Russo-Magno P, O'Brien A, Panciera T, et al. Compliance with CPAP therapy in older men with obstructive sleep apnea. J Am Geriatr Soc 2001;49(9):1205–11.

44. Martinez-Garcia MA, Soler-Cataluna JJ, Ejarque-Martinez L, et al. Continuous positive airway pressure treatment reduces mortality in patients with ischemic stroke and obstructive sleep apnea: a 5-year follow-up study. Am J Respir Crit Care Med 2000;180(1):36 41.

45. Likar LL, Panciera TM, Erickson AD, et al. Group education sessions and compliance with nasal CPAP therapy. Chest 1997;111(5):1273–7.

46. Richards D, Bartlett DJ, Wong K, et al. Increased adherence to CPAP with a group cognitive behavioral treatment intervention: a randomized trial. Sleep 2007;30(5):635–40.

47. Chervin RD, Theut S, Bassetti C, et al. Compliance with nasal CPAP can be improved by simple interventions. Sleep 1997;20(4):284–9.

48. Jean WH, Boethel C, Phillips B, et al. CPAP compliance: video education may help!. Sleep Med 2005;6(2):171–4.

49. Aloia MS, Arnedt JT, Riggs RL, et al. Clinical management of poor adherence to CPAP: motivational enhancement. Behav Sleep Med 2004;2(4):205–22.

50. Stepnowsky CJ, Palau JJ, Gifford AL, et al. A self-management approach to improving continuous positive airway pressure adherence and outcomes. Behav Sleep Med 2007;5(2):131–46.

51. Stepnowsky CJ, Palau JJ, Marler MR, et al. Pilot randomized trial of the effect of wireless telemonitoring on compliance and treatment efficacy in obstructive sleep apnea. J Med Internet Res 2007;9(2):e14.

52. Smith I, Nadig V, Lasserson TJ. Educational, supportive and behavioural interventions to improve usage of continuous positive airway pressure machines for adults with obstructive sleep apnoea. Cochrane Database Syst Rev 2009;2:CD007736.

53. Pepin JL, Leger P, Veale D, et al. Side effects of nasal continuous positive airway pressure in sleep apnea syndrome. Study of 193 patients in two French sleep centers. Chest 1995;107(2):375–81.

54. Rakotonanahary D, Pelletier-Fleury N, Gagnadoux F, et al. Predictive factors for the need for additional humidification during nasal continuous positive airway pressure therapy. Chest 2001;119(2):460–5.

55. Mador MJ, Krauza M, Pervez A, et al. Effect of heated humidification on compliance and quality of life in patients with sleep apnea using nasal continuous positive airway pressure. Chest 2005;128(4):2151–8.

56. Neill AM, Wai HS, Bannan SP, et al. Humidified nasal continuous positive airway pressure in obstructive sleep apnoea. Eur Respir J 2003;22(2):258–62.

57. Ryan S, Doherty LS, Nolan GM, et al. Effects of heated humidification and topical steroids on compliance, nasal symptoms, and quality of life in patients with obstructive sleep apnea syndrome using nasal continuous positive airway pressure. J Clin Sleep Med 2009;5(5):422–7.

58. Morgenthaler TI, Kapen S, Lee-Chiong T, et al. Practice parameters for the medical therapy of obstructive sleep apnea. Sleep 2006;29(8):1031–5.

59. Chai CL, Pathinathan A, Smith B. Continuous positive airway pressure delivery interfaces for obstructive sleep apnoea. Cochrane Database Syst Rev 2006;4:CD005308.

60. Dolan DC, Okonkwo R, Gfullner F, et al. Longitudinal comparison study of pressure relief (C-Flex) vs. CPAP in OSA patients. Sleep Breath 2009;13(1):73–7.

61. Marshall NS, Neill AM, Campbell AJ. Randomised trial of compliance with flexible (C-Flex) and standard continuous positive airway pressure for severe obstructive sleep apnea. Sleep Breath 2008;12(4):393–6.

62. Nilius G, Happel A, Domanski U, et al. Pressure-relief continuous positive airway pressure vs constant continuous positive airway pressure: a comparison of efficacy and compliance. Chest 2006;130(4):1018–24.

63. Smith I, Lasserson TJ. Pressure modification for improving usage of continuous positive airway pressure machines in adults with obstructive sleep apnoea. Cochrane Database Syst Rev 2009;4:CD003531.

64. Ballard RD, Gay PC, Strollo PJ. Interventions to improve compliance in sleep apnea patients previously non-compliant with continuous positive airway pressure. J Clin Sleep Med 2007;3(7):706–12.

65. Gay PC, Herold DL, Olson EJ. A randomized, double-blind clinical trial comparing continuous positive airway pressure with a novel bilevel pressure system for treatment of obstructive sleep apnea syndrome. Sleep 2003;26(7):864–9.

66. Reeves-Hoche MK, Hudgel DW, Meck R, et al. Continuous versus bilevel positive airway pressure for obstructive sleep apnea. Am J Respir Crit Care Med 1995;151:443–9.

67. Meurice JC, Marc I, Series F. Efficacy of auto-CPAP in the treatment of obstructive sleep apnea/hypopnea syndrome. Am J Respir Crit Care Med 1996;153(2):794–8.

68. Massie CA, McArdle N, Hart RW, et al. Comparison between automatic and fixed positive airway pressure therapy in the home. Am J Respir Crit Care Med 2003;167(1):20–3.

69. Morgenthaler TI, Aurora RN, Brown T, et al. Practice parameters for the use of autotitrating continuous positive airway pressure devices for titrating pressures and treating adult patients with obstructive sleep apnea syndrome: an update for 2007. An American Academy of Sleep Medicine report. Sleep 2008;31(1):141–7.

70. Drake CL, Day R, Hudgel D, et al. Sleep during titration predicts continuous positive airway pressure compliance. Sleep 2003;26(3):308–11.

71. Lettieri CJ, Collen JF, Eliasson AH, et al. Sedative use during continuous positive airway pressure titration improves subsequent compliance: a randomized, double-blind, placebo-controlled trial. Chest 2009;136(5):1263–8.

72. Lettieri CJ, Quast TN, Eliasson AH, et al. Eszopiclone improves overnight polysomnography and continuous positive airway pressure titration: a prospective, randomized, placebo-controlled trial. Sleep 2008;31(9):1310–6.

73. Bradshaw DA, Ruff GA, Murphy DP. An oral hypnotic medication does not improve continuous positive airway pressure compliance in men with obstructive sleep apnea. Chest 2006;130(5):1369–76.

74. Lettieri CJ, Shah AA, Holley AB, et al. Effects of a short course of eszopiclone on continuous positive airway pressure adherence: a randomized trial. Ann Intern Med 2009;151(10):696–702.

CPAP and BPAP Titration

Kannan Ramar, MD[a], Clete A. Kushida, MD, PhD[b],*

KEYWORDS

- Positive airway pressure • CPAP • BPAP
- Sleep-related breathing disorders • Obstructive sleep apnea

Positive airway pressure (PAP) devices such as continuous positive airway pressure (CPAP) and bilevel positive airway pressure (BPAP) are used to treat sleep-disordered breathing (SDB). Unfortunately, adherence in use of these PAP devices can be low,[1] with pressure-related side effects and difficulty adjusting to mask interfaces being the most commonly cited reasons. At an optimal pressure, PAP devices eliminate SDB events without creating pressure-related side effects.

The gold standard method for identifying the optimal pressure is attended overnight laboratory-based polysomnography during which a sleep technologist manually titrates the PAP devices to eliminate SDB events, such as apneas, hypopneas, respiratory effort-related arousals (RERAs), and snoring. The American Academy of Sleep Medicine (AASM) published a new scoring manual that defines the various SDB events that are used in the diagnostic portion of the polysomnogram.[2] Apnea is defined as a drop in the peak thermal sensor (using a thermistor or a thermocouple) excursion by more than 90% of baseline, lasting at least 10 seconds.[2] Hypopnea is defined as a drop in the nasal pressure signal excursions by more than 30% of baseline, lasting at least 10 seconds, and associated with a 4% or greater oxyhemoglobin desaturation (recommended definition).[2] A RERA is defined as a sequence of breaths lasting at least 10 seconds characterized by increasing respiratory effort or flattening of the nasal pressure signal, leading to an arousal, after exclusion of apneas and hypopneas.[2]

Using a nasal pressure transducer or a thermistor/thermocouple during the titration portion of the polysomnography may not be feasible because of problems obtaining a good seal with the mask interfaces. Therefore, during a titration study, recordings from the airflow signal generated by the PAP device, or estimating the airflow through measuring the pressure difference between the mask and the outlet machine using a transducer, are acceptable methods to detect apneas, hypopneas, and RERAs.[3]

Titration protocols to identify the optimal pressure for PAP devices to treat sleep-related breathing disorders (SRBDs) vary widely among sleep centers.[4] In fact, in a survey of 51 accredited sleep centers conducted by Stepanski and colleagues,[5] PAP titration varied widely, with 22% of these centers not having a written protocol and, of those that did, only 14% of the protocols mentioned SDB events as reasons to consider pressure changes. Therefore, it is very likely that the same patient undergoing a titration study at different accredited centers may end up with different optimal pressures. With very few PAP titration protocols published to guide sleep centers and help standardize the current practice, the AASM recently published clinical guidelines (evidence- and consensus-based statements) for the manual titration of PAP in patients with obstructive sleep apnea (OSA)[3] but not other SRBDs. This article describes the CPAP/BPAP titration protocols for SRBDs only in adults and not in the pediatric population.

PATHOGENESIS OF SRBD

OSA is the most common SRBD for which CPAP/BPAP titrations are performed. Briefly reviewing

a Center for Sleep Medicine, Division of Pulmonary, Sleep and Critical Care Medicine, Mayo Clinic, Rochester, MN, USA
b Stanford University Center of Excellence for Sleep Disorders, Stanford, CA 94305, USA
* Corresponding author. Stanford Sleep Disorders Clinic, 450 Broadway Street, Pavilion B, 2nd Floor, MC 5730, Redwood City, CA 94063-5730.
E-mail address: clete@stanford.edu

Sleep Med Clin 5 (2010) 335–346
doi:10.1016/j.jsmc.2010.05.007

the pathogenesis of OSA will help in understanding the role of PAP devices in treating OSA. OSA is a common disorder characterized by sleep fragmentation from repeated arousals and disruptions of normal sleep architecture secondary to partial or complete airway closure during sleep. The critical narrowing of the upper airway during sleep in OSA develops because of a dysfunctional interplay of anatomic factors narrowing the airway and compensatory neuromuscular mechanisms insufficient to maintain upper airway patency.[6] The pressure at which the upper airway closure just begins is called the critical closing pressure (P_{crit}). P_{crit} is a measure of upper airway collapsibility.[7] For those without OSA, a negative pressure must be exerted to cause airway closure (negative P_{crit}). Elevated or positive P_{crit} is seen in patients with OSA and occurs from a synergistic combination of obesity, craniofacial anomalies, and pharyngeal collapsibility.[8] PAP is required to overcome the positive P_{crit} in OSA. The degree of respiratory control instability can be quantified by loop gain. Loop gain is measured as a ratio of corrective response to a disturbance, in this case, an apnea. If the response is robust, the loop gain is greater than 1 and results in an unstable respiratory system with periodic breathing. This effect is certainly seen in central sleep apnea (CSA), but its role in OSA pathogenesis is being studied. Loop gain is abnormally elevated in patients with OSA, but whether this is a consequence of OSA or a pathogenetic mechanism for OSA is still debated. Arousals can increase loop gain, and although traditionally thought to rescue patients with OSA through opening the upper airway, it may also cause OSA through increasing loop gain, destabilizing respiratory control, and promoting upper airway collapse during the terminal phase of the hyperpnea.[9]

Most apneic events tend to occur at end exhalation when the positive pressure within the upper airway lumen is at a minimum and the pharynx is most susceptible to collapse.[10] PAP therapy has evolved to include targeted treatment of both inspiratory and expiratory events to eliminate SDB events. CPAP provides the same magnitude of pressure during the inspiratory and expiratory phases of the ventilatory cycle, whereas BPAP permits independent adjustment of the inspiratory and expiratory positive airway pressures (IPAP and EPAP, respectively).

OPTIMAL PRESSURE

The optimal pressure for PAP devices to treat SRBD is the effective pressure that eliminates SDB events without creating any untoward pressure-related side effects for the patient. Pressures lower than the optimal pressure, apart from inadequately treating the SDB, may also result in mouth breathing and claustrophobic symptoms. Pressures exceeding the optimal pressure may lead to air leaks, mouth breathing, worsening of nasal congestion, and rhinorrhea; exacerbate central apneas; and of course lead to difficulty tolerating the PAP, resulting in decreased overall adherence. The optimal pressure should be effective in all sleep positions and sleep stages.

The optimal pressure identified for one patient may not be same or adequate for another patient. Several factors may influence identification of the optimal pressure, such as sleep position, rapid eye movement (REM) sleep, sleep duration,[11] the degree of respiratory effort, and the length of the soft palate.[12] The correlation between the optimal pressure of PAP and the severity of SRBD or obesity is unclear, with some suggesting that no correlation exists[12] (ie, that higher optimal pressure is needed for severe OSA or higher body mass index [BMI]), whereas others suggest the opposite.[13]

Several mathematical equations were developed to identify the optimal pressure, using variables such as BMI, OSA severity using the apnea-hypopnea index (AHI), and neck circumference.[13,14] However, studies have failed to confirm the accuracy,[15,16] and these mathematical equations are currently not part of routine clinical practice.

SPLIT-NIGHT VERSUS FULL-NIGHT TITRATION STUDY

A PAP titration study could be accomplished either by a full-night or split-night polysomnography study. The current recommended procedure on initiating the split-night protocol for titration is based on the AHI from the diagnostic study. The criteria that is typically used is an AHI of 40 or more per hour with a minimum of 120 minutes of sleep, or an AHI of 20 to 40 per hour in certain cases.[17] Some sleep centers may use different criteria based on the AHI, minimum oxygen saturation, and total sleep time.

Initiating the split-night study may also be guided by third-party payors, such as the regional carriers for the Center for Medicare & Medicaid services (CMS). Based on their recent 2009 requirements for CPAP reimbursement, CMS requires either the documentation of an AHI of 15 or more per hour with a minimum of 30 events, or an AHI of 5 to 14 per hour with a minimum of 10 events, along with documentation of one of the following: excessive sleepiness, impaired cognition, mood disorder, insomnia, hypertension, ischemic heart disease, or history of stroke. When one of the aforementioned criteria are met, the night can be split to perform the titration study.

Although split-night studies may be cost-effective and time-saving in delivering care for SRBDs, they also present significant challenges in accomplishing the titration within a short period compared with a full-night titration study. One significant challenge in a split-night polysomnography is obtaining adequate duration of sleep, specifically supine and REM sleep during the titration. Despite these challenges, results from studies comparing the adherence and acceptance of CPAP from split-night versus full-night titration were not significantly different.[18–20] Although the optimal pressure obtained by a split-night titration might be lower than that obtained from a full-night titration, especially for patients with mild to moderate OSA[21]; however, the overall mean optimal CPAP requirement seemed to be the same, especially in patients with severe OSA.[21,22] Similar data assessing adherence and adequacy of prescribed BPAP in split-night versus full night titration, or data for other SRBDs, are not available.

GOALS OF PAP TITRATION

The goal of PAP titration is to identify the optimal pressure that eliminates SDB events (apneas, hypopneas, RERAs, oxygen desaturation, and snoring), restores normal respiratory patterns, and improves the patient's quality of sleep. The optimal pressure from PAP that accomplishes all this should be adequate during all stages of sleep and in all sleep positions (particularly supine position), because the severity of OSA is commonly worse during sleep in the supine position, and during REM sleep, whereas the severity of CSA might be worse during supine and non-REM sleep. Also, patients with chronic obstructive pulmonary disease (COPD) and progressive neuromuscular disorders may exhibit worsening of SDB during supine REM sleep.

During PAP titration, if the patient attains a particular stage (eg, REM in OSA, COPD, and neuromuscular disorders; neuromuscular disorders in CSA) of sleep, but not in the supine position, the patient may be awakened to change sleep position. Disrupting sleep to change sleep position should be carefully considered before implementation because it affects sleep quality and efficiency. Improvement in sleep efficiency during CPAP titration compared with during the diagnostic study has been shown to increase CPAP adherence.[23]

The titration goal with PAP devices is to attain an AHI of less than 5 per hour with the optimal

pressure, with no oxygen desaturation below 88% and with minimal leak around the mask interface.

A grading system has been proposed for the various goals of titration. Optimal titration is obtained when the AHI is less than 5 per hour for at least 15 minutes and includes supine REM sleep at the optimal pressure.[3,24] A good titration reduces the AHI to less than 10 per hour or by 50% if the baseline is less than 15 per hour and includes supine REM sleep at the selected pressure on the PAP device.[3,24] Adequate titration is obtained when the AHI cannot be reduced to less than 10 per hour, but is reduced by 75% from baseline (especially in severe SDB), or when the titration grading of optimal and good are obtained even though supine REM sleep did not occur.[3,24] An unacceptable titration occurs if any one of the above grades are not met, at which time a repeat titration is necessary.[3,24] Repeat full titration is also needed if only adequate titration was obtained, especially if it was part of a split-night protocol.

PREPARATION FOR PAP TITRATION

Before the diagnostic polysomnogram, eligible patients must be prepared in advance for the titration study if a possibility exists that a split-night will be performed. Currently, these preparations are not conducted routinely or uniformly across all centers.

The AASM practice parameters recommend that all eligible patients receive adequate PAP education, hands-on demonstration, careful mask fitting, and acclimatization to the PAP device before titration.[25] PAP education before titration could be in the form of a video describing sleep apnea, consequences of untreated sleep apnea, rationale for the use of PAP, the process involved during the diagnostic and PAP titration polysomnogram, and side effects related to the PAP and mask interfaces. Also, showing and explaining the device along with its parts and equipment, and having the patient try on the mask interface to experience the pressure generated by the device, are all important steps before implementing PAP titration.

Mask fitting by an experienced technician or health care worker familiar with these interfaces is vital for identifying a mask that will be comfortable for the patient with minimal leak issues before titration. Some patients may experience claustrophobia and this must be addressed, if possible, before the titration, to enhance the study quality and PAP adherence.

Potential side effects of the mask interface and procedures that could be undertaken if problems arise during the titration should be explained to the patient. Different mask interfaces should be available during the titration, in case the patient experiences problems with the mask that was fitted earlier. Chin straps and full-face mask interfaces may be needed in case of mouth breathing. Heated humidification might also help with comfort and nasal stuffiness during titration. After titration, discussions on cleaning the equipment and purchasing or rental options should be discussed, if applicable. Providers must be aware that most patients may have never purchased medical equipment before this PAP device.

Follow-up appointments, preferably in a month or earlier, should be set up to address any issues that may arise when the patient starts using the PAP at home. Also, it is very helpful for providers to be aware of durable medical equipment insurance to help address any issues that may arise. To continue coverage for a CPAP device, current CMS regulations require a face-to-face visit with a physician no sooner than the 31st day but no later than the 91st day after initiating CPAP therapy for clinical reevaluation that documents adherence from the download, indicating minimum use of 4 hours per night for 70% of the nights during a consecutive 30-day period, and documents that the patient is benefiting from the CPAP use. Similar CMS regulations are available for BPAP use.

CPAP TITRATION
Indications for CPAP

The most common indication for CPAP use is for the treatment of OSA. Most patients with OSA can be effectively treated with CPAP, which serves as a passive pneumatic splint to keep the upper airway from collapsing during sleep.[26,27] It also tends to increase lung volumes and exerts tracheal traction (tracheal tug mechanism) to prevent collapsibility of the upper airway. It is beyond the scope of this article to discuss the benefits of CPAP use in the treatment of OSA and other sleep disorders, such as CSA. The AASM has published practice parameters on the indications for CPAP/BPAP in the treatment of SDB.[25]

CPAP may also be effective in treating CSA. According to the *International Classification of Sleep Disorders, Second* Edition[28] (ICSD-II) CSA syndromes encompass primary CSA and CSA caused by Cheyne-Stokes breathing pattern (CSA/CSR), high-altitude periodic breathing, or drug or substance use such as opioids. Several case-control, randomized crossover, and randomized controlled trials have shown the effectiveness of CPAP in reducing CSA (particularly in CSA/CSR

and primary CSA) as measured using the AHI, with some studies showing improvement in the left ventricular ejection fraction and daytime alertness as measured by the Epworth sleepiness scale (ESS).[29–32] Therefore, performing a CPAP titration for CSA is reasonable to assess for effectiveness before switching to a different PAP device, such as BPAP in the spontaneous timed mode (BPAP-ST) or adaptive servoventilators. In fact, the current CMS regulations will not cover BPAP-ST unless CPAP has been shown to be ineffective in treating CSA. CPAP may not be effective in treating CSA caused by opioid use.[33] The titration protocol explained below is for OSA and CSA using CPAP and not for SRBD related to COPD and neuromuscular disorders.

Titration

CPAP titration for OSA is shown in **Fig. 1**. At the start of CPAP titration, pressure is usually initiated at 4 to 5 cm H_2O. In patients who are intolerant even at 5 cm H_2O, pressure is initiated at 4 cm H_2O, which is the minimum recommended starting pressure.[3] Some patients may experience insufficient pressure at the start of titration, even with pressure at 5 cm H_2O. In these cases, the pressure can be increased until the patient is comfortable and then, once the patient falls asleep, the pressure is reduced in decrements of 1 cm H_2O at 5-minute intervals until SDB returns or the patient awakens. If the patient tolerates the initial pressure before sleep onset, further titration is not performed until the patient falls asleep.

CPAP is then increased incrementally by 1 cm H_2O at intervals of no less than 5 minutes until all SDB events are eliminated.[3] CPAP increments are performed in the presence of at least two obstructive apneas, or at least three hypopneas, or at least five RERAs, or at least 3 minutes of loud or unambiguous snoring.[3] The recommended maximum pressure to titrate CPAP is 20 cm H_2O,[3] at which time BPAP titration will need to be considered if SDB events are still occurring. Adding supplemental oxygen for sleep-related hypoxemia or hypoventilation may also need to be considered. Titration of supplemental oxygen is discussed in a separate section.

If the SDB events are not controlled with CPAP because of patient complaints of increased pressure side effects (even at CPAP <20 cm H_2O), then adding a humidifier for nasal congestion or instituting a pressure-relief mechanism at end expiration, such as with C-flex or expiration pressure relief, should be considered.[34–36] If SDB events are persistent, one may then need to proceed with BPAP. Ideally, the optimal pressure

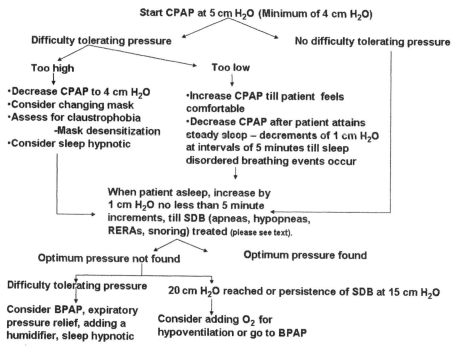

Fig. 1. CPAP titration algorithm for the treatment of OSA.

is attained in the supine position and REM sleep for at least 15 minutes if possible.[3] If this is not attainable, a repeat titration study should be considered. If the patient is unwilling to undergo or insurance does not cover another night titration, clinicians could consider prescribing the best pressure attained on the titration with a follow-up overnight oximetry on the optimal CPAP settings. Some prescribers might advocate an auto-CPAP in these situations. A follow-up study is usually required on auto-CPAP to ascertain whether the SDB is well controlled.

Titration is usually started with a nasal interface. If the patient exhibits open-mouth breathing, either a chin strap or a full-face mask should be considered. Some clinicians may advocate use of oxymetazoline nasal spray to help with nasal congestion and prevent open-mouth breathing. If the spray works, long-term use can be accomplished with the use of a nasal steroid spray.

The titration protocol using CPAP for CSA/CSR is a bit different from that for OSA. Titration with CPAP can be started at 4 to 5 cH_2O, and then titrated upwards by 1 cm H_2O every 5 minutes until CSA/CSR is eliminated. CPAP beyond 10 cm H_2O is unlikely to be helpful in controlling CSA/CSR,[37,38] although exploring higher pressures may sometimes help identify the optimal pressure for treating CSA/CSR. Persistent or worsening

CSA on CPAP titration will necessitate BPAP titration. Also, although CPAP can decrease the AHI to less than 5 per hour in OSA, this may not occur in CSA/CSR.[37,38]

Treatment-Emergent CSA

Some patients may have central apneas that become apparent after CPAP alleviates OSA during CPAP titration. This event is commonly referred to as *treatment-emergent CSA*, or *complex sleep apnea*. The exact prevalence and underlying mechanism behind this phenomenon remain unclear. However, treatment with adaptive servoventilation that stabilizes the upper airway obstruction and addresses the respiratory center dysfunction through providing 90% of the calculated ventilatory assistance to minimize hypo- and hyperventilation may provide some clues about the underlying pathophysiology. The term *complex sleep apnea* and its treatment are debatable[39,40] and are beyond the scope of this article. However, treatment-emergent CSA may contribute to repeated oxyhemoglobin desaturation along with sleep fragmentation. No established protocol exists to address treatment-emergent CSA, and the treatment options and protocol discussed in this article are the authors' own proposed guidelines until further research can guide treatment.

One option is to proceed directly to adaptive servoventilation to address treatment-emergent CSA on CPAP to treat OSA. This approach may lead to the use of an expensive device without proven long-term benefits. Another approach is to decrease CPAP by 1 to 2 cm H_2O and monitor for 5 to 10 minutes. If central apneas persist, pressure can be decreased further by 1 to 2 cm H_2O as long as no recurrence of OSA is seen. This downward titration can be attempted until the centrals disappear as long as OSA does not recur. If centrals persist or OSA recurs at a lower pressure, then proceeding with one of the other approaches discussed is advisable.

A third approach is to perform an upward titration with CPAP, not beyond 5 cm H_2O above the pressure that eliminated the OSA. This upward titration may help in certain cases, especially when the central apneas may have been misclassified as OSA. If central apneas worsen with this upward titration, the pressure should be lowered to the previous level that alleviated OSA. BPAP may also be tried (as discussed in next section). Data suggest that these central apneas dissipate over time with CPAP use.[41] Therefore, some providers may choose to treat these patients with CPAP for 2-to 3-months before repeating another titration study. If central apneas persist on CPAP with the repeat titration study, then treatment should proceed using other modalities, such as adaptive servoventilation. The selected approach may vary depending on the sleep center, provider preference based on experience and understanding of this syndrome, patient preference and attitude, underlying comorbidities, and cost issues. The hope is that further research in this area will soon elucidate which approach would be most effective.

BPAP TITRATION

Although BPAP uses the same patient interface as CPAP, it permits independent adjustment of the IPAP and EPAP to target the SDB events. Upper-airway instability in OSA tends to occur during not only the inspiratory phase[42–44] but also the expiratory phase[45,46]; hence the rationale in using BPAP.[47,48] The EPAP tends to stabilize the upper airway at end expiration so that the airway is sufficiently patent to permit the patient to trigger delivery of IPAP by generating low-level inspiratory volume or flow during the subsequent effort. The IPAP level is set to prevent upper-airway closure and partial obstruction (hypopnea) during the inspiratory phase of breathing.[47,48]

Different types of BPAP devices are available, with the most common ones being the conventional spontaneous mode (S-mode) and the backup rate mode (ST-mode). In the BPAP-S mode, patients may breathe with their own frequency, with the BPAP supporting both phases of respiration based on the pressure settings of IPAP and EPAP. The BPAP-ST mode guarantees a certain number of pressure cycles (or breaths) per minute, which changes to the higher pressure (IPAP) if the patient does not initiate a breath within a specified period. Inspiratory time must be set on the BPAP-ST machines, which tells the machine the maximum time allowed for inspiration. If an inspiratory time is not specified, the machine will use default settings.

Indications for BPAP Use

OSA
OSA is commonly treated with CPAP, which splints the airway open with continuous positive airflow. Experts have suggested that BPAP, through stabilizing the upper airway during both the inspiratory and expiratory phases of respiration, might be more effective in treating OSA, although studies have not conclusively proven this theory. Several studies comparing the effectiveness of BPAP and CPAP, with and without coexisting respiratory disorders, showed no differences in the improvement of AHI, ESS, or sleep quality.[49,50] Similarly, no differences have been seen in adherence or comfort level among BPAP and CPAP users in the treatment of OSA without coexisting respiratory disorders.[49,51] Some data suggest that a subset of patients with OSA who have comorbid obesity and daytime hypercapnia prefer BPAP over CPAP in the treatment of OSA.[52,53] Despite the overall lack of evidence, BPAP still tends to be considered for OSA treatment, even in patients without comorbid respiratory disorders, particularly when they are uncomfortable or unable to tolerate CPAP because of a high pressure requirement or have persistent OSA on CPAP even at a pressure of 20 cm H_2O.[3]

COPD
BPAP has been used in disorders other than OSA, including COPD. The use of BPAP is well defined in patients presenting with acute respiratory failure related to COPD exacerbation. Use of BPAP in these conditions has clearly reduced the mortality rate and the need for invasive mechanical ventilatory support.[54] The role of BPAP during sleep in patients with stable chronic COPD and chronic hypercapnic respiratory failure is less well defined.[55–58] Because of the variable results in the literature on the use of BPAP for stable patients with hypercapnia caused by COPD, guidelines have been published based on a consensus report.[59] According to these guidelines, BPAP can be considered in the presence of symptoms

such as fatigue, morning headache, or daytime hypersomnolence, and one of the following: (1) $Paco_2$ greater than 55 mm Hg, (2) $Paco_2$ of 50 to 54 mm Hg and nocturnal desaturation (overnight oximetry showing oxygen saturation of 88% or less for 5 minutes while receiving oxygen therapy of >2 L/min), or (3) $Paco_2$ of 50 to 54 mm Hg and hospitalization related to recurrent episodes (≥ 2 in a 12-month period) of hypercapnic respiratory failure.[59] Recent CMS regulations to cover BPAP in patients with stable COPD are as follows: (1) daytime $Paco_2$ is 52 mm Hg or greater while the patient is awake and breathing the usual Fio_2; (2) sleep oximetry shows oxygen saturation of 88% or less for at least five continuous minutes, performed while breathing oxygen at 2 L/min or the patient's usual Fio_2; and (3) OSA has been considered and ruled out.

Neuromuscular disorders and chest wall deformities

The use of BPAP in patients with chronic hypercapnic respiratory failure caused by neuromuscular disorders and chest wall restriction such as kyphoscoliosis, has shown improvement in daytime gas exchange,[60–62] daytime respiratory muscle strength,[60,62] and daytime sleepiness as measured with the multiple sleep latency test (MSLT).[63] In a small prospective, controlled trial of 20 patients with amyotrophic lateral sclerosis (ALS), the use of BPAP showed a significant improvement in 1-year mortality.[64] Current CMS regulations for BPAP coverage in patients with restrictive thoracic disorders are as follows: (1) documentation exists of a progressive neuromuscular disorders or severe thoracic cage abnormality; (2) either (a) an arterial blood gas $Paco_2$ of greater than 45 mm Hg while the patient is awake and breathing the usual Fio_2 or (b) sleep oximetry shows an oxygen saturation of 88% of less for at least 5 continuous minutes, performed while the patient is breathing the usual Fio_2, or (c) for a progressive neuromuscular disorders (only), maximal inspiratory pressure is less than 60 cm H_2O or forced vital capacity is less than 50% predicted; and (3) COPD does not contribute to the patient's pulmonary limitation.[65]

CSA

According to the ICSD-II,[28] the CSA syndromes encompass primary CSA and CSA caused by Cheyne-Stokes breathing pattern, high-altitude periodic breathing, and drugs or substances such as opioids. BPAP in the ST mode is useful to treat patients with CSA syndromes, specifically primary CSA and CSA/CSR, with various randomized controlled and crossover trials confirming the

effectiveness.[29,66–69] Apart from effectively treating CSA based on the AHI, the BPAP-ST mode has been effective in improving the left ventricular ejection fraction[29,66,67,69] and daytime alertness measured with the ESS.[66,68] BPAP-ST can also be used in CSA caused by opioids.[70] Current CMS regulations cover BPAP in both the S and the ST mode in the treatment of CSA and complex-CSA, as long as documentation of the diagnosis exists, with CPAP found to be ineffective and BPAP reported to significantly improve CSA.[65]

Titration

BPAP use is indicated for several sleep disorders. Initial BPAP settings and titration strategies will vary depending on the underlying patient's diagnosis. In all cases, optimum BPAP settings should be observed in non-REM and REM stages of sleep on the back and off-back positions for at least 15 minutes.

BPAP for OSA

BPAP titration for OSA is shown in **Fig. 2**. Patients requiring BPAP to treat OSA normally do not require an ST mode; the S mode is usually sufficient. In fact, CMS does not reimburse for BPAP-ST for treating OSA. If a patient is switched from CPAP to BPAP, the EPAP is started at the CPAP level at which the obstructive apneas were eliminated.[3] However, the EPAP may initially be set 1 to 4 cm H_2O below optimal CPAP to optimize patient comfort. Otherwise, the EPAP is started at 4 cm H_2O and increased in increments of 1 cm H_2O at intervals no shorter than 5 minutes until the obstructive apneic events are eliminated. In some situations, as in retitration studies or patients with an elevated BMI, the EPAP may be started higher than 4 cm H_2O.[3] The IPAP in all these situations is usually started 4 cm H_2O higher than the EPAP, and titrated upward along with the EPAP in increments of 1 cm H_2O, maintaining the IPAP–EPAP difference at 4 cm H_2O until the obstructive apneic events are treated. Increases in IPAP and EPAP are performed if at least two obstructive apneas are observed. Once the optimal EPAP is obtained to eliminate the obstructive apneic events, the IPAP is then increased in increments of 1 cm H_2O every 5 minutes in the presence of at least three hypopneas or five5 RERAs, or at least 3 minutes of loud or unambiguous snoring.[3]

According to the consensus among the AASM task force members, the maximum recommended IPAP is 30 cm H_2O in adults because of reports of increased risk for barotrauma when IPAP exceeds 30 cm H_2O. The minimum IPAP–EPAP differential is 4 cm H_2O and the maximum IPAP–EPAP differential is 10 cm H_2O.[3]

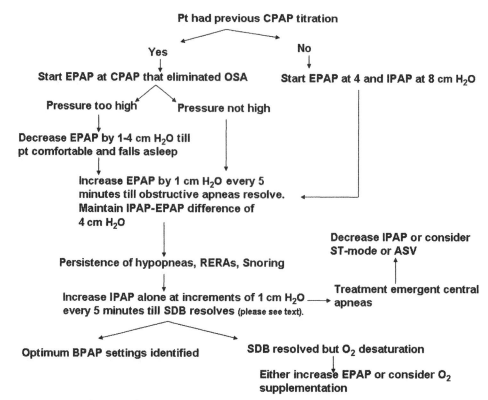

Fig. 2. BPAP titration algorithm for the treatment of OSA.

The AASM task force recommends not adjusting the BPAP settings in the event of oxygen desaturation-resaturation as long as they are not associated with any obstructive events.[3] The members do not recommend exploration by increasing the IPAP above the optimal pressure that achieved control of SDB events. If a patient develops treatment-emergent central apneas, decreasing the IPAP could be attempted. If this does not help, changing to the ST mode with backup rate might be helpful. The titration protocol with BPAP-ST for treatment-emergent CSA and complex-CSA is the same as that for CSA (explained later).

BPAP for CSA

Most if not all patients require a BPAP-ST mode rather than an S mode to treat CSA. CSA may also worsen with BPAP-ST,[71] and hence requires close monitoring during titration. If CSA worsens with BPAP, changing to adaptive servoventilation should be considered. The following are general guidelines that the authors propose for BPAP titration in patients with CSA.

If OSA is mixed with CSA during the diagnostic polysomnogram, the EPAP is usually started at the CPAP level that eliminated the OSA events.

Otherwise, the EPAP is usually started at 4 cm H_2O, with the IPAP at 4 cm H_2O higher than EPAP along with ST backup rate. The backup rate is usually started below the patient's spontaneous awake breathing rate and then increased slowly after the patient falls asleep. If central apneic episodes persist, the backup rate is increased by 1 to 2 breaths every 5 minutes to a maximum of 16 breaths per minute or until the trigger artifact from the BPAP-ST results in a flow signal. If there is a trigger artifact from the ST backup rate with very minimal flow, the IPAP is increased at increments of 1 cm H_2O every 5 minutes until the hypopneic events are corrected. Once the airflow improves or apneic events are controlled, the ST backup rate and IPAP are not titrated further. If the patient is uncomfortable with the increase in respiratory rate, the rate is decreased slowly to 12 breaths per minute or to a rate that the patient is comfortable, without necessarily compromising the titration.

In the presence of obstructive apneic events in patients with CSA, the EPAP is increased by 1 cm H_2O every 5 minutes, maintaining an IPAP–EPAP difference, until the obstructive apneic events are corrected. Subsequent titration of IPAP is based on the presence of hypopneas and central apneas and is explained earlier. Although it is unlikely, the authors do not recommend the maximum IPAP to exceed 20 cm H_2O and recommend maintaining the minimum IPAP–EPAP at 4 cm H_2O. Also, increasing the IPAPEPAP differential has the potential to worsen CSA by decreasing $Paco_2$. Every effort should be made to assess/titrate BPAP and identify the optimal BPAP settings during supine and non-REM sleep, because CSA tends to worsen during these situations. If CSA events are persistent after the maximum IPAP of 20 cm H_2O is reached, other modalities should be considered, such as adaptive servoventilation to treat CSA.

BPAP for COPD

The following are general guidelines that the authors propose for BPAP titration in patients with COPD. BPAP is started in the S mode (CMS does not cover for a BPAP-ST mode unless the S mode has been tried for 3 months; this may change with the new regulations). BPAP use for COPD in the setting of acute respiratory failure used high inspiratory pressure in the range of 15 to 20 cm H_2O, to help with gas exchange.

The difference between the IPAP and EPAP gives pressure support to the breath that the patient initiates. Increasing the pressure support increases tidal breathing, resulting in increased minute ventilation and improvement in hypercapnia. Usually the EPAP is set low at 4 to 6 cm H_2O, with the IPAP generally set 4 cm H_2O higher than the EPAP to give a pressure support breath of 4 cm H_2O. Presence of OSA with apneic episodes should be treated by adjusting the EPAP to eliminate apneas while maintaining an IPAPEPAP difference of 4 cm H_2O. EPAP and IPAP are increased in increments of 1 cm H_2O every 5 minutes. If OSA is not a concern and no apneic episodes occur, the EPAP is usually left alone and the IPAP is slowly increased by increments of 1 cm H_2O every 5 minutes to correct hypopneas and hypoventilation in patients with COPD. Maximum IPAP–EPAP difference exceeding 15 cm H_2O may become uncomfortable for patients.

Every effort should be made to assess and titrate BPAP during REM sleep because patients with COPD are most vulnerable to hypoventilation during this stage. Some may require a backup rate with the ST mode during REM sleep. With the machine-triggered breaths, a pressure support of 4 cm H_2O (IPAPEPAP difference) may not be sufficient to deliver adequate tidal volume. In these situations, the IPAP will need to be increased to deliver adequate tidal volume. Despite obtaining adequate BPAP settings to treat hypoventilation, occasionally supplemental oxygen is required (for sleep-related hypoxemia) if oxyhemoglobin desaturations persist. An arterial blood gas is obtained within a few minutes of waking to assess $Paco_2$ levels.

BPAP for neuromuscular disorders

The following are general guidelines proposed for BPAP titration in patients with neuromuscular disorders. BPAP is usually started in the ST mode with a rate at or near the patient's spontaneous breathing rate (generally at least 10–12 breaths per minute) for patients with neuromuscular disorders. The rate may need to be increased based on patient's respiratory rate during sleep. If OSA is not a concern, the EPAP is initially set low (4–6 cm H_2O) with the IPAP generally 4 cm H_2O higher. Patients with neuromuscular disorders patients may find higher EPAP settings to be uncomfortable due to difficulty exhaling. Therefore the titration of EPAP and IPAP may need to proceed slowly. The EPAP is increased in increments of 1 cm H_2O in intervals no shorter than 15 minutes to eliminate apneic events. During such titration for obstructive apneic events, the IPAP-EPAP difference is maintained at a minimum of 4 cm H_2O. Once the optimal EPAP is obtained based on elimination of apneic episodes at a pressure that is comfortable for the patient, the IPAP is then adjusted by increments of 1 cm H_2O in intervals no shorter than 15 minutes to eliminate hypopneas and hypoventilation. In patients with only neuromuscular disorders, it is unlikely that they will need supplemental oxygen. The predominant underlying pathophysiology is hypoventilation during sleep, which normally should be corrected by BPAP alone. Use of supplemental oxygen alone (without BPAP) in patients with neuromuscular disorders may depress the drive to breathe. Similar to COPD patients, every effort should be made to assess/titrate BPAP during REM sleep since patients with neuromuscular disorders are most vulnerable to hypoventilation during this stage. The initial requirement for the back up rate occurs during REM sleep when hypoventilation is the worst resulting in the patient not triggering the BPAP. As neuromuscular disorders progress and the hypoventilation worsens, most if not all patients require back up rate in all stages of sleep. Obtaining an arterial blood gas within a few minutes of waking up the following morning of the titration is also recommended to assess $Paco_2$ levels.

SUPPLEMENTAL OXYGEN TITRATION

If the patient's awake supine baseline oxyhemoglobin saturation is less than 88%, supplemental oxygen is usually initiated at 1 L/min at the start of the PAP titration and titrated upward by 1 L/min at intervals no shorter than 15 minutes.[3] Supplemental oxygen should be started during the titration study if the patient's oxyhemoglobin saturation is less 88% for 5 or more minutes in the absence of OSA events.[3] Supplemental oxygen is titrated up at a rate of 1 L/min at intervals no shorter than 15 minutes to maintain oxyhemoglobin saturation of more than 88%.[3]

Patients who have persistent sleep-related hypoxemia or hypoventilation that is not effectively treated with a PAP device will need supplemental oxygen to maintain oxyhemoglobin saturation of more than 88%. In these situations, supplemental oxygen is connected to the PAP device outlet and not the mask.[3] Furthermore, patients who were on supplemental oxygen before PAP titration are likely to need a higher amount of oxygen with the PAP device because of higher flow rates reducing the effective oxygen concentration for a given supplemental oxygen flow.[3,72,73] Ideally in those patients who required supplemental oxygen or upward titration of the previously used oxygen, an arterial blood gas is performed the following day, usually within a few minutes of waking, to assess for hypercapnia.

SUMMARY

The recently published guidelines from the AASM on the manual titration of PAP in patients with OSA[3] are the first step toward standardizing titration protocols in the sleep center. Standardizing titration protocols brings uniformity to the whole titration process so that patients, when recommended an optimum pressure on a PAP device at a certain sleep center, are likely to get the same (or very close to the same) recommended optimum pressure if the titration study was repeated at a different sleep center. This standardization will significantly improve reliability of treatment and overall quality of care. Further work is needed, specifically to discuss and establish titration protocols for sleep disorders other than OSA and for different modes of PAP (and ventilatory) devices. Based on the current available literature (which is limited) and experience, the authors advanced several recommendations to titrate for SRBDs other than OSA. More importantly, further research is required to not only establish titration protocols for other SRBDs but also address barriers that might prevent implementation of these recommendations in sleep centers.

REFERENCES

1. Weaver TE, Grunstein RR. Adherence to continuous positive airway pressure therapy: the challenge to effective treatment. Proc Am Thorac Soc 2008;5(2): 173–8.

2. Iber C, Ancoli-Israel S, Chesson A, et al. The AASM manual for the scoring of sleep and associated events: rules, terminology and technical specifications. 2nd edition. Westchester (IL): American Academy of Sleep Medicine; 2007.

3. Kushida CA, Chediak A, Berry RB, et al. Clinical guidelines for the manual titration of positive airway pressure in patients with obstructive sleep apnea. J Clin Sleep Med 2008;4(2):157–71.

4. Stepanski EJ. The need for a standardized CPAP titration protocol and follow-up procedures. J Clin Sleep Med 2005;1(3):311.

5. Stepanski EJ, Dull R, Basner R. CPAP titration protocols among accredited sleep disorder centers. J Sleep Res 1996;25:374.

6. White DP. Pathogenesis of obstructive and central sleep apnea. Am J Respir Crit Care Med 2005; 172(11):1363–70.

7. Schwartz AR, Smith PL, Wise RA, et al. Induction of upper airway occlusion in sleeping individuals with subatmospheric nasal pressure. J Appl Physiol 1988;64(2):535–42.

8. Watanabe T, Isono S, Tanaka A, et al. Contribution of body habitus and craniofacial characteristics to segmental closing pressures of the passive pharynx in patients with sleep-disordered breathing. Am J Respir Crit Care Med 2002;165(2):260–5.

9. Younes M, Ostrowski M, Thompson W, et al. Chemical control stability in patients with obstructive sleep apnea. Am J Respir Crit Care Med 2001;163(5): 1181–90.

10. Schwab RJ, Gupta KB, Gefter WB, et al. Upper airway and soft tissue anatomy in normal subjects and patients with sleep-disordered breathing. Significance of the lateral pharyngeal walls. Am J Respir Crit Care Med 1995;152(5 Pt 1):1673–89.

11. Sullivan CE, Issa FG, Berthon-Jones M, et al. Home treatment of obstructive sleep apnoea with continuous positive airway pressure applied through a nose-mask. Bull Eur Physiopathol Respir 1984; 20(1):49–54.

12. Sforza E, Krieger J, Bacon W, et al. Determinants of effective continuous positive airway pressure in obstructive sleep apnea. Role of respiratory effort. Am J Respir Crit Care Med 1995;151(6):1852–6.

13. Miljeteig H, Hoffstein V. Determinants of continuous positive airway pressure level for treatment of obstructive sleep apnea. Am Rev Respir Dis 1993; 147(6 Pt 1):1526–30.

14. Hoffstein V, Mateika S. Predicting nasal continuous positive airway pressure. Am J Respir Crit Care Med 1994;150(2):486–8.

15. Gokcebay N, Iqbal S, Yang K, et al. Accuracy of CPAP predicted from anthropometric and polysomnographic indices. Sleep 1996;19(7):600–1.

16. Rowley JA, Tarbichi AG, Badr MS. The use of a predicted CPAP equation improves CPAP titration success. Sleep Breath 2005;9(1):26–32.

17. Kushida CA, Littner MR, Morgenthaler T, et al. Practice parameters for the indications for polysomnography and related procedures: an update for 2005. Sleep 2005;28(4):499–521.

18. McArdle N, Grove A, Devereux G, et al. Split-night versus full-night studies for sleep apnoea/hypopnoea syndrome. Eur Respir J 2000;15(4):670–5.

19. Sanders MH, Kern NB, Costantino JP, et al. Prescription of positive airway pressure for sleep apnea on the basis of a partial-night trial. Sleep 1993;16(Suppl 8):S106–7.

20. Strollo PJ Jr, Sanders MH, Costantino JP, et al. Split-night studies for the diagnosis and treatment of sleep-disordered breathing. Sleep 1996;19(10 Suppl): S255–9.

21. Yamashiro Y, Kryger MH. CPAP titration for sleep apnea using a split-night protocol. Chest 1995; 107(1):62–6.

22. Sanders MH, Kern NB, Costantino JP, et al. Adequacy of prescribing positive airway pressure therapy by mask for sleep apnea on the basis of a partial-night trial. Am Rev Respir Dis 1993; 147(5):1169–74.

23. Drake CL, Day R, Hudgel D, et al. Sleep during titration predicts continuous positive airway pressure compliance. Sleep 2003;26(3):308–11.

24. Hirshkowitz M, Sharafkhaneh A. Positive airway pressure therapy of OSA. Semin Respir Crit Care Med 2005;26(1):68–79.

25. Kushida CA, Littner MR, Hirshkowitz M, et al. Practice parameters for the use of continuous and bilevel positive airway pressure devices to treat adult patients with sleep-related breathing disorders. Sleep 2006;29(3):375–80.

26. Strohl KP, Redline S. Nasal CPAP therapy, upper airway muscle activation, and obstructive sleep apnea. Am Rev Respir Dis 1986;134(3):555–8.

27. Sullivan CE, Issa FG, Berthon-Jones M, et al. Reversal of obstructive sleep apnoea by continuous positive airway pressure applied through the nares. Lancet 1981;1(8225):862–5.

28. American Academy of Sleep Medicine. International classification of sleep disorders: diagnostic and coding manual. 2nd edition. Westchester (IL): American Academy of Sleep Medicine; 2005.

29. Dohi T, Kasai T, Narui K, et al. Bi-level positive airway pressure ventilation for treating heart failure with central sleep apnea that is unresponsive to continuous positive airway pressure. Circ J 2008;72(7): 1100–5.

30. Hu K, Li QQ, Yang J, et al. The role of high-frequency jet ventilation in the treatment of Cheyne-Stokes respiration in patients with chronic heart failure. Int J Cardiol 2006;106(2):224–31.

31. Philippe C, Stoica-Herman M, Drouot X, et al. Compliance with and effectiveness of adaptive servoventilation versus continuous positive airway pressure in the treatment of Cheyne-Stokes respiration in heart failure over a six month period. Heart 2006; 92(3):337–42.

32. Ruttanaumpawan P, Logan AG, Floras JS, et al. Effect of continuous positive airway pressure on sleep structure in heart failure patients with central sleep apnea. Sleep 2009;32(1):91–8.

33. Javaheri S, Malik A, Smith J, et al. Adaptive pressure support servoventilation: a novel treatment for sleep apnea associated with use of opioids. J Clin Sleep Med 2008;4(4):305–10.

34. Aloia MS, Stanchina M, Arnedt JT, et al. Treatment adherence and outcomes in flexible vs standard continuous positive airway pressure therapy. Chest 2005;127(6):2085–93.

35. Mulgrew AT, Cheema R, Fleetham J, et al. Efficacy and patient satisfaction with autoadjusting CPAP with variable expiratory pressure vs standard CPAP: a two-night randomized crossover trial. Sleep Breath 2007;11(1):31–7.

36. Ruhle KH, Domanski U, Happel A, et al. [Analysis of expiratory pressure reduction (C-Flex method) during CPAP therapy]. Pneumologie 2007;61(2): 86–9 [in German].

37. Bradley TD, Logan AG, Kimoff RJ, et al. Continuous positive airway pressure for central sleep apnea and heart failure. N Engl J Med 2005;353(19):2025–33.

38. Teschler H, Dohring J, Wang YM, et al. Adaptive pressure support servo-ventilation: a novel treatment for Cheyne-Stokes respiration in heart failure. Am J Respir Crit Care Med 2001;164(4):614–9.

39. Gay PC. Complex sleep apnea: it really is a disease. J Clin Sleep Med 2008;4(5):403–5.

40. Malhotra A, Bertisch S, Wellman A. Complex sleep apnea: it isn't really a disease. J Clin Sleep Med 2008;4(5):406–8.

41. Dernaika T, Tawk M, Nazir S, et al. The significance and outcome of continuous positive airway pressure-related central sleep apnea during split-night sleep studies. Chest 2007;132(1):81–7.

42. Remmers JE, deGroot WJ, Sauerland EK, et al. Pathogenesis of upper airway occlusion during sleep. J Appl Physiol 1978;44(6):931–8.

43. Smith PL, Wise RA, Gold AR, et al. Upper airway pressure-flow relationships in obstructive sleep apnea. J Appl Physiol 1988;64(2):789–95.

44. Suratt PM, Wilhoit SC, Cooper K. Induction of airway collapse with subatmospheric pressure in awake patients with sleep apnea. J Appl Physiol 1984; 57(1):140–6.

45. Sanders MH, Moore SE. Inspiratory and expiratory partitioning of airway resistance during sleep in patients with sleep apnea. Am Rev Respir Dis 1983;127(5):554–8.

46. Sanders MH, Rogers RM, Pennock BE. Prolonged expiratory phase in sleep apnea. A unifying hypothesis. Am Rev Respir Dis 1985;131(3):401–8.

47. Resta O, Guido P, Picca V, et al. The role of the expiratory phase in obstructive sleep apnoea. Respir Med 1999;93(3):190–5.

48. Sanders MH, Kern N. Obstructive sleep apnea treated by independently adjusted inspiratory and expiratory positive airway pressures via nasal mask. Physiologic and clinical implications. Chest 1990;98(2):317–24.

49. Gay PC, Herold DL, Olson EJ. A randomized, double-blind clinical trial comparing continuous positive airway pressure with a novel bilevel pressure system for treatment of obstructive sleep apnea syndrome. Sleep 2003;26(7):864–9.

50. Resta O, Guido P, Foschino Barbaro MP, et al. Sleep-related breathing disorders in acute respiratory failure assisted by non-invasive ventilatory treatment: utility of portable polysomnographic system. Respir Med 2000;94(2):128–34.

51. Reeves-Hoche MK, Hudgel DW, Meck R, et al. Continuous versus bilevel positive airway pressure for obstructive sleep apnea. Am J Respir Crit Care Med 1995;151(2 Pt 1):443–9.

52. Resta O, Guido P, Picca V, et al. Prescription of nCPAP and nBIPAP in obstructive sleep apnoea syndrome: Italian experience in 105 subjects. A prospective two centre study. Respir Med 1998; 92(6):820–7.

53. Schafer H, Ewig S, Hasper E, et al. Failure of CPAP therapy in obstructive sleep apnoea syndrome: predictive factors and treatment with bilevel-positive airway pressure. Respir Med 1998;92(2): 208–15.

54. Keenan SP, Kernerman PD, Cook DJ, et al. Effect of noninvasive positive pressure ventilation on mortality in patients admitted with acute respiratory failure: a meta-analysis. Crit Care Med 1997;25(10): 1685–92.

55. Gay PC, Hubmayr RD, Stroetz RW. Efficacy of nocturnal nasal ventilation in stable, severe chronic obstructive pulmonary disease during a 3-month controlled trial. Mayo Clin Proc 1996;71(6):533–42.

56. Krachman SL, Quaranta AJ, Berger TJ, et al. Effects of noninvasive positive pressure ventilation on gas exchange and sleep in COPD patients. Chest 1997;112(3):623–8.

57. Lin CC. Comparison between nocturnal nasal positive pressure ventilation combined with oxygen therapy and oxygen monotherapy in patients with severe COPD. Am J Respir Crit Care Med 1996; 154(2 Pt 1):353–8.

58. Meecham Jones DJ, Paul EA, Jones PW, et al. Nasal pressure support ventilation plus oxygen compared with oxygen therapy alone in hypercapnic COPD. Am J Respir Crit Care Med 1995;152(2):538–44.

59. Clinical indications for noninvasive positive pressure ventilation in chronic respiratory failure due to restrictive lung disease, COPD, and nocturnal hypoventilation–a consensus conference report. Chest 1999;116(2):521–34.

60. Ellis ER, Grunstein RR, Chan S, et al. Noninvasive ventilatory support during sleep improves respiratory failure in kyphoscoliosis. Chest 1988;94(4):811–5.

61. Hill NS, Eveloff SE, Carlisle CC, et al. Efficacy of nocturnal nasal ventilation in patients with restrictive thoracic disease. Am Rev Respir Dis 1992;145(2 Pt 1):365–71.

62. Piper AJ, Sullivan CE. Effects of long-term nocturnal nasal ventilation on spontaneous breathing during sleep in neuromuscular and chest wall disorders. Eur Respir J 1996;9(7):1515–22.

63. Guilleminault C, Philip P, Robinson A. Sleep and neuromuscular disease: bilevel positive airway pressure by nasal mask as a treatment for sleep disordered breathing in patients with neuromuscular disease. J Neurol Neurosurg Psychiatry 1998; 65(2):225–32.

64. Pinto AC, Evangelista T, Carvalho M, et al. Respiratory assistance with a non-invasive ventilator (Bipap) in MND/ALS patients: survival rates in a controlled trial. Journal of the neurological sciences. J Neurol Sci 1995;129(Suppl):19–26.

65. Department of Health and Human Services. Medicare part B fee-for-service claims data 2005. Available at: www.cms.hhs.gov. Accessed May 13, 2010

66. Fietze I, Blau A, Glos M, et al. Bi-level positive pressure ventilation and adaptive servo ventilation in patients with heart failure and Cheyne-Stokes respiration. Sleep Med 2008;9(6):652–9.

67. Kasai T, Narui K, Dohi T, et al. Efficacy of nasal bilevel positive airway pressure in congestive heart failure patients with Cheyne-Stokes respiration and central sleep apnea. Circ J 2005;69(8):913–21.

68. Kohnlein T, Welte T, Tan LB, et al. Assisted ventilation for heart failure patients with Cheyne-Stokes respiration. Eur Respir J 2002;20(4):934–41.

69. Noda A, Izawa H, Asano H, et al. Beneficial effect of bilevel positive airway pressure on left ventricular function in ambulatory patients with idiopathic dilated cardiomyopathy and central sleep apnea hypopnea: a preliminary study. Chest 2007;131(6):1694–701.

70. Alattar MA, Scharf SM. Opioid-associated central sleep apnea: a case series. Sleep Breath 2009; 13(2):201–6.

71. Johnson KG, Johnson DC. Bilevel positive airway pressure worsens central apneas during sleep. Chest 2005;128(4):2141–50.

72. Schwartz AR, Kacmarek RM, Hess DR. Factors affecting oxygen delivery with bi-level positive airway pressure. Respir Care 2004;49(3):270–5.

73. Yoder EA, Klann K, Strohl KP. Inspired oxygen concentrations during positive pressure therapy. Sleep Breath 2004;8(1):1–5.

Positive Airway Pressure Treatment of Adult Patients with Obstructive Sleep Apnea

Tapan Desai, MD, Meena Khan, MD, Nitin Y. Bhatt, MD*

KEYWORDS

- Positive airway pressure
- Obstructive sleep apnea
- Therapy

Obstructive sleep apnea/hypopnea syndrome (OSA) is a disorder that is characterized by intermittent and recurrent upper airway closure during sleep that results in sleep fragmentation, intermittent hypoxemia/hypercapnia, and increased sympathetic nervous system activation. OSA is associated with daytime sleepiness, cognitive defects, increased risk of cardiovascular disease, hypertension, stroke, and glucose intolerance. In addition, OSA has a cost to society in economic terms as well as public safety.[1–3] As a result, the Centers for Disease Control and Prevention has emphasized the role of sleep disorders including OSA in the development and management of chronic diseases. The care of chronic illness accounts for a significant portion of total health care expenditures each year and diseases associated with or affected by OSA, including hypertension, heart disease, diabetes, asthma, and mood disorders, account for approximately one-half of United States health care spending.[4,5] Positive airway pressure (PAP) therapy, and in particular continuous positive airway pressure (CPAP) therapy, has been shown to be effective in the management of OSA.[6] For many reasons, difficulty with patient adherence to PAP therapy remains a problem. Like these other chronic diseases, long-term management of OSA and PAP therapy require a structured, multidisciplinary approach to monitoring and treatment.

Nasal continuous positive airway pressure (nCPAP) therapy for sleep apnea was first described in 1981 by Sullivan and colleagues.[7] In their case series report, 5 patients who had severe OSA were treated with CPAP applied through the nares. Their use of lower pressure levels completely prevented upper airway occlusion and allowed uninterrupted sleep.[8] PAP therapy is both safe and effective, and can be used in all forms of sleep-disordered breathing.[9] Furthermore, high-quality evidence exists from multiple randomized studies showing benefit of PAP therapy regarding subjective daytime sleepiness, alertness, and improvement in overall quality of life.[10,11] Treatment with PAP should ideally be approached on a case-by-case basis. A multidisciplinary approach should be used in the management of these patients. Patients should be educated about the function, care, and maintenance of their equipment, the benefits of PAP therapy, and potential problems.[12] PAP therapy goes beyond CPAP alone. Bilevel PAP, end-expiratory pressure relief, and autotitrating PAP (APAP) devices may also be used in the management of OSA. Adaptive servo-ventilation (ASV) may also be used but is typically reserved for

Division of Pulmonary, Allergy, Critical Care, and Sleep Medicine, The Ohio State University, 201 Davis Heart and Lung Research Institute, 473 West 12th Avenue, Columbus, OH 43210, USA
* Corresponding author.
E-mail address: nitin.bhatt@osumc.edu

Sleep Med Clin 5 (2010) 347–359
doi:10.1016/j.jsmc.2010.05.003
1556-407X/10/$ – see front matter © 2010 Elsevier Inc. All rights reserved.

complicated central sleep apnea and/or Cheyne-Stokes respiration.

The indication for treatment of OSA is dependent on a thorough clinical history and clinical signs along with objective evaluation via a polysomnogram.[12] The severity of sleep apnea is defined by the apnea/hypopnea index (AHI), which is the total number of apneas plus hypopneas divided by the hours of sleep, or the respiratory disturbance index (RDI), the total of apneas, hypopneas, and respiratory event-related arousals divided by the hours of sleep. Mild sleep apnea is defined as an AHI or RDI of from 5 to 15, moderate is 15 to 29, and severe is 30 or greater. Nasally applied CPAP is now the established treatment for OSA syndrome. CPAP acts as a pneumatic splint to prevent the collapse of the pharyngeal airway, achieving this by reversing the transmural pressure gradient across the pharyngeal airway. CPAP is currently the "gold standard" for treatment of moderate to severe OSA (AHI >15). It also can be used as adjunctive therapy in the management of blood pressure that is difficult to control. Current guidelines recommend that treatment of OSA should be advised and offered when the following criteria on polysomnography have been met[13]:

1. AHI or a RDI greater than or equal to 15 events per hour; OR
2. AHI (or RDI) greater than or equal to 5, and less than 15 events per hour with documentation demonstrating any of the following symptoms:
   Excessive daytime sleepiness, as documented by either a score of greater than 10 on the Epworth Sleepiness Scale (ESS) or inappropriate daytime napping (eg, during driving, conversation, or eating) or sleepiness that interferes with daily activities; or
   Impaired cognition or mood disorders; or
   Hypertension; or
   Ischemic heart disease or history of stroke; or
   Cardiac arrhythmias, or
   Pulmonary hypertension.

Despite the benefit that may be obtained from a fixed pressure device, CPAP compliance remains a major issue.[14] Factors including the amount of pressure itself, interface, social stigma, affordability, relatives who have OSA, education level, and severity of disease all can adversely affect compliance.[15–17] Given the inherent nature of CPAP and its fixed pressure, it has been thought that APAP may eliminate issues with compliance by varying the pressure throughout the night needed to maintain airway patency. APAP has been investigated both as a means to establish the required level of therapeutic "fixed" CPAP for long-term use as an alternative to sleep laboratory technician-titrated CPAP, and as a long-term therapeutic alternative to fixed CPAP. APAP devices use an algorithm to increase the pressure in response to snoring, airflow limitation, apneas, and hypopneas, and decrease the pressure when no events are detected.[18] There have been similarities shown regarding improvement in awakening/arousal index, daytime sleepiness, nocturnal oxygen saturation, and AHI.[19,20] APAP should not be used to diagnose OSA, nor be used in a split-night polysomnogram. APAP can be used as an unattended treatment or as a way to determine a fixed CPAP pressure in patients with moderate to severe OSA without significant comorbidities such as congestive heart failure, chronic obstructive pulmonary disease (COPD), central sleep apnea syndromes, or hypoventilation syndromes.[21]

Expiratory pressure relief CPAP (C-Flex; Respironics, Murrysville, PA), differs from conventional CPAP in that the devices lower the pressure at the onset of expiration. The magnitude of the reduction in pressure depends on the expiratory flow and can be preset in 3 different steps. The reduction of pressure at the beginning of expiration is intended to reduce the sensation of breathing against high pressure without causing the upper airways to collapse.[22]

Bilevel PAP devices cycle between a predetermined inspiratory PAP phase and a preset expiratory PAP phase. The backup rate feature on some of these machines ensures that the patient will receive a set minimum number of breaths per minute should the patient stop breathing spontaneously. Bilevel PAP devices can also be used to augment spontaneous patient respirations, as part of the treatment plan for certain pulmonary conditions, and can also be used for complicated OSA. In patients with coexisting disease comorbidities such as COPD, neuromuscular disease, and thoracic restrictive diseases, bilevel ventilation may be beneficial.[23] The use of these noninvasive positive pressure (NIPPV) respiratory assist devices for the treatment of patients with severe COPD is considered medically necessary when ALL of the following are met:

- An arterial blood gas $PaCO_2$, done while awake and breathing the individual's usual FIO_2, is ≥ 52 mm Hg; and
- Sleep oximetry demonstrates oxygen saturation $\leq 88\%$ for at least 5 continuous minutes, done while breathing oxygen at

2 L/min. or the individual's usual FIO_2 (whichever is higher); and

In patients with OSA and neuromuscular disease, the following criteria may be used for bilevel ventilation initiation[23,24]:

- The patient has been diagnosed with a progressive neuromuscular disease (eg, amyotrophic lateral sclerosis) or a severe thoracic cage abnormality (eg, postthoracoplasty for tuberculosis); and

- COPD does not contribute significantly to the individual's pulmonary limitation; and ONE or more of the following criteria are met:
  An arterial blood gas $PaCO_2$ level is ≥ 45 mm Hg, done while awake and breathing the patient's usual FIO_2 (fractionated inspired oxygen concentration); or
  Sleep oximetry demonstrates an oxygen saturation $\leq 88\%$ for at least 5 continuous minutes, done while breathing the patient's usual FIO_2; or
  Maximal inspiratory pressure is <60 cm H_2O or forced vital capacity is <50% of predicted for patients with a progressive neuromuscular disease.

NIPPV can also play a role in the management of patients diagnosed with OSA in the perioperative setting with the aforementioned comorbidities and/or in whom CPAP is not indicated or has failed.[25] Another large group that may benefit from NIPPV is those with obesity-hypoventilation syndrome (OHS). The American Academy of Sleep Medicine's International Classification of Sleep Disorders categorizes sleep-related hypoventilation syndromes based on etiology: these may be idiopathic in origin, due to pulmonary parenchymal or vascular pathology, due to lower airway obstruction, or due to neuromuscular and chest wall disorders. This last group, for which obesity is the only identifiable cause of hypoventilation, includes OHS.[26] OHS is a diagnosis of exclusion. Clinical features of OHS include symptoms of daytime hypercapnia (such as fatigue and morning headache), right-sided heart failure/cor pulmonale, $PaCO_2$ of 45 mm Hg or more, hypoxia during wakefulness and sleep (arterial oxygen saturation <90%), a greater than 10 mm Hg increase in the $PaCO_2$ during sleep (the primary manifestation), and respiratory acidosis (pH <7.3) during sleep. There is increased risk that OSA/OHS can lead to chronic respiratory failure in these individuals. Although CPAP may be used to also treat many OHS patients, some will require bilevel PAP.[27,28]

Sleep-disordered breathing is a general term that incorporates OSA and central sleep apnea (CSA). In recent years, many studies have demonstrated significant associations between sleep-disordered breathing and multiple cardiovascular disease processes including systemic hypertension, pulmonary hypertension, coronary artery disease, cerebrovascular accidents, and arrhythmias.[29] Cheyne-Stokes respiration (CSR) is a subtype of CSA constituted by periodic breathing in which central apneas (and hypopneas) alternate with periods of hyperventilation in a crescendo/decrescendo ventilatory pattern. Even though it is classically taught that CSA-CSR is found most commonly in association with systolic heart failure, it is important to remember that the majority of patients who have central apneas can also have some obstructive physiology. There is also an entity called complex sleep apnea. In this condition, patients most often have classic OSA on diagnostic polysomnography but exhibit disruptive central apneas when CPAP is initiated.[30] At present there is no consensus regarding the management of complex sleep apnea or CSA-CSR. In terms of CSR, the best data come from the Canadian Positive Airway Pressure (CANPAP) trial in which 258 patients who had heart failure and CSA syndrome were randomly assigned to receive CPAP or no CPAP for 2 years. The CPAP group had a greater reduction in the AHI, as well as greater improvements in mean nocturnal arterial oxyhemoglobin saturation, left ventricular ejection fraction, and the 6-minute walk distance than the control group. However, there were no differences in the number of hospitalizations, quality of life, or transplant-free survival. Based on an early divergence of the transplantation-free survival curves favoring the control group, an enrollment rate that was only 50% of the predicted rate, and a falling rate of death and heart transplantation, the study was terminated early. CPAP is not recommended for patients who have CSA and heart failure.[31]

ASV uses an automatic, minute ventilation-targeted device that performs breath-to-breath analysis and adjusts its settings accordingly. Depending on either flow or minute ventilation, the device will automatically adjust the amount of pressure support it delivers to maintain a certain flow or minute ventilation. ASV has been shown to be more effective than CPAP in treating patients with CSR and CSA both in the short term and over several months.[32] ASV has also been shown to be effective in patients with complex sleep apnea. At present there are several ongoing trials comparing ASV with CPAP in the management of CSA/CSR and complex sleep apnea syndrome.

Despite the efficacy of PAP in treating sleep apnea, compliance with therapy remains a significant problem. Compliance with any therapy such as PAP is a multistep process, beginning with acceptance of the therapy. In most studies, acceptance of the need for CPAP and prescription of therapy for the use of PAP therapy at home ranges from 70% to 80% of patients.[33,34] Adherence to PAP is the ongoing use of PAP at home and tolerance of potential side effects associated with usage.[33,35] Currently accepted measures of adequate adherence are the use of PAP for at least 4 hours a night on 70% of the nights. In general, patients overestimate their use of PAP therapy by over an hour per night.[36] Patterns of patient adherence to PAP therapy develop early in the course of treatment, typically within the first week.[37,38] These patterns are predictive of long-term use of PAP therapy. A study of patterns of PAP use over the first 3 months of treatment found that about half of the patients consistently used PAP therapy for greater than 90% of the nights and averaged over 6 hours of use per night. The other half of the patients were much more variable in their use, ranging anywhere from 2% to 79% of the nights, and averaging approximately 3.5 hours per night. These 2 patterns of use developed by the fourth night of PAP use. No specific predictors of PAP adherence have been consistently reported that identify patients prior to beginning PAP in terms of age, gender, education, marital status, physiologic parameters, severity of sleep apnea or nocturnal hypoxemia, ESS score, or CPAP pressures. The presence of self-reported daytime sleepiness[39–41] as well as subjective improvement in sleep quality and daytime sleepiness[42–44] may correlate with increased PAP adherence. The lack of symptoms may predict poor compliance to PAP therapy.[45] Depression, anxiety, and stress have not consistently correlated with PAP therapy compliance.[43] The presence of a type D personality with a negative affect and social inhibition was associated with lower PAP adherence.[46]

Improvements in measures of daytime sleepiness, quality of life, and mortality have been reported with use below the recommended levels. Furthermore, different levels of PAP adherence are associated with improvement in different outcome measures. A threshold of 4 hours was found for the ESS, 6 hours for the Multiple Sleep Latency Test, and 7.5 hours for the Functional Outcomes associated with Sleepiness Questionnaire (FOSQ). PAP use above this threshold did not result in further improvements in the respective outcome measures. In addition, a linear dose-response relationship was found between increased use of PAP therapy and achieving normal levels of objective and subjective daytime sleepiness; this plateaued at 7 hours of use for measures of functional status.[47] Symptoms can recur with a single missed night.[48] In the long term, up to 25% of patients may discontinue PAP therapy in the first year.[40]

Problems with compliance are not unique to PAP therapy, and affect any medical therapy. Studies of multiple medications ranging from antihypertensives, inhalers, home oxygen, antiepileptics, and others have shown compliance rates of 50% to 80%.[49] A meta-analysis of patient adherence to various treatment regimens found an average nonadherence rate of approximately 25%. The highest adherence rates were 80% or more for human immunodeficiency virus disease, arthritis, gastrointestinal disorders, and cancer. The lowest rates (<70%) were for pulmonary disease, diabetes, and sleep.[50] A recent study investigated the compliance of patients with severe OSA based on their adherence and persistence with PAP and 3 medication categories: antihypertensives, statins, and antiplatelet agents. These patients were selective in their compliance to various therapies, and medication adherence and persistence during the 2-year period for the cardiovascular medications were not different in patients who were nonadherent to CPAP.[34] Other studies have shown the "healthy user" effect in that patients more compliant with medications were more compliant with CPAP. In a recent study, those with low medication adherence demonstrated a 40.1% probability of using CPAP for 4 hours a day or longer compared with 55.2% for subjects with adequate (≥80%) medication adherence. Married patients were more adherent to medications and CPAP.[51]

A task force of the American Academy of Sleep Medicine (AASM) recently published guidelines for the evaluation, management, and long-term care of OSA in adults.[12] The guidelines recommended a multidisciplinary approach to patient care involving a sleep specialist, nursing, respiratory therapy, sleep technicians, and the patient's primary care physician. Different modifications of CPAP have been developed to improve patient comfort and compliance with minimal success. Improving patient perception and acceptance of therapy via education and cognitive therapy is a promising way to promote good compliance. An all-encompassing approach to therapy is needed, which includes educating patients on OSA, emphasizing the importance of CPAP therapy, monitoring response to therapy, and troubleshooting side effects.

Up to 50% of patients have been shown to abandon CPAP therapy.[52] Many will do so after the titration study or within 2 weeks of receiving CPAP, often before they are scheduled to follow up with their physician.[52] Patterns of adherence develop within the first week,[37,38] and discontinuing CPAP is associated with lower hours of use early in the course of treatment.[40,52,53] This finding suggests that to promote good compliance, patients should receive some contact within the first week of receiving CPAP to evaluate hours of use, improvement or lack of improvement in symptoms, potential side effects of treatment, and any necessary interventions. In addition, patients who have difficulty with PAP therapy on the night of the titration, who do not believe that they can tolerate the device long term, or who did not notice any benefit on the initial night of use are at higher risk for noncompliance and can often be identified after the PAP titration.[42] This group may benefit from more directed follow-up during the first few days to the first week than those who did notice benefit. This approach has been made more practical with the development of technology to remotely monitor PAP use or direct telephone contact with the patient.[15,54–56]

Early adherence to PAP therapy is important, as patterns of adherence in the short term can predict long-term compliance.[36,40,57,58] Therefore, if sleep physicians can help their patients obtain good patient compliance early in the treatment course, it is reasonable to assume that this will be maintained in the long term. A study of a population-based CPAP program achieved compliance rates of 84% at 6 months. These patients underwent an educational session before starting CPAP, telephone contact daily during the first week, and clinic visits at weeks 2 and 4 and months 3 and 6.[56] Another study showed that CPAP use can increase over time with regular follow-up at 9, 18, and 30 months.[52] Some patients will decide to stop using CPAP after a year,[40,53] and regular follow-up may deter this. Therefore, regular long-term follow-up is important as well. Current recommendations are for follow-up visits annually, based on the patient's early adherence, tolerance, and improvement in symptoms.[59]

During the follow-up evaluation, possible side effects that affect tolerance and adherence should be addressed. Side effects include mask discomfort, claustrophobia, pressure discomfort, nasal obstruction, and dryness. It is important to ask patients about these side effects, especially if compliance is low. Not all patients will tell their physician they are experiencing these problems.

Mask discomfort is a common issue.[60,61] The types of interfaces are nasal, oronasal, and oral.

The nasal mask is the traditional way to deliver CPAP. Complaints associated with the nasal mask are nasal congestion, nasal dryness, epistaxis, dry nose or mouth, pressure from the mask or straps, frequent mask dislodgment, abrasion to the bridge of the nose, sneezing, nasal drip, sinusitis, and claustrophobia.[61–63] Mask leak can lead to drying of eyes and discomfort. In addition, tightening of head gear to compensate for air leak can lead to contact dermatitis, skin breakdown, and possible infection.[63] To combat these issues, alternatives to the traditional nasal mask have been developed and include the full face mask, nasal pillows, and the oral mask.[64] The full face mask may help with those who have nasal congestion or mouth leak.[64] Nasal pillows are smaller and less bulky, and thus may be more comfortable and reduce pressure sores on the bridge of the nose. The oral mask might be a good alternative for those with mouth leak or nasal congestion who cannot tolerate a full face mask. There are limited studies comparing effectiveness and compliance between the different interfaces. CPAP delivered via nasal mask versus nasal pillow or full face mask is equally effective in decreasing the AHI.[65–67] The face mask alleviates mouth leak and improves airway dryness compared with the nasal mask; however, there are more complaints of claustrophobia and discomfort.[62] Most patients prefer a nasal mask to a full face mask, and one study did show that the ESS score was lower and compliance was 1 hour more per night at 4 weeks with the nasal mask.[62,68] Another study showed that the number of days used was higher for the nasal pillow than for the nasal mask, but not mean hours of use.[67] Fewer side effects in terms of less leakage and claustrophobia, better sleep quality, and more satisfaction were noted with nasal pillows.[67] Studies of nasal interface versus oral mask found no difference in compliance, therapeutic pressure needs, symptomatic improvement, and overall patient satisfaction.[63,69] Side effects of the oral mask are dry mouth or throat, excessive salivation, and sore gums or lips.[63,69] One study comparing nasal, oronasal, and oral masks showed that most patients preferred the nasal mask to the oronasal and oral mask.[70] Another way to combat mouth leak and still use a nasal mask is the use of a chin strap. The chin strap has been shown to subjectively improve dryness as well as objectively reduce mouth leak and arousals, although these were not eliminated.[71] Addressing issues concerning the interface is important for patient comfort. However, compliance and effectiveness has not been shown to be superior for any one type of interface.

Claustrophobia can also be an issue. One way to combat this is by choosing a less bulky and obtrusive interface such as a nasal pillow or even an oral mask. In addition, some success has been described with desensitization for claustrophobic patients. Edinger and Radtke[72] described this in a case report of a male patient who failed CPAP because of claustrophobia, who then went through a desensitization process. He was able to use CPAP on a regular basis at 6.5 years' follow-up. Means and colleagues[73,74] reported a case series of patients who were not adherent to CPAP because of claustrophobia. The patients were put through a graded desensitization process with the aid of a clinical psychologist. This process was successful in increasing the nights of CPAP use and hours used per night.

Devices such as bilevel PAP, APAP, and expiratory pressure relief have been used to improve patient comfort in the expectation that adherence may improve. None have been shown to improve compliance conclusively compared with traditional CPAP, but still may be used as an option in those who complain of pressure intolerance. Bilevel PAP was thought to be a good alternative to CPAP, based on the idea that less pressure is needed to maintain airway patency during expiration as compared with inspiration. Bilevel PAP can be achieved by independently varying the expiratory PAP (EPAP) and inspiratory PAP (IPAP) pressures whereby the EPAP maintains upper airway patency during expiration and IPAP maintains upper airway patency during inspiration.[75] Sanders and Kern[75] showed that when comparing nasal CPAP to bilevel PAP titration, the effective IPAP pressure is the same as the effective CPAP pressure but the EPAP was lower. The reduction in AHI was similar for bilevel PAP and CPAP. Thus, bilevel PAP can effectively treat OSA with lower levels of pressure during expiration as compared with CPAP. Randomized clinical studies have demonstrated similar improvement in AHI, ESS, and FOSQ; however, no difference in compliance was found at 30 days or at 1 year.[76,77] These trials were done in patients new to PAP therapy. Bilevel PAP may be a viable option in patients who have failed CPAP due to pressure intolerance.

APAP machines were designed based on the idea that CPAP pressure requirements can vary during the night depending on sleep posture, sleep stage, alcohol, and nasal congestion.[19,20,78,79] A patient may require more pressure during supine rapid eye movement (REM) than during non-REM.[64] APAP is designed to analyze upper airway patency and increase the pressure to open the airway as needed, and then decrease the pressure if no events are detected. The purpose is to effectively treat OSA with a lower mean nightly pressure, which may improve pressure tolerance and increase compliance. With APAP, mean airway pressures have been reported to be less than those with fixed CPAP.[19,79–84] There are also similar improvements in AHI, ESS scores, sleep architecture,[19,20,79,80,82–84] quality of life,[79,83] oxygen saturation,[20,85] cognitive impairment,[80] and vigilance testing.[86] Whereas several studies have shown better compliance with APAP compared with fixed CPAP,[80,84,87] many studies looking at compliance from 1 month to 6 months have shown no difference in compliance.[19,79,82,83,88] A meta-analysis also showed similar adherence between APAP and fixed CPAP.[81] Some studies support a patient preference of APAP over fixed CPAP, but this did not translate to better compliance.[19,20,88] APAP titration was not shown to increase acceptance of CPAP therapy compared with a manual titration.[85] In those patients requiring water pressure of 10 cm or greater, one study showed that those on APAP had an increased compliance of 35 minutes per night, better quality of sleep, and greater improvement in quality of life and mental health scores at 6 weeks.[89,90] While APAP devices have not been shown to convincingly increase compliance or acceptance of CPAP therapy, APAP may have a role in those who complain of pressure intolerance, particularly in those with high pressures. In addition, as APAP has been shown to treat OSA as effectively as a fixed CPAP pressure determined during a formal in-laboratory titration, it has a potential use as an attended or unattended titration study to determine fixed CPAP pressure or as a way to quickly start treatment.[91,92] However, APAP is not recommended for split-night titration, or as an unattended study in those with congestive heart failure, COPD, CSA, or hypoventilation.[21]

Expiratory pressure relief was developed as a way to improve patient comfort by reducing airway pressure briefly during early exhalation in proportion to the patient's expiratory flow on a breath-by-breath basis.[93] The hope is to improve patient comfort and, in effect, adherence. Studies have shown an equal reduction in AHI, snoring, arousals, and ESS and FOSQ scores in expiratory pressure relief and standard CPAP.[22,93–95] One nonrandomized study showed improved compliance of 1.7 hours a night on expiratory pressure relief versus standard CPAP at 3 months.[93] However, randomized studies have not shown a significant difference in compliance between expiratory pressure relief and standard CPAP for up to 180 days.[22,94,95] However, expiratory pressure relief may have a role in those with complaints of pressure intolerance.

Nasal obstruction is a common reason given for stopping CPAP.[60] Measures of nasal resistance have been associated with lower rates of CPAP acceptance and compliance.[96,97] Patients often cannot tolerate nasal CPAP due to difficulty in breathing entirely through the nasal route, which can be due to rhinitis, deviated septum, or turbinate hypertrophy. It has been shown that correction of nasal obstruction can reduce CPAP pressure requirement, which results in fewer side effects.[98,99] CPAP compliance was shown to increase by 32 minutes in those with OSA and receiving radiofrequency treatment for turbinate hypertrophy versus placebo at 4 weeks.[100] Surgical treatment of nasal obstruction may be a useful method to improve CPAP compliance. However, physicians must educate patients that these surgeries do not effectively reduce the RDI or improve saturations and are adjunctive to, and not in lieu of, CPAP.[98,99] The use of nasal steroids may aid in increasing CPAP compliance by reducing nasal congestion. Fluticasone was shown to reduce AHI in those with OSA and rhinitis, although significant sleep apnea still remained.[101]

Dry throat and dry nose is a reported side effect in as many as 44% of those using CPAP.[60,102] Some studies show that this interferes with CPAP use.[103] Relative humidity of inspired air is decreased when using nasal CPAP.[68] This reduction can be perpetuated by mouth leak, which causes unidirectional flow over nasal and oral mucosa, leading to nasal dryness.[104,105] It has been shown that normal awake individuals using CPAP with their mouth open have increased nasal mucosa blood flux, nasal resistance, and feelings of dryness and nasal congestion that improve with heated humidification.[104,105] Based on these studies, cold and heated humidity has been used to try to alleviate dryness and nasal congestion. In general, with humidity patients have overall more satisfaction.[106] Many studies show improved nasal symptoms of dryness, congestion, sneezing, and mouth and throat dryness with heated humidity.[106–109] Cold humidity has not been shown to improve compliance.[106] Heated humidity has been shown to be associated with increased compliance in a few studies[106,107] whereas other studies have shown no difference in compliance,[108,109] nor a difference in acceptance, preference, subjective sleep quality, improvement of symptoms, treatment satisfaction, or comfort between heated humidity and no humidity.[107,108,110,111] These studies mostly looked at those patients naïve to CPAP.

Rakotonanahary and colleagues[112] investigated whether compliance improved with the addition of humidification in those with nasal symptoms. Compliance increased with the use of heated humidification but not with cold humidification. The current AASM practice parameters do recommend that in those with nasal symptoms, heated humidification is an appropriate intervention to improve CPAP compliance.[113]

The aforementioned interventions address side effects of CPAP therapy. However, none of them clearly and convincingly improve CPAP compliance. Furthermore, there is not always a correlation of side effects and compliance.[36,61,114] A patient's perception of the benefit and need for treatment plays an important role in discontinuing CPAP.[40,44] Weaver and colleagues[115] showed that 50% of patients did not perceive the risks associated with OSA. Perception, acceptance, and compliance can be improved via education. Patients should be educated about OSA, its clinical significance and associated health concerns, what to expect with CPAP therapy, and potential problems and methods to address these problems.[64] While some studies did not support the suggestion that increased education improves CPAP compliance,[114,116] most studies do show increased compliance with various educational interventions. Reviewing sleep study results, symptoms, and compliance data with patients along with education on treatment of OSA and troubleshooting of issues results in more compliant patients as compared with minimal education at 12 weeks.[117] Written education materials improved compliance by 2.5 hours more per night compared with standard verbal CPAP education.[15] Group education and support has been shown to increase hours of use that can be sustained for 3 years.[118] The addition of a 15-minute video tape of 2 male patients discussing OSA and CPAP to standard education resulted in an increased follow-up rate at 1 month of 72.9% for the video group versus 48.9% for the standard group. This result was inferred as better compliance by the investigators; however, hours of use were not reported.[119] Additional intensive support via home visits and additional titration nights showed increased compliance compared with standard education.[120] Intense education in the form of written materials, educational videos, and group sessions are cost-effective methods that have been shown to improve compliance. Education that allows the patient to understand and take an active role in care should be part of the initial visit, to be reinforced at follow-up visits.

In addition to patient education, patient perception and acceptance of CPAP may also improve with cognitive behavioral therapy (CBT). CBT is based on psychosocial theories such as the transtheoretical model and social cognitive theory, which describe how patients who perceive more benefit have higher outcome expectation, and with more knowledge will likely be more compliant.[121] Richards and colleagues[122] performed a randomized study of the effects of cognitive behavioral therapy in addition to standard education on compliance. CBT was used to give a positive outlook to treatment and to correct distorted beliefs about OSA and CPAP in two 1-hour sessions with an additional 15-minute video of CPAP users and their experience, as well as written educational material. The CBT intervention group used CPAP for 2.9 hours longer per night at 28 days compared with the standard group. In the intervention group 77% was using CPAP for 4 hours or longer per night compared with 31% in the standard group. CPAP refusal was 8% in the intervention group compared with 30% in the standard group. Enhancing patient perception via education and cognitive therapy therefore seems to be a promising way to improve adherence.

At follow-up visits, patients should be assessed for several OSA outcomes in addition to adherence and tolerance of PAP therapy. These outcomes include resolution of sleepiness and snoring, OSA-specific quality of life measures, patient and (equally important) spouse satisfaction with the therapy and response to therapy, avoidance of factors known to worsen OSA, obtaining adequate sleep and proper sleep hygiene, as well as weight loss/management in overweight patients. As described previously, some patients may have improvement in their symptoms with less than the accepted degree of adherence. Other patients may have symptoms of ongoing sleepiness despite adequate PAP adherence. These patients should be evaluated for other causes of daytime sleepiness including insufficient sleep or poor sleep hygiene, mood disorders, comorbid illness and associated medication effects, as well as the possible presence of other sleep disorders. Some patients will experience residual sleepiness despite adequate therapy,[47,123] and may be candidates for pharmacologic therapy with modafinil.[124]

Of the risk factors associated with the development of OSA, obesity is the strongest.[125–127] A 10% gain in body weight increased the odds of developing moderate to severe OSA by 6-fold and each 1% change in body weight was associated with a 3% change in AHI. As a result, weight loss is the best long-term therapy for OSA in conjunction with PAP therapy. Patients seen in follow-up should be evaluated for progress in weight loss and management. Studies of weight loss in the management of OSA have been lacking.[128] A recent study investigated lifestyle intervention and weight reduction as the initial approach to mild OSA. Patients with mild OSA underwent a 12-week very low calorie diet and supervised lifestyle counseling. At the end of 3 months there was statistically significant weight loss, with improvement in symptoms of OSA and AHI. These changes were maintained at 1 year.[129] A similar study investigated the benefits of a 16-week diet and exercise program in patients with AHI of 10 to 50 events per hour and a body mass index (BMI; weight in kilograms divided by height in meters, squared) of greater than 30. Of note, those with significant comorbidities, including insulin-dependent diabetes or the inability to exercise, were excluded. The results showed a significant weight loss that was maintained at 12 months, and improvement in other neurobehavioral and cardiometabolic measures; however, AHI was not significantly changed.[130] A larger study of a 9-week, open-label, randomized controlled trial compared a liquid, very low energy diet combined with lifestyle counseling with weight maintenance in 63 obese men (BMI 30–40) with at least moderate OSA who were all using CPAP. The investigators found that weight loss and AHI in the intervention group was significantly greater than in the control group. Weight loss reduced the AHI to mild severity in 50% of patients and eradicated it in another 17%.[131] A large randomized study compared the effects of an intensive lifestyle intervention (ILI) with diabetes support and education over a year. Patients in the ILI group had a greater weight loss and decrease in AHI, and total remission of their OSA.[132] In some patients, evaluation for bariatric surgery may represent a better option.[133,134] It has also been well described that in general, weight loss improves OSA; however, some patients may have persistent OSA despite weight loss.[135,136] As a result, current guidelines recommend reassessment of OSA and the need for ongoing PAP therapy by polysomnography after significant weight loss.[59]

Sleep apnea represents a chronic disease and like many of its associated comorbid conditions such as heart disease, diabetes, and obesity, requires a multidisciplinary approach to proper care. The goal is to improve patent care through the development of a disease care model for treatment of OSA. This model includes the appropriate identification of those requiring treatment and those who are more likely to have difficulty with PAP therapy, evidence-based practice guidelines, collaborative practice models that include the patient's sleep and primary care physicians, and support-service providers such as nurses, sleep technicians, and respiratory therapists, with the aim of developing a process that measures and monitors outcomes and management. The goal of the process is to educate patients on their underlying disease and provide them with the information to be involved in self-management of their disease and, using these outcome measures, develop more effective treatment strategies over time.

REFERENCES

1. George CF. Sleep apnea, alertness, and motor vehicle crashes. Am J Respir Crit Care Med 2007;176:954.
2. Young T, Peppard PE, Gottlieb DJ. Epidemiology of obstructive sleep apnea: a population health perspective. Am J Respir Crit Care Med 2002; 165:1217.
3. Kapur V, Blough DK, Sandblom RE, et al. The medical cost of undiagnosed sleep apnea. Sleep 1999;22:749.
4. Hoffman C, Rice D, Sung HY. Persons with chronic conditions. Their prevalence and costs. JAMA 1996;276:1473.
5. Druss BG, Marcus SC, Olfson M, et al. Comparing the national economic burden of five chronic conditions. Health Aff (Millwood) 2001;20:233.
6. Gay P, Weaver T, Loube D, et al. Evaluation of positive airway pressure treatment for sleep related breathing disorders in adults. Sleep 2006;29:381.
7. Sullivan CE, Issa FG, Berthon-Jones M, et al. Reversal of obstructive sleep apnoea by continuous positive airway pressure applied through the nares. Lancet 1981;1:862.
8. Dyken ME, Yamada T, Glenn CL, et al. Obstructive sleep apnea associated with cerebral hypoxemia and death. Neurology 2004;62:491.
9. Jenkinson C, Davies RJ, Mullins R, et al. Comparison of therapeutic and subtherapeutic nasal continuous positive airway pressure for obstructive sleep apnoea: a randomised prospective parallel trial. Lancet 1999;353:2100.
10. Giles TL, Lasserson TJ, Smith BH, et al. Continuous positive airways pressure for obstructive sleep apnoea in adults. Cochrane Database Syst Rev 2006;3:CD001106.
11. Patel SR, White DP, Malhotra A, et al. Continuous positive airway pressure therapy for treating sleepiness in a diverse population with obstructive sleep apnea: results of a meta-analysis. Arch Intern Med 2003;163:565.
12. Epstein LJ, Kristo D, Strollo PJ Jr, et al. Clinical guideline for the evaluation, management and long-term care of obstructive sleep apnea in adults. J Clin Sleep Med 2009;5:263.
13. Sleep-related breathing disorders in adults: recommendations for syndrome definition and measurement techniques in clinical research. The report of an American Academy of Sleep Medicine Task Force. Sleep 1999;22:667.
14. Alarcon A, Leon C, Maimo A, et al. [Compliance with nasal continuous positive airway pressure (CPAP) treatment in sleep apnea-hypopnea syndrome]. Arch Bronconeumol 1995;31:56 [in Spanish].
15. Chervin RD, Thout S, Baccotti C, et al. Compliance with nasal CPAP can be improved by simple interventions. Sleep 1997;20:284.
16. Meurice JC, Dore P, Paquereau J, et al. Predictive factors of long-term compliance with nasal continuous positive airway pressure treatment in sleep apnea syndrome. Chest 1994;105:429.
17. Krieger J, Kurtz D, Petiau C, et al. Long-term compliance with CPAP therapy in obstructive sleep apnea patients and in snorers. Sleep 1996;19:S136.
18. Littner M, Hirshkowitz M, Davila D, et al. Practice parameters for the use of auto-titrating continuous positive airway pressure devices for titrating pressures and treating adult patients with obstructive sleep apnea syndrome. An American Academy of Sleep Medicine report. Sleep 2002;25:143.
19. d'Ortho MP, Grillier-Lanoir V, Levy P, et al. Constant vs automatic continuous positive airway pressure therapy: home evaluation. Chest 2000;118:1010.
20. Sharma S, Wali S, Pouliot Z, et al. Treatment of obstructive sleep apnea with a self-titrating continuous positive airway pressure (CPAP) system. Sleep 1996;19:497.
21. Morgenthaler TI, Aurora RN, Brown T, et al. Practice parameters for the use of autotitrating continuous positive airway pressure devices for titrating pressures and treating adult patients with obstructive sleep apnea syndrome: an update for 2007. An American Academy of Sleep Medicine report. Sleep 2008;31:141.
22. Nilius G, Happel A, Domanski U, et al. Pressure-relief continuous positive airway pressure vs constant continuous positive airway pressure: a comparison of efficacy and compliance. Chest 2006;130:1018.
23. Bonekat HW. Noninvasive ventilation in neuromuscular disease. Crit Care Clin 1998;14:775.
24. Bradley WG, Anderson F, Bromberg M, et al. Current management of ALS: comparison of the ALS CARE Database and the AAN Practice Parameter. The American Academy of Neurology. Neurology 2001;57:500.
25. Gross JB, Bachenberg KL, Benumof JL, et al. Practice guidelines for the perioperative management of patients with obstructive sleep apnea: a report by the American Society of Anesthesiologists Task Force on Perioperative Management of patients with obstructive sleep apnea. Anesthesiology 2006;104:1081.

26. American Academy of Sleep Medicine. International classification of sleep disorders. In: Diagnostic and coding manual. 2nd edition. Westchester (IL): American Academy of Sleep Medicine; 2005. p. 74–5.

27. Piper AJ, Wang D, Yee BJ, et al. Randomised trial of CPAP vs bilevel support in the treatment of obesity hypoventilation syndrome without severe nocturnal desaturation. Thorax 2008;63:395.

28. Mokhlesi B, Kryger MH, Grunstein RR. Assessment and management of patients with obesity hypoventilation syndrome. Proc Am Thorac Soc 2008;5:218.

29. Nieto FJ, Young TB, Lind BK, et al. Association of sleep-disordered breathing, sleep apnea, and hypertension in a large community-based study. Sleep Heart Health Study. JAMA 2000;283:1829.

30. Morgenthaler TI, Kagramanov V, Hanak V, et al. Complex sleep apnea syndrome: is it a unique clinical syndrome? Sleep 2006;29:1203.

31. Bradley TD, Logan AG, Kimoff RJ, et al. Continuous positive airway pressure for central sleep apnea and heart failure. N Engl J Med 2005;353:2025.

32. Teschler H, Dohring J, Wang YM, et al. Adaptive pressure support servo-ventilation: a novel treatment for Cheyne-Stokes respiration in heart failure. Am J Respir Crit Care Med 2001;164:614.

33. Collard P, Pieters T, Aubert G, et al. Compliance with nasal CPAP in obstructive sleep apnea patients. Sleep Med Rev 1997;1:33.

34. Villar I, Izuel M, Carrizo S, et al. Medication adherence and persistence in severe obstructive sleep apnea. Sleep 2009;32:623.

35. Grunstein RR. Sleep-related breathing disorders. 5. Nasal continuous positive airway pressure treatment for obstructive sleep apnoea. Thorax 1995; 50:1106.

36. Kribbs NB, Pack AI, Kline LR, et al. Objective measurement of patterns of nasal CPAP use by patients with obstructive sleep apnea. Am Rev Respir Dis 1993;147:887.

37. Weaver TE, Kribbs NB, Pack AI, et al. Night-to-night variability in CPAP use over the first three months of treatment. Sleep 1997;20:278.

38. Budhiraja R, Parthasarathy S, Drake CL, et al. Early CPAP use identifies subsequent adherence to CPAP therapy. Sleep 2007;30:320.

39. Edinger JD, Carwile S, Miller P, et al. Psychological status, syndromatic measures, and compliance with nasal CPAP therapy for sleep apnea. Percept Mot Skills 1994;78:1116.

40. McArdle N, Devereux G, Heidarnejad H, et al. Long-term use of CPAP therapy for sleep apnea/hypopnea syndrome. Am J Respir Crit Care Med 1999;159:1108.

41. Engleman HM, Wild MR. Improving CPAP use by patients with the sleep apnoea/hypopnoea syndrome (SAHS). Sleep Med Rev 2003;7:81.

42. Drake CL, Day R, Hudgel D, et al. Sleep during titration predicts continuous positive airway pressure compliance. Sleep 2003;26:308.

43. Wells RD, Freedland KE, Carney RM, et al. Adherence, reports of benefits, and depression among patients treated with continuous positive airway pressure. Psychosom Med 2007;69:449.

44. Wolkove N, Baltzan M, Kamel H, et al. Long-term compliance with continuous positive airway pressure in patients with obstructive sleep apnea. Can Respir J 2008;15:365.

45. Barbe F, Mayoralas LR, Duran J, et al. Treatment with continuous positive airway pressure is not effective in patients with sleep apnea but no daytime sleepiness. A randomized, controlled trial. Ann Intern Med 2001;134:1015.

46. Brostrom A, Stromberg A, Martensson J, et al. Association of Type D personality to perceived side effects and adherence in CPAP-treated patients with OSAS. J Sleep Res 2007;16:439.

47. Weaver TE, Maislin G, Dinges DF, et al. Relationship between hours of CPAP use and achieving normal levels of sleepiness and daily functioning. Sleep 2007;30:711.

48. Kribbs NB, Pack AI, Kline LR, et al. Effects of one night without nasal CPAP treatment on sleep and sleepiness in patients with obstructive sleep apnea. Am Rev Respir Dis 1993;147:1162.

49. Osterberg L, Blaschke T. Adherence to medication. N Engl J Med 2005;353:487.

50. DiMatteo MR. Variations in patients' adherence to medical recommendations: a quantitative review of 50 years of research. Med Care 2004;42:200.

51. Platt AB, Kuna ST, Field SH, et al. Adherence to sleep apnea therapy and use of lipid-lowering drugs: a study of the healthy-user effect. Chest 2010;137:102.

52. Grote L, Hedner J, Grunstein R, et al. Therapy with nCPAP: incomplete elimination of sleep related breathing disorder. Eur Respir J 2000;16:921.

53. Johnson MK, Carter R, Nicol A, et al. Long-term continuous positive airway pressure (CPAP) outcomes from a sleep service using limited sleep studies and daycase CPAP titration in the management of obstructive sleep apnoea/hypopnoea syndrome. Chron Respir Dis 2004;1:83.

54. Taylor Y, Eliasson A, Andrada T, et al. The role of telemedicine in CPAP compliance for patients with obstructive sleep apnea syndrome. Sleep Breath 2006;10:132.

55. Stepnowsky CJ, Palau JJ, Marler MR, et al. Pilot randomized trial of the effect of wireless telemonitoring on compliance and treatment efficacy in obstructive sleep apnea. J Med Internet Res 2007;9:e14.

56. Sin DD, Mayers I, Man GC, et al. Long-term compliance rates to continuous positive airway pressure

in obstructive sleep apnea: a population-based study. Chest 2002;121:430.

57. Rosenthal L, Gerhardstein R, Lumley A, et al. CPAP therapy in patients with mild OSA: implementation and treatment outcome. Sleep Med 2000;1:215.

58. Popescu G, Latham M, Allgar V, et al. Continuous positive airway pressure for sleep apnoea/hypopnoea syndrome: usefulness of a 2 week trial to identify factors associated with long term use. Thorax 2001:56:727.

59. Kushida CA, Littner MR, Morgenthaler T, et al. Practice parameters for the indications for polysomnography and related procedures: an update for 2005. Sleep 2005;28:499.

60. Nino-Murcia G, McCann CC, Bliwise DL, et al. Compliance and side effects in sleep apnea patients treated with nasal continuous positive airway pressure. West J Med 1989;150:165.

61. Pepin JL, Leger P, Veale D, et al. Side effects of nasal continuous positive airway pressure in sleep apnea syndrome. Study of 193 patients in two French sleep centers. Chest 1995;107:375.

62. Mortimore IL, Whittle AT, Douglas NJ. Comparison of nose and face mask CPAP therapy for sleep apnoea. Thorax 1998;53:290.

63. Khanna R, Kline LR. A prospective 8 week trial of nasal interfaces vs a novel oral interface (Oracle) for treatment of obstructive sleep apnea hypopnea syndrome. Sleep Med 2003;4:333.

64. Berry RB. Improving CPAP compliance—man more than machine. Sleep Med 2000;1:175.

65. Prosise GL, Berry RB. Oral-nasal continuous positive airway pressure as a treatment for obstructive sleep apnea. Chest 1994;106:180.

66. Sanders MH, Kern NB, Stiller RA, et al. CPAP therapy via oronasal mask for obstructive sleep apnea. Chest 1994;106:774.

67. Massie CA, Hart RW. Clinical outcomes related to interface type in patients with obstructive sleep apnea/hypopnea syndrome who are using continuous positive airway pressure. Chest 2003;123:1112.

68. Martins De Araujo MT, Vieira SB, Vasquez EC, et al. Heated humidification or face mask to prevent upper airway dryness during continuous positive airway pressure therapy. Chest 2000;117:142.

69. Anderson FE, Kingshott RN, Taylor DR, et al. A randomized crossover efficacy trial of oral CPAP (Oracle) compared with nasal CPAP in the management of obstructive sleep apnea. Sleep 2003;26:721.

70. Beecroft J, Zanon S, Lukic D, et al. Oral continuous positive airway pressure for sleep apnea: effectiveness, patient preference, and adherence. Chest 2003;124:2200.

71. Bachour A, Hurmerinta K, Maasilta P. Mouth closing device (chinstrap) reduces mouth leak during nasal CPAP. Sleep Med 2004;5:261.

72. Edinger JD, Radtke RA. Use of in vivo desensitization to treat a patient's claustrophobic response to nasal CPAP. Sleep 1993;16:678.

73. Edinger JD, Means MK, Stechuchak KM, et al. A pilot study of inexpensive sleep-assessment devices. Behav Sleep Med 2004;2:41.

74. Means MK, Edinger JD. Graded exposure therapy for addressing claustrophobic reactions to continuous positive airway pressure: a case series report. Behav Sleep Med 2007;5:105.

75. Sanders MH, Kern N. Obstructive sleep apnea treated by independently adjusted inspiratory and expiratory positive airway pressures via nasal mask. Physiologic and clinical implications. Chest 1990;98:317.

76. Reeves-Hoche MK, Hudgel DW, Meck R, et al. Continuous versus bilevel positive airway pressure for obstructive sleep apnea. Am J Respir Crit Care Med 1995;151:443.

77. Gay PC, Herold DL, Olson EJ. A randomized, double-blind clinical trial comparing continuous positive airway pressure with a novel bilevel pressure system for treatment of obstructive sleep apnea syndrome. Sleep 2003;26:864.

78. Oksenberg A, Silverberg DS, Arons E, et al. The sleep supine position has a major effect on optimal nasal continuous positive airway pressure: relationship with rapid eye movements and non-rapid eye movements sleep, body mass index, respiratory disturbance index, and age. Chest 1999;116:1000.

79. Hukins C. Comparative study of autotitrating and fixed-pressure CPAP in the home: a randomized, single-blind crossover trial. Sleep 2004;27:1512.

80. Meurice JC, Marc I, Series F. Efficacy of auto-CPAP in the treatment of obstructive sleep apnea/hypopnea syndrome. Am J Respir Crit Care Med 1996;153:794.

81. Ayas NT, Patel SR, Malhotra A, et al. Auto-titrating versus standard continuous positive airway pressure for the treatment of obstructive sleep apnea: results of a meta-analysis. Sleep 2004;27:249.

82. Teschler H, Wessendorf TE, Farhat AA, et al. Two months auto-adjusting versus conventional nCPAP for obstructive sleep apnoea syndrome. Eur Respir J 2000;15:990.

83. Senn O, Brack T, Matthews F, et al. Randomized short-term trial of two autoCPAP devices versus fixed continuous positive airway pressure for the treatment of sleep apnea. Am J Respir Crit Care Med 2003;168:1506.

84. Hudgel DW, Fung C. A long-term randomized, cross-over comparison of auto-titrating and standard nasal continuous positive airway pressure. Sleep 2000;23:645.

85. Stradling JR, Barbour C, Pitson DJ, et al. Automatic nasal continuous positive airway pressure titration in the laboratory: patient outcomes. Thorax 1997;52:72.

86. Ficker JH, Wiest GH, Lehnert G, et al. Evaluation of an auto-CPAP device for treatment of obstructive sleep apnoea. Thorax 1998;53:643.

87. Konermann M, Sanner BM, Vyleta M, et al. Use of conventional and self-adjusting nasal continuous positive airway pressure for treatment of severe obstructive sleep apnea syndrome: a comparative study. Chest 1998;113:714.

88. Randerath WJ, Schraeder O, Galetke W, et al. Autoadjusting CPAP therapy based on impedance efficacy, compliance and acceptance. Am J Respir Crit Care Med 2001;163:652.

89. Fukamachi K, Harasaki H, Massiello AL, et al. In vitro evaluation of automatic control performance of a total artificial heart with changes in pump orientation. ASAIO J 1996;42:M589.

90. Massie CA, McArdle N, Hart RW, et al. Comparison between automatic and fixed positive airway pressure therapy in the home. Am J Respir Crit Care Med 2003;167:20.

91. Berry RB, Parish JM, Hartse KM. The use of autotitrating continuous positive airway pressure for treatment of adult obstructive sleep apnea. An American Academy of Sleep Medicine review. Sleep 2002;25:148.

92. d'Ortho MP. Auto-titrating continuous positive airway pressure for treating adult patients with sleep apnea syndrome. Curr Opin Pulm Med 2004;10:495.

93. Aloia MS, Stanchina M, Arnedt JT, et al. Treatment adherence and outcomes in flexible vs standard continuous positive airway pressure therapy. Chest 2005;127:2085.

94. Wenzel M, Kerl J, Dellweg D, et al. [Expiratory pressure reduction (C-Flex Method) versus fix CPAP in the therapy for obstructive sleep apnoea]. Pneumologie 2007;61:692 [in German].

95. Dolan DC, Okonkwo R, Gfullner F, et al. Longitudinal comparison study of pressure relief (C-Flex) vs CPAP in OSA patients. Sleep Breath 2009;13:73.

96. Li HY, Engleman H, Hsu CY, et al. Acoustic reflection for nasal airway measurement in patients with obstructive sleep apnea-hypopnea syndrome. Sleep 2005;28:1554.

97. Sugiura T, Noda A, Nakata S, et al. Influence of nasal resistance on initial acceptance of continuous positive airway pressure in treatment for obstructive sleep apnea syndrome. Respiration 2007;74:56.

98. Friedman M, Tanyeri H, Lim JW, et al. Effect of improved nasal breathing on obstructive sleep apnea. Otolaryngol Head Neck Surg 2000;122:71.

99. Balcerzak J, Niemczyk K, Arcimowicz M, et al. [The role of functional nasal surgery in the treatment of obstructive sleep apnea syndrome]. Otolaryngol Pol 2007;61:80 [in Polish].

100. Powell NB, Zonato AI, Weaver EM, et al. Radiofrequency treatment of turbinate hypertrophy in subjects using continuous positive airway pressure: a randomized, double-blind, placebo-controlled clinical pilot trial. Laryngoscope 2001;111:1783.

101. Kiely JL, Nolan P, McNicholas WT. Intranasal corticosteroid therapy for obstructive sleep apnoea in patients with co-existing rhinitis. Thorax 2004;59:50.

102. Hoffstein V, Viner S, Mateika S, et al. Treatment of obstructive sleep apnea with nasal continuous positive airway pressure. Patient compliance, perception of benefits, and side effects. Am Rev Respir Dis 1992;145:841.

103. Engleman HM, Martin SE, Douglas NJ. Compliance with CPAP therapy in patients with the sleep apnoea/hypopnoea syndrome. Thorax 1994;49:263.

104. Hayes MJ, McGregor FB, Roberts DN, et al. Continuous nasal positive airway pressure with a mouth leak: effect on nasal mucosal blood flux and nasal geometry. Thorax 1995;50:1179.

105. Richards GN, Cistulli PA, Ungar RG, et al. Mouth leak with nasal continuous positive airway pressure increases nasal airway resistance. Am J Respir Crit Care Med 1996;154:182.

106. Massie CA, Hart RW, Peralez K, et al. Effects of humidification on nasal symptoms and compliance in sleep apnea patients using continuous positive airway pressure. Chest 1999;116:403.

107. Neill AM, Wai HS, Bannan SP, et al. Humidified nasal continuous positive airway pressure in obstructive sleep apnoea. Eur Respir J 2003;22:258.

108. Mador MJ, Krauza M, Pervez A, et al. Effect of heated humidification on compliance and quality of life in patients with sleep apnea using nasal continuous positive airway pressure. Chest 2005;128:2151.

109. Worsnop CJ, Miseski S, Rochford PD. The routine use of humidification with nasal continuous positive airway pressure. Intern Med J 2009. [Epub ahead of print]. DOI:10.1111/j.1445-5994.2009.01969.x. Available at: http://www3.interscience.wiley.com/journal/122380781/abstract. Accessed May 13, 2010.

110. Wiest GH, Harsch IA, Fuchs FS, et al. Initiation of CPAP therapy for OSA: does prophylactic humidification during CPAP pressure titration improve initial patient acceptance and comfort? Respiration 2002;69:406.

111. Duong M, Jayaram L, Camfferman D, et al. Use of heated humidification during nasal CPAP titration in obstructive sleep apnoea syndrome. Eur Respir J 2005;26:679.

112. Rakotonanahary D, Pelletier-Fleury N, Gagnadoux F, et al. Predictive factors for the need for additional humidification during nasal continuous positive airway pressure therapy. Chest 2001;119:460.

113. Kushida CA, Littner MR, Hirshkowitz M, et al. Practice parameters for the use of continuous and bilevel positive airway pressure devices to treat adult patients with sleep-related breathing disorders. Sleep 2006;29:375.

114. Fletcher EC, Luckett RA. The effect of positive reinforcement on hourly compliance in nasal continuous positive airway pressure users with obstructive sleep apnea. Am Rev Respir Dis 1991;143:936.

115. Weaver TE, Maislin G, Dinges DF, et al. Self-efficacy in sleep apnea: instrument development and patient perceptions of obstructive sleep apnea risk, treatment benefit, and volition to use continuous positive airway pressure. Sleep 2003;26:727.

116. Hui DS, Chan JK, Choy DK, et al. Effects of augmented continuous positive airway pressure education and support on compliance and outcome in a Chinese population. Chest 2000;117:1410.

117. Aloia MS, Di Dio L, Ilniczky N, et al. Improving compliance with nasal CPAP and vigilance in older adults with OAHS. Sleep Breath 2001;5:13.

118. Likar LL, Panciera TM, Erickson AD, et al. Group education sessions and compliance with nasal CPAP therapy. Chest 1997;111:1273.

119. Jean Wiese H, Boethel C, Phillips B, et al. CPAP compliance: video education may help! Sleep Med 2005;6:171.

120. Hoy CJ, Vennelle M, Kingshott RN, et al. Can intensive support improve continuous positive airway pressure use in patients with the sleep apnea/hypopnea syndrome? Am J Respir Crit Care Med 1999;159:1096.

121. Stepnowsky CJ Jr, Marler MR, Ancoli-Israel S. Determinants of nasal CPAP compliance. Sleep Med 2002;3:239.

122. Richards D, Bartlett DJ, Wong K, et al. Increased adherence to CPAP with a group cognitive behavioral treatment intervention: a randomized trial. Sleep 2007;30:635.

123. Guilleminault C, Philip P. Tiredness and somnolence despite initial treatment of obstructive sleep apnea syndrome (what to do when an OSAS patient stays hypersomnolent despite treatment). Sleep 1996;19:S117.

124. Pack AI, Black JE, Schwartz JR, et al. Modafinil as adjunct therapy for daytime sleepiness in obstructive sleep apnea. Am J Respir Crit Care Med 2001;164:1675.

125. Young T, Skatrud J, Peppard PE. Risk factors for obstructive sleep apnea in adults. JAMA 2004; 291:2013.

126. Young T, Shahar E, Nieto FJ, et al. Predictors of sleep-disordered breathing in community-dwelling adults: the Sleep Heart Health Study. Arch Intern Med 2002;162:893.

127. Peppard PE, Young T, Palta M, et al. Longitudinal study of moderate weight change and sleep-disordered breathing. JAMA 2000;284:3015.

128. Shneerson J, Wright J. Lifestyle modification for obstructive sleep apnoea. Cochrane Database Syst Rev 2001;1:CD002875.

129. Tuomilehto HP, Seppa JM, Partinen MM, et al. Lifestyle intervention with weight reduction: first-line treatment in mild obstructive sleep apnea. Am J Respir Crit Care Med 2009;179:320.

130. Barnes M, Goldsworthy UR, Cary BA, et al. A diet and exercise program to improve clinical outcomes in patients with obstructive sleep apnea—a feasibility study. J Clin Sleep Med 2009;5:409.

131. Johansson K, Neovius M, Lagerros YT, et al. Effect of a very low energy diet on moderate and severe obstructive sleep apnoea in obese men: a randomised controlled trial. BMJ 2009;339:b4609.

132. Foster GD, Borradaile KE, Sanders MH, et al. A randomized study on the effect of weight loss on obstructive sleep apnea among obese patients with type 2 diabetes: the Sleep AHEAD study. Arch Intern Med 2009;169:1619.

133. NIH conference. Gastrointestinal surgery for severe obesity. Consensus Development Conference Panel. Ann Intern Med 1991;115:956.

134. Kiernan M, Winkleby MA. Identifying patients for weight-loss treatment: an empirical evaluation of the NHLBI obesity education initiative expert panel treatment recommendations. Arch Intern Med 2000;160:2169.

135. Pillar G, Peled R, Lavie P. Recurrence of sleep apnea without concomitant weight increase 7.5 years after weight reduction surgery. Chest 1994;106:1702.

136. Lettieri CJ, Eliasson AH, Greenburg DL. Persistence of obstructive sleep apnea after surgical weight loss. J Clin Sleep Med 2008;4:333.

APAP and Alternative Titration Methods

Omer Ahmed, MD[a], Sairam Parthasarathy, MD[b,c],*

KEYWORDS

- Obstructive sleep apnea
- Continuous positive airway pressure • Adherence
- Compliance • Artificial respiration

INTRODUCTION AND HISTORICAL PERSPECTIVE

Ever since the first report of continuous positive airway pressure (CPAP) for treatment of obstructive sleep apnea (OSA) was made in 1981, the methodologies and end points for titration of the CPAP level was quickly brought to the forefront.[1] Publications on the alternatives to manual in-laboratory polysomnography-based titrations of positive airway pressure (PAP) did not occur until a decade later.[2–4] Intelligent devices with in-built microprocessors for detection and treatment of sleep-disordered breathing (SDB) events have gone by different names, including self-adjusting, automatic, auto-adjusting, smart CPAP, and auto-titrating PAP (APAP).

The purpose of APAP devices varied and included the replacement of in-laboratory manual titration, reducing mean pressures to achieve better adherence, and adapting CPAP levels to changes in severity of OSA in response to changes in weight, sleep state, body position, and alcohol ingestion. Today the purpose of automation has expanded toward detecting and ameliorating central apneas and hypoventilation. This article provides an up-to-date synthesis of APAP technology, scientific evidence in support of APAP use, and issues surrounding the regulation, reimbursement, and health services aspects of APAP therapy.

TECHNOLOGY

The functioning of APAP devices can be broken down into three components: sensing of SDB events (sensors), automated computing and analysis of the sensed signals (analysis), and a hierarchal set of algorithms that will determine the action taken by the APAP device in response to the conditions exposed (effectors).

In the older generation of APAP devices, the sensors were simplistic and measured only the pressure inflections (vibrations) of a certain frequency and amplitude that were caused by snoring. The next generation of APAP devices became more sophisticated and were able to sense flow-based changes, such as apnea, hypopnea, or inspiratory flow limitation based on the inspiratory flow contour (ie, flattening of the inspiratory flow waveform). More recently, devices have been developed to differentiate central from obstructive apneas (using forced oscillation technique or rapid injection of air), identify Cheyne-Stokes respiration (through breath-by-breath changes in peak flow), identify hypoventilation (through measuring tidal volume or minute ventilation using calibrated flow sensors), compensate

This work was supported by Grant No. HL095748 from the National Institutes of Health. Dr Parthasarathy received $200,000 of research grant funding between 2006–2007 from Respironics, Inc. Dr Ahmed does not have any conflicts of interest to disclose.

[a] Pulmonary and Critical Care Medicine, Department of Medicine, University of Arizona, 1501 North Campbell, Avenue, Room 2342B, PO Box 245030, Tucson, AZ 85724, USA

[b] Research Service Line, Southern Arizona Veterans Administration Healthcare System, 3601 South Sixth Avenue, Mail Stop 0-151, Tucson, AZ 85723, USA

[c] Department of Medicine, University of Arizona, Tucson, AZ 85724, USA

* Corresponding author. Research Service Line, Southern Arizona Veterans Administration Healthcare System, 3601 South Sixth Avenue, Mail Stop 0-151, Tucson, AZ 85723.
E-mail address: spartha@arc.arizona.edu

Sleep Med Clin 5 (2010) 361–368
doi:10.1016/j.jsmc.2010.05.010
1556-407X/10/$ – see front matter. Published by Elsevier Inc.

sleep.theclinics.com

for air-leaks (using sophisticated flow-based algorithms), and measure both upper and lower airway resistance (using forced oscillation techniques).[5] These signals are computed and analyzed instantaneously by a built-in microprocessor with a preset hierarchical set of algorithms that determine the rate and magnitude of pressure response.

APAP devices may increase the pressure in response to events such as apneas and hypopneas. Some devices are programmed not to increase the pressure beyond an arbitrarily identified pressure if the apneas do not respond to pressure changes in a predictable fashion (ie, change from apneas to obstructive "flow-limited" hypopneas). Other devices can be programmed to not increase the pressure in response to nonobstructive hypopneas (namely, hypopneas without inspiratory flow limitation).[6]

Newer-generation devices can differentiate obstructive from central apneas, and thereby be programmed not to raise pressure in response to central apneas, but to increase the pressure only in response to obstructive apneas. Algorithms are designed to not only increase but also decrease the pressure on certain occasions. The APAP device may reduce the pressure when the inspiratory flow curve has the convexity facing upwards or if no events of SDB are detected over a certain period. These algorithms are proprietary and providers should probably be well informed about their characteristics before prescribing these types of APAP devices.[7]

The *effector* arm of the APAP device also has undergone radical changes. Newer-generation devices can increase not only the CPAP level but also the inspiratory PAP (IPAP) alone to ameliorate obstructive events (auto bi-level PAP), correct hypoventilation (averaged volume assured pressure support [AVAPS], or auto variable positive airway pressure), or combat central apneas in patients with complex sleep apnea or CPAP-emergent central apneas (servoventilation).[8–11] Devices may also introduce a back-up rate to prevent central apneas and, although generally are not referred to as APAP devices, function using similar principles and can be judged as the latest generation of APAP devices.[10,11]

SCIENTIFIC EVIDENCE

The scientific evidence governing autotitrating and other alternative methods for titrating PAP devices continue to evolve. Both bench and clinical studies must be considered in assessing these autotitrating methods. However, although the bench studies provide valuable information on the performance of APAP devices through controlling their exposure to artificially simulated apneas and hypopneas, only clinical trials with measured benefits to patient outcomes should guide practice.

Bench Studies

Numerous bench studies have been performed comparing the devices made by different manufacturers across different generations of devices.[6,12–15] These studies have consistently shown that for a given set of events characterizing SDB, devices from different manufacturers have different responses. One particular study showed the scatter in pressure response of four older-generation APAP devices to be as wide as 10 cm H_2O.[6] These changes may be attributable to the APAP devices' ability to sense the event or the preprogrammed algorithms that determine the rate of pressure change and magnitude of step change in pressure.[7] Moreover, bench studies have shown that air-leak deleteriously affected the performance of APAP devices,[6,13,15] and that some devices were less likely to be influenced by air-leak than others.[6] In addition, humidifiers may act as a capacitor and muffle some of the snoring pressure waveforms before they reach the sensors in the APAP device. Predictably, in at least one bench study, humidifiers resulted in a small reduction (2 cm H_2O) in pressure response over a 5-minute run.[6]

Despite these bench studies, no published clinical studies have identified the clinical implications of the effects of air-leak or humidifiers on APAP device performance. These clinical studies are needed in place of extrapolating findings from bench studies to the clinical realm. Limitations of bench studies include the brief duration of simulations, highly controlled conditions, apnea simulators that do not respond to changes in pressure administered by the APAP device (referred to as "open loop" system), or failure to account for patient comorbidities that may influence pressure response (nasal congestion, palatal surgery, or morbid obesity).

Clinical Effectiveness

A large body of clinical trials aimed at assessing the efficacy of APAP and other alternative methods to titrate APAP devices has accumulated over the past decade. This article focuses primarily on randomized controlled trials (RCT).

Dating back to the first publications of prospective RCTs of APAP in 1996, most if not all have shown that APAP devices can be used to determine the fixed treatment pressure that is comparable to the gold standard (attended manually titrated CPAP during polysomnography).[16,17] Subsequently, using older generation APAP devices, investigators have shown that the fixed CPAP pressure determined by APAP therapy can either be the same, greater, or less than that derived from attended polysomnography.[17–20]

Such a simplistic comparison, however, should probably not be made, considering that the gold standard itself has inherent limitations, such as cost, inconvenience of electrode placements, laboratory versus home environment, and limited "one-night" sampling. A better benchmark would be to consider patient outcomes, such as patient preference, patient comfort, treatment adherence, and improvements in other clinical end points (eg, sleepiness, health-related quality of life [HR-QOL], cardiovascular and neurocognitive measures). Most of these RCTs recruited CPAP-naïve patients with moderate to severe OSA and avoided comorbid conditions that would deleteriously affect performance of APAP devices.[21] Some of the exclusionary criteria were nasal obstruction, palatal surgery, and morbid obesity with hypoventilation, central sleep apnea, coexistent heart failure, or chronic obstructive pulmonary disease (COPD).

In a large European study, Masa and colleagues[22] randomized 360 CPAP-naïve patients to either APAP, CPAP titration during full-night polysomnography, or a prediction formula-based CPAP level in a multicenter RCT. In this study, APAP was initiated at home after the patient received instructions and mask-fitting in an outpatient setting. Over a 3-month period, improvements in subjective sleepiness, disease-specific HR-QOL measures, and apnea-hypopnea index (AHI) were similar across the groups. No differences in adherence to CPAP treatment or the dropout rates were seen during the follow-up period. Some general HR-QOL measures that were not tailored for assessing patients with SDB improved to a slightly lesser magnitude in the APAP group when compared with polysomnography or formula-based methods for determining treatment CPAP level (effect size ≤ 0.5).

Another very recent study identified patients with OSA using either polysomnography or limited polysomnography, and then randomized the subjects and crossed them over to receive either APAP or polysomnography-derived CPAP therapy.[23] Patients in the APAP group reported greater improvement in subjective sleepiness and greater objective evidence of PAP adherence, although these differences are small and their clinical benefits unclear. In this rather large study, involving more than 180 patients, objective measures of vigilance (Osler test) and HR-QOL were not different between the groups. Study limitations included issues surrounding the crossover design (namely a strong order effect), a short assessment period (6-weeks), and perhaps a failure to choose a patient population most likely to benefit from APAP therapy.[23]

Noseda and colleagues,[24] however, did select and study patients who were more likely to benefit form APAP therapy, namely those with a high within-night variability in APAP-titrated pressure levels. However, they failed to show any difference in PAP adherence or mean pressure levels when compared with a polysomnography-derived CPAP trial over an 8-week treatment period. Although subjective ratings for sleepiness were better with APAP therapy, these improvements were not clearly explained by group differences in pressure or adherence levels.[24]

Similarly, Massie and colleagues[25] selected patients requiring a CPAP pressure level of 10 cm H_2O or more, and reported that APAP therapy resulted in greater improvements in HR-QOL and self-reported sleep quality than conventional laboratory polysomnography-determined fixed CPAP pressure. One study, however, reported that APAP therapy failed to reduce AHI as much as conventional polysomnography-derived CPAP settings.[26] In this study, Patruno and colleagues[26] showed that blood pressure and insulin resistance improved to a lesser degree in the APAP group than in the group receiving conventional polysomnography-derived CPAP therapy. However, this study had rather lenient exclusion criteria that did not exclude patients with significant comorbid conditions.

Moreover, in a study using APAP device technology, intensive home support with monthly visits over a 6-month period was more effective in achieving adherence to PAP therapy than the relatively more expensive APAP device technology.[27] Considering the expenditure of provider time in issuing APAP, downloading and interpreting the APAP device outputs, and monitoring patients after initiation of APAP therapy, cost-effectiveness analysis of APAP therapy versus conventional treatment methodologies is direly needed to justify their use.

Forced oscillation technology (FOT) has been used to measure upper airway impedance. A proposed advantage of this technology is the ability to determine whether the upper airway is open or closed, and thereby prevent inappropriate increments in pressure during central events with an open airway. An RCT involving 38 patients compared FOT-based APAP with laboratory polysomnography-derived CPAP and found that the pressure recommendation between these methodologies were comparable, and observed similar reductions in AHI and self-reported sleepiness over a 6-week period.[28]

The use of APAP therapy in patients who have not undergone conventional polysomnography to establish the diagnosis of OSA has also seen tremendous growth. Berry and colleagues[29] performed an RCT in which patients underwent portable testing for OSA based on a tonometry- and actigraphy-based system. In 106 patients with daytime sleepiness and a high likelihood of having OSA, administration of APAP versus polysomnography-derived CPAP did not result in any differences in adherence to PAP therapy, improvement in sleepiness, improvement in HR-QOL, or patient satisfaction levels. Although limitations included the possibility of being underpowered to show group differences and a population that was all male with high pretest probability for OSA, this study highlighted the ability of APAP to achieve benefits comparable to polysomnography-derived CPAP levels when used with home study testing without electroencephalography.[29]

In another study that did not use polysomnography, Mulgrew and colleagues[30] showed that polysomnography-derived CPAP titration did not confer any advantage over APAP therapy initiated after OSA was identified through sequential application of the Epworth Sleepiness Scale (ESS) score, Sleep Apnea Clinical Score, and overnight oximetry. In fact, patients randomized to the APAP group were more adherent to PAP therapy than those in the conventional polysomnography-derived CPAP pressure group.[30] One limitation of this study is that it was designed as a superiority trial; large studies designed as noninferiority trials are still needed.

Another very recent study has moved further down this aggressive path by using only a Berlin questionnaire to diagnose OSA in a U.S. veteran population.[31] Patients with high likelihood of OSA (n = 109) who were awaiting diagnostic polysomnography were randomized to remain in the conventional pathway or assigned to APAP therapy, which was initiated on an outpatient basis. In this study by Drummond and colleagues,[31] patients with two or more positive responses in the Berlin questionnaire, APAP therapy resulted in improvements in self-reported symptoms and disease-specific HR-QOL measures that were comparable to those in patients in the conventional group. Limitations to the generalizability of this finding are the high pretest probability and the all-male population, with 66% of eligible patients being excluded because of the presence of comorbid conditions such as heart failure and COPD.

A large noninferiority trial encompassing 619 subjects, the largest published RCT involving APAP therapy, showed that nurse-led home-based initiation of APAP therapy had outcomes equivalent to those for treatment by sleep physicians using conventional polysomnography.[32] In this study, Antic and colleagues[32] also showed lower costs in the nurse-led group. These large noninferiority trials must be replicated in the United States for change in practice to occur.

Clinical comparisons between different APAP devices have been made in a randomized controlled manner. In a crossover study design with three conditions and a 1-month period of therapy, Senn and colleagues[33] used two different APAP devices and CPAP therapy based on pressure level determined after 2-weeks of APAP therapy. Patients underwent the three treatments in a random manner over three consecutive 1-month periods. All three treatment modalities achieved comparable improvements in symptoms, quality-of-life domains, and AHI.

Series and colleagues[34] performed a similar trial with a 10-day washout period between three different APAP devices. Each patient underwent therapy for a 1-week home trial. They found that the median pressure value during therapy with one manufacturer's device (5.9 cm H_2O) was significantly lower than that during therapy with the other two devices (7.4 cm H_2O). These clinical results parallel the bench study findings of the precursor devices from the same manufacturers.[6] The results suggest that bench study results may be extrapolated to the clinical realm. Despite the inherent limitations of this extrapolation, bench testing may have value considering that devices constantly undergo upgrades and enhancements that outdate, and thereby minimize, the value of comprehensive clinical trial testing.[7,35] In a survey of board-certified sleep physicians, only 37% who prescribed APAP preferred a particular brand.[36] These data may underscore the incongruence between scientific evidence and day-to-day practice, and calls for better dissemination of study findings.

A study (N = 83) comparing polysomnography-derived CPAP and four different APAP devices administered to patients with severe OSA over a 6-month period showed no differences in adherence, clinical symptoms, or HR-QOL.[37] Despite differences in the mean CPAP pressure delivered by the different devices, significant clinical differences were seen over the 6-month treatment period. However, this study was not adequately powered to prove equivalence, but raises interesting questions concerning the clinical significance of small differences in therapeutic pressure administered.[37]

The comparative effectiveness research (CER) strategic framework calls for generation, synthesis, and dissemination of alternate methods to treat and monitor complex medical conditions (such as OSA) requiring complex interventions (such as medical devices in OSA).[38] The development of alternate methods to titrate and treat OSA, or other forms of SDB such as obesity hypoventilation and central sleep apnea, is based on this call. More work on how and where these therapies are being delivered, by pragmatic studies analyzing outcomes in patients with complex co-morbid medical conditions subjected to APAP therapy, may be needed to increase the reach and universal acceptance of these alternate methods of titration. Specifically, most if not all of the RCTs have excluded patients with significant comorbid conditions that could cause hypoventilation (morbid obesity and COPD) and central apneas (heart failure). Reports from large databases including patients with these comorbidities are needed for the field to advance and results to be made generalizable to patients with OSA.

ADVANCED METHODS OF TITRATION

Advanced automation in titration that could tackle central apneas has been developed and is currently marketed. Small RCTs have shown that servoventilation developed by different manufacturers can successfully detect and treat central apneas.[10,11,39,40] Some of these studies have shown improvement in objectively measured sleepiness and urinary measures of catecholamines.[40] However, large studies have not been published on the effects of these devices on other patient outcomes, such as HR-QOL, cardiac function, and adherence to PAP therapy.

During servoventilation, the expiratory PAP is set at a level to treat obstructive apneas and hypopneas before central hypopneas manifest, but some interobserver variability may occur in determining such a pressure level. Combining APAP and servoventilation, with APAP determining the EPAP level automatically and the servoventilation controlling periodic breathing and central apneas, was recently reported to be effective in ameliorating SDB.[41] However, RCTs using this device are awaited.

Advanced titration methods for patients with hypoventilation target minute ventilation and tidal volume rather than events of sleep-disordered breathing such as apneas and hypopneas.[8,9] Although better ventilation and gas exchange have been observed, studies using these devices have failed to show advantages over conventional bilevel PAP settings in terms of sleep quality improvement.[8,9]

OTHER TITRATION METHODS

A small randomized, single-blind, two-period crossover trial of CPAP treatment at the laboratory polysomnography-determined optimal pressure versus at-home self-adjusted CPAP (starting pressure based on prediction equation) showed comparable patient outcomes between the arms.[42] The prediction formula was derived from readily available parameters, namely body mass index, neck circumference, and AHI.[43] Patients were subsequently encouraged to adjust the pressure as necessary to maximize comfort and perceived efficacy.[42] After the 5-week treatment period, adherence to PAP therapy, subjective and objective sleepiness, sleep apnea severity, and sleep architecture were all similar between the groups. However, this was a small study.

In a much larger study, Masa and colleagues[22] subjected one-third of the patients to the prediction formula (predicted pressure = [0.16 × body mass index] + [0.13 × neck circumference] + [0.04 × AHI] − 5.12 up to a maximum of 9 cm H_2O), and the other two groups were either managed using the conventional laboratory polysomnography-derived pressure or APAP-derived pressure. Patients who exceeded a requirement of 9 cm H_2O based on the formula were prescribed only 9 cm H_2O and asked to self-adjust the pressure upwards in 1- or 2-cm H_2O increments based on the observations of their bed partner. Although the CPAP level based on the predicted formula was slightly lower than that achieved by APAP, the predicted formula achieved comparable pressure levels when compared with laboratory polysomnography-derived CPAP levels. No difference was seen among all 3 groups with respect to AHI, subjective sleepiness, or PAP adherence levels.[22] Other prediction formulas exist but have not been studied in a RCT.[44]

REGULATION, REIMBURSEMENT, AND THE PROVIDER

APAP devices, like CPAP devices, are undergoing constant change and evolution. The sophisticated APAP devices of today are the result of multiple incremental changes over many years since the inception of the "auto" concept. This advancement is a natural process that pertains to any device, and represents a much different process from that for drug development. This constant evolution, which is performed through a 510(k) clearance process, has advantages and disadvantages.[35] The disadvantage to these constant changes is that before a clinical trial of a particular device is completed and published, the device has undergone numerous modifications by the manufacturer. These changes undermine the relevance of the eventual publication of the clinical trial findings. Although the perfect clinical study after development of the perfect APAP device will probably never occur, prescribing physicians should pay close attention to changes and characteristics of the APAP devices they prescribe. Changes in device regulation are afoot and may alter the landscape of device innovation and afore-mentioned opinions regarding clinical research involving these devices.[35]

Although APAP devices are generally categorized as low-risk devices by the U.S. Food and Drug Administration, their performance in an individual patient may depend on how they are set, where they are set up, how patients are selected and instructed, and how patients are monitored.[45] The concern is that physicians in busy practices may be unable to keep up with the changes in technology. Unlike pharmaceutical products, physicians do not receive information regarding postapproval trials, nor do they receive education by a cadre of pharmaceutical representatives. In a 2004 survey of board-certified sleep physicians, only 30% of physicians correctly identified the contraindications for administration of APAP devices.[36] Moreover, 30% of sleep physicians never prescribed APAP devices. Physicians who never prescribed APAP devices tended to interpret fewer sleep studies and to prescribe fewer PAP devices per month than physicians who prescribed APAP devices, suggesting that patient volumes were indicative of physician confidence in prescribing these devices.[36] Moreover, 90% of physicians who prescribed auto-PAP devices reported that they reviewed the data downloaded from the device for pressure, leak, and adherence information. However, physician time spent in interpreting the downloads for leak, appropriate pressure level, and troubleshooting during care delivery in an ambulatory APAP program is not reimbursed. Future policy changes for reimbursement should consider provider compensation for this care delivery if APAP is to be embraced by providers.

SUMMARY

Rapid developments have occurred in both the technology and clinical evidence supporting APAP and other alternate methods of titration. Although the results of at least three large noninferiority trials are earnestly anticipated in this area, the future of APAP and alternative modes of titration in daily practice remains in the hands of policy makers, regulatory bodies, and expert consensus.[35,45,46] Future research must move this field ahead from scientific evidence derived from RCTs to development and dissemination of CER that addresses the incorporation of such APAP titration methods into complex medical systems of health care delivery.

REFERENCES

1. Sullivan CE, Issa FG, Berthon-Jones M, et al. Reversal of obstructive sleep apnoea by continuous positive airway pressure applied through the nares. Lancet 1981;1(8225):862–5.
2. Chediak AD, Lipson E, Demirozu MC, et al. The second generation of nasal continuous positive airway pressure devices. Are they created equal? Sleep 1993;16(7):662–7.
3. Miles LE, Buschek GD, McClintock DP, et al. Development and application of automatic nasal CPAP calibration procedures for use in the unsupervised home environment. Sleep 1993;16(Suppl 8):S118–119.
4. Berthon-Jones M. Feasibility of a self-setting CPAP machine. Sleep 1993;16(Suppl 8):S120–1 [discussion: S121–3].
5. Ficker JH, Clarenbach CF, Neukirchner C, et al. Auto-CPAP therapy based on the forced oscillation technique. Biomed Tech (Berl) 2003;48(3):68–72.
6. Coller D, Stanley D, Parthasarathy S. Effect of air leak on the performance of auto-PAP devices: a bench study. Sleep Breath 2005;9(4):167–75.
7. Brown LK. Autotitrating CPAP: how shall we judge safety and efficacy of a black box. Chest 2006; 130(2):312–4.
8. Ambrogio C, Lowman X, Kuo M, et al. Sleep and non-invasive ventilation in patients with chronic respiratory insufficiency. Intensive Care Med 2009; 35(2):306–13.
9. Storre JH, Seuthe B, Fiechter R, et al. Average volume-assured pressure support in obesity hypoventilation: a randomized crossover trial. Chest 2006;130(3):815–21.
10. Morgenthaler TI, Gay PC, Gordon N, et al. Adaptive servoventilation versus noninvasive positive pressure ventilation for central, mixed, and complex sleep apnea syndromes. Sleep 2007;30(4):468–75.
11. Teschler H, Dohring J, Wang YM, et al. Adaptive pressure support servo-ventilation: a novel treatment for Cheyne-Stokes respiration in heart failure. Am J Respir Crit Care Med 2001;164(4):614–9.
12. Lofaso F, Desmarais G, Leroux K, et al. Bench evaluation of flow limitation detection by automated continuous positive airway pressure devices. Chest 2006;130(2):343–9.
13. Farre R, Montserrat JM, Rigau J, et al. Response of automatic continuous positive airway pressure devices to different sleep breathing patterns: a bench study. Am J Respir Crit Care Med 2002; 166(4):469–73.

14. Hirose M, Honda J, Sato E, et al. Bench study of auto-CPAP devices using a collapsible upper airway model with upstream resistance. Respir Physiol Neurobiol 2008;162(1):48–54.

15. Rigau J, Montserrat JM, Wohrle H, et al. Bench model to simulate upper airway obstruction for analyzing automatic continuous positive airway pressure devices. Chest 2006;130(2):350–61.

16. Sharma S, Wali S, Pouliot Z, et al. Treatment of obstructive sleep apnea with a self-titrating continuous positive airway pressure (CPAP) system. Sleep 1996;19(6):497–501.

17. Teschler H, Berthon-Jones M, Thompson AB, et al. Automated continuous positive airway pressure titration for obstructive sleep apnea syndrome. Am J Respir Crit Care Med 1996;154(3 Pt 1):734–40.

18. Lloberes P, Ballester E, Montserrat JM, et al. Comparison of manual and automatic CPAP titration in patients with sleep apnea/hypopnea syndrome. Am J Respir Crit Care Med 1996; 154(6 Pt 1):1755–8.

19. Teschler H, Wessendorf TE, Farhat AA, et al. Two months auto-adjusting versus conventional nCPAP for obstructive sleep apnoea syndrome. Eur Respir J 2000;15(6):990–5.

20. Lloberes P, Rodriguez B, Roca A, et al. Comparison of conventional nighttime with automatic or manual daytime CPAP titration in unselected sleep apnea patients: study of the usefulness of daytime titration studies. Respir Med 2004;98(7):619–25.

21. To KW, Chan WC, Choo KL, et al. A randomized cross-over study of auto-continuous positive airway pressure versus fixed-continuous positive airway pressure in patients with obstructive sleep apnoea. Respirology 2008;13(1):79–86.

22. Masa JF, Jimenez A, Duran J, et al. Alternative methods of titrating continuous positive airway pressure: a large multicenter study. Am J Respir Crit Care Med 2004;170(11):1218–24.

23. Vennelle M, White S, Riha RL, et al. Randomized controlled trial of variable-pressure versus fixed-pressure continuous positive airway pressure (CPAP) treatment for patients with obstructive sleep apnea/hypopnea syndrome (OSAHS). Sleep 2010; 33(2):267–71.

24. Noseda A, Kempenaers C, Kerkhofs M, et al. Constant vs auto-continuous positive airway pressure in patients with sleep apnea hypopnea syndrome and a high variability in pressure requirement. Chest 2004;126(1):31–7.

25. Massie CA, McArdle N, Hart RW, et al. Comparison between automatic and fixed positive airway pressure therapy in the home. Am J Respir Crit Care Med 2003;167(1):20–3.

26. Patruno V, Aiolfi S, Costantino G, et al. Fixed and autoadjusting continuous positive airway pressure treatments are not similar in reducing cardiovascular risk factors in patients with obstructive sleep apnea. Chest 2007;131(5):1393–9.

27. Damjanovic D, Fluck A, Bremer H, et al. Compliance in sleep apnoea therapy: influence of home care support and pressure mode. Eur Respir J 2009; 33(4):804–11.

28. Galetke W, Randerath WJ, Stieglitz S, et al. Comparison of manual titration and automatic titration based on forced oscillation technique, flow and snoring in obstructive sleep apnea. Sleep Med 2009;10(3): 337–43.

29. Berry RB, Hill G, Thompson L, et al. Portable monitoring and autotitration versus polysomnography for the diagnosis and treatment of sleep apnea. Sleep 2008;31(10):1423–31.

30. Mulgrew AT, Fox N, Ayas NT, et al. Diagnosis and initial management of obstructive sleep apnea without polysomnography: a randomized validation study. Ann Intern Med 2007;146(3):157–66.

31. Drummond F, Doelken P, Ahmed QA, et al. Empiric auto-titrating continuous positive airway pressure in obstructive sleep apnea suspects. J Clin Sleep Med 2010;6(2):140–5.

32. Antic NA, Buchan C, Esterman A, et al. A randomized controlled trial of nurse-led care for symptomatic moderate-severe obstructive sleep apnea. Am J Respir Crit Care Med 2009;179(6):501–8.

33. Senn O, Brack T, Matthews F, et al. Randomized short-term trial of two autoCPAP devices versus fixed continuous positive airway pressure for the treatment of sleep apnea. Am J Respir Crit Care Med 2003;168(12):1506–11.

34. Series F, Plante J, Lacasse Y. Reliability of home CPAP titration with different automatic CPAP devices. Respir Res 2008;9:56.

35. Garber AM. Modernizing device regulation. N Engl J Med 2010;362(13):1161–3.

36. Parthasarathy S, Habib M, Quan SF. How are automatic positive airway pressure and related devices prescribed by sleep physicians? A web-based survey. J Clin Sleep Med 2005;1(1):27–34.

37. Meurice JC, Cornette A, Philip-Joet F, et al. Evaluation of autoCPAP devices in home treatment of sleep apnea/hypopnea syndrome. Sleep Med 2007;8(7–8):695–703.

38. VanLare JM, Conway PH, Sox HC. Five next steps for a new national program for comparative-effectiveness research. N Engl J Med 2010; 362(11):970–3.

39. Arzt M, Wensel R, Montalvan S, et al. Effects of dynamic bilevel positive airway pressure support on central sleep apnea in men with heart failure. Chest 2008;134(1):61–6.

40. Pepperell JC, Maskell NA, Jones DR, et al. A randomized controlled trial of adaptive ventilation for Cheyne-Stokes breathing in heart failure. Am J Respir Crit Care Med 2003;168(9):1109–14.

41. Randerath WJ, Galetke W, Kenter M, et al. Combined adaptive servo-ventilation and automatic positive airway pressure (anticyclic modulated ventilation) in co-existing obstructive and central sleep apnea syndrome and periodic breathing. Sleep Med 2009;10(8):898–903.

42. Fitzpatrick MF, Alloway CE, Wakeford TM, et al. Can patients with obstructive sleep apnea titrate their own continuous positive airway pressure? Am J Respir Crit Care Med 2003;167(5):716–22.

43. Hoffstein V, Mateika S. Predicting nasal continuous positive airway pressure. Am J Respir Crit Care Med 1994;150(2):486–8.

44. Loredo JS, Berry C, Nelesen RA, et al. Prediction of continuous positive airway pressure in obstructive sleep apnea. Sleep Breath 2007;11(1):45–51.

45. Morgenthaler TI, Aurora RN, Brown T, et al. Practice parameters for the use of autotitrating continuous positive airway pressure devices for titrating pressures and treating adult patients with obstructive sleep apnea syndrome: an update for 2007. An American Academy of Sleep Medicine report. Sleep 2008;31(1):141–7.

46. Garber AM, Tunis SR. Does comparative-effectiveness research threaten personalized medicine? N Engl J Med 2009;360(19):1925–7.

Adjunctive Therapy to CPAP: Sedative Hypnotics, Heated Humidification, and Supplemental Oxygen

W. McDowell Anderson, MD[a,b,*],
Sherwin M. Mina, MS, MD[c]

KEYWORDS

- CPAP • Hypnotics and sedatives • Oxygen
- Heated humidification • Adherence • Compliance

Untreated obstructive sleep apnea (OSA) has been associated with an increased incidence of heart disease, hypertension, and cerebrovascular accident.[1] Recently, uncontrolled OSA was implicated as a cause of increased incidence and difficulty in controlling diabetes mellitus because of increased insulin resistance.[2] Furthermore, daytime sleepiness and fatigue associated with OSA may be factors leading to motor vehicle accidents.[3]

The gold standard for OSA treatment has been the use of nocturnal continuous positive airway pressure (CPAP). However, as many as 50% of patients do not tolerate CPAP and discontinue its use within the first year.[4] One of the challenges of a sleep physician is to encourage patients to continue using CPAP and reduce the incidence of the adverse consequences of untreated OSA. This article examines adjunctive measures that may help increase adherence to therapy among patients with OSA and the use of supplemental oxygen when conditions warrant its use (note: for the purpose of this article the terms adherence and compliance are used interchangeably).

HYPNOTICS AND SEDATIVES

Various hypnotics and sedatives are available for treating insomnia (**Table 1**). However, their long-term effectiveness and safety in patients with OSA is unknown. Several studies examine how these medications may affect sleep-disordered breathing.[5] Hanly and Powles[5] debate the use of hypnotics in patients with sleep apnea in a summary from a meeting of the Canadian Sleep Society. In this discussion, Hanly acknowledged that benzodiazepines are thought to decrease arousal from sleep, reduce upper airway muscle tone, and decrease the ventilatory response to hypoxia.[2,6] He supports this by citing a case report in which 30 mg of flurazepam precipitated OSA,[7] and another study that showed an increase in the apnea-hypopnea index (AHI) from 33 to 42 in a group of three patients.[8]

Dolly and Block[9] studied the effects of flurazepam, 30 mg, on sleep-disordered breathing. They noted that this dose of flurazepam increased the number of apneas and their duration but did not significantly affect the number of episodes of hypopnea or desaturation (although the degree

[a] James A Haley Veterans Affairs Hospital, 13000 Bruce B Downs Boulevard, Room 111C, Tampa, FL 33612, USA
[b] Sleep Medicine Sleep Disorder Center, Tampa General Hospital, Tampa, FL, USA
[c] University of South Florida, 13000 Bruce B Downs Boulevard, Room 111C, Tampa, FL, USA
* Corresponding author. James A Haley Veterans Affairs Hospital, 13000 Bruce B Downs Boulevard, Room 111C, Tampa, FL 33612.
E-mail address: William.Anderson4@va.gov

Table 1
Commonly used sedatives and hypnotics

Drug	Recommended Dosage	Indications/Specific Comments
Benzodiazepine receptor agonists		
Eszopiclone	2–3 mg hs	Primarily used for sleep onset and maintenance insomnia
	1 mg hs in elderly or debilitated; maximum 2 mg	Intermediate-acting
	1 mg hs in severe hepatic impairment; maximum 2 mg	No short-term use restrictions
Zolpidem	10 mg hs; maximum 10 mg	Primarily used for sleep-onset insomnia
	5 mg hs in elderly	Short- to intermediate-acting
Zolpidem extended-release	12.5 mg hs extended-release	Primarily used for sleep-onset and maintenance insomnia
	6.25 mg hs extended-release in elderly	Controlled release; swallow whole, not divided, crushed, or chewed
Zaleplon	10 mg hs; maximum 20 mg	Primarily used for sleep-onset insomnia
	5 mg hs in elderly, debilitated, mild to moderate hepatic impairment	Short-acting
Benzodiazepines		
Estazolam	1–2 mg hs	Short- to intermediate-acting
	0.5 mg hs in elderly or debilitated	
Flurazepam	15–30 mg hs	Long-acting
	15 mg hs in elderly or debilitated	Risk of residual daytime drowsiness
Temazepam	15–30 mg hs	Short- to intermediate-acting
	7.5 mg in elderly or debilitated	
Triazolam	0.25 mg hs; maximum 0.5 mg	Short-acting
	0.125 mg hs in elderly or debilitated; maximum 0.25 mg	
Melatonin receptor agonists		
Ramelteon	8 mg hs	Primarily used for sleep-onset insomnia
		Short-acting
		No short-term use restrictions
Melatonin	1–3 mg hs	Over-the-counter herbal supplement
		Not regulated by U.S. Food and Drug Administration
		Helpful in circadian rhythm disorders
Psychotropics		
Trazodone	Starting dose, 25–100 mg hs	Mainly for depression
	Up to 150–200 mg hs for a hypnotic	May be prescribed for long-term use
Quetiapine	Starting dose, 25–50 mg hs	Used primarily for schizophrenia and bipolar disorder
	Up to 300 mg hs for insomnia	
Antihistamines		
Diphenhydramine	25–50 mg hs	Primarily for transient insomnia
Doxylamine	25–50 mg hs	Efficacy in chronic insomnia is poor
		Short- to intermediate-acting
		Tolerance may occur
		Anticholinergic effects

Abbreviation: hs, bedtime.

of desaturation was found to be greater). Berry and colleagues[10] found that triazolam, 0.25 mg, showed a modest prolongation of apneic events (26.8 ± 1.7 vs 23.8 ± 1.2 seconds). However,

Hanly[5] adds that many conflicting studies exist on the effect of benzodiazepines. He then cites a study by Cirignotta and colleagues,[11] which showed that neither 0.25 mg of britzolam nor

30 mg of flurazepam worsened respiratory distur-bance index (RDI) or mean oxygen saturation.[11]

A study by Ancoli-Israel and colleagues[12] showed that although 45 mg of flurazepam increased the number of apneas from 15 to 29 during non–rapid eye movement (REM) sleep, this was not found to be statistically significant. Sateia and colleagues[13] compared the use of the short-acting benzodiazepine midazolam, 15 mg, with longer-acting flurazepam, 15 mg and 30 mg, and with placebo and found no increase in sleep apneas during the treatment period for any group.

More recent studies have examined the effects of non–benzodiazepine receptor agonists.[14,15] Berry and Patel[14] showed that zolpidem, 10 mg, did not increase the AHI (**Fig. 1**) or amount of oxygen desaturation, and did not significantly affect sleep architecture except for a reduction in sleep latency and slight reduction in the mean arousal index on 16 patients using zolpidem and placebo on different nights (**Tables 2** and **3**). In fact, the effect of non–benzodiazepine receptor agonists has been studied in the setting of polysomnography and CPAP titration.[16] Eszopiclone and zolpidem (when compared to patients who did not receive a non-benzodiazepine receptor agonist) was shown to improve the quality of polysomnography and improve CPAP titration by improving sleep efficiency (84% ± 9% vs 78% ± 11%), increasing total sleep time (345 ± 42 vs 314 ± 51 minutes), and lowering RDI on the final CPAP pressure (6.1 ± 7 events per hour vs 9.8 ± 14.6).[16]

Lettieri and colleagues[17] examined the effect on short-term compliance of giving eszopiclone as a one-time dose during CPAP titration. At 4 to 6 weeks follow-up, the study showed that patients

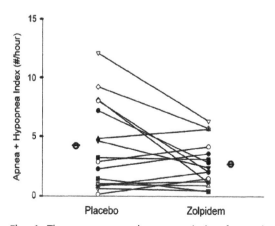

Fig. 1. The mean apnea-hypopnea index for each subject on placebo and zolpidem nights. The mean values for the entire group are shown lateral to the individual values. The mean values on placebo and zolpidem nights did not differ. (*From* Berry RB. Sleep 2006;29(8):1052–6; with permission.)

treated with eszopiclone had improved compliance, defined as use of CPAP for more than 70% of all nights for more than 4 hours (75.9% ± 20% vs 60.1% ± 24.3%).[17,18] However, patients were not extensively screened for comorbid sleep problems, and despite randomization, the eszopiclone group was largely composed of women compared with the placebo group.[17] The implication of this study is that short-term compliance with CPAP may be a predictor of long-term compliance.[17] This finding is supported by a study by Drake and colleagues,[19] who showed that patients' initial experience with CPAP treatment, most reflected by an improvement in sleep efficiency from baseline polysomnography to titration polysomnography, plays an important role in long-term compliance.

Bradshaw and colleagues[20] found that adminis-tration of zolpidem did not improve initial CPAP compliance in men with OSA. The zolpidem group did not show significant differences in total days used (20.58 ± 7.4 vs 17.83 ± 9.33 days).[20] In his letter to the editor, Pelayo[21] questions several aspects of the Bradshaw study, including small sample size, inclusion of only men with OSA, number of days zolpidem was administered to the study group (14 of 28 days), and proper use of humidification. Pelayo proposes that "data from this study should not at present be extrapo-lated to general clinical practice." He also noted that patients in this study were given only passive humidifiers. Heated humidifiers can significantly reduce mouth dryness,[22] one of the key complaints of CPAP use.

A practical application of hypnotics would be in patients who experience claustrophobia. Claus-trophobia, a fear of closed spaces, involves the fear of suffocation and restriction. Chasens and colleagues[23] showed that patients with poor adherence to CPAP had higher claustrophobia scores, as measured by a 15-item subscale adap-ted from the Fear and Avoidance Scale (FAAS) (**Fig. 2**).[24] The corollary from this data is that the modified FAAS may be useful in screening patients who will be nonadherent to CPAP because of claustrophobia. Therapy may be initiated to include benzodiazepines, which are an adjunct therapy for anxiety related to claustrophobia.[25] This role of the non–benzodiazepine receptor agonists such as zolpidem and eszopiclone, which have many of the properties of benzodiazepines but lack the muscle relaxant effect,[25] have not been well defined in this setting. However, they also lack the anxiolytic of benzodiazepines. Lettieri and colleagues[17] showed that use of eszopiclone during CPAP titration improved short-term adherence to therapy, but long-term studies of these medications must be performed before

Table 2
Sleep architecture: zolpidem versus placebo

	Placebo (n = 16)	Zolpidem (n = 16)	P value
Sleep period time, min	428.3 ± 12.5	434.2 ±13.8	NS
Total sleep time, min	384.7 ± 15	401.9 ± 14.2	NS
WASO, min	43.6 ± 5.8	32.3 ± 7.6	NS
Stage 1, min	20.1 ± 2.1	19.3 ± 2.4	NS
Stage 2, min	225.6± 17.2	234.0 ± 9.4	NS
Stage 3/4, min	66.6 ± 9.3	75.9 ± 10.1	NS
Stage REM. min	71.2 ± 8	70.8 ± 7.3	NS
WASO[a]	10.5 ± 1.6	7.4 ± 1.6	NS
Stage 1[a]	4.8 ± 0.5	4.6 ± 0.6	NS
Stage 2[a]	52.3 ± 3.2	54.2 ± 2.0	NS
Stage 3,4[a]	15.5 ± 2.0	17.4 ± 2.2	NS
Stage REM[a]	16.7 ± 1.8	16.0 ± 1.5	NS
Arousal index, no/h	19.0 ± 1.6	16.5 ± 1.2	<.03
Sleep latency, min	23.5 ± 4.7	13.1 ± 3.3	<.02
REM latency, min	128.4 ± 16.9	129.5 ± 8.3	NS
PLM index, no/h	4.9 ± 2.8	9.3 ± 4.1	NS

[a] Sleep stage as a percentage of the sleep period time.
Data from Berry RB, Patel PB. Effect of zolpidem on the efficacy of continuous positive airway pressure as treatment for obstructive sleep apnea. Sleep 2006;29(8):1052–6.

they can be prescribed for claustrophobia-related nonadherence.

Significant data are lacking on the effect of other categories of hypnotics or sedatives on sleep-disordered breathing. Among the categories of drugs not discussed in this article are antihistamines, which include doxylamin and diphenhydramine (which are the main components in many over-the-counter sleep-aids), hydroxyzine, melatonin and the melatonin receptor agonists, other herbal supplements, and other drugs with sedative properties, such as mirtazapine, and gamma-aminobutyric acid (GABA) receptor agonists, such as gabapentin.

Several studies examine the use of medications that improve overall sleep quality in patients with OSA and sleep-disordered breathing.[26–29] Most studies did not show a significant improvement with these medications.[26,29] Although only Carley and colleagues[27] showed that mirtazapine improved AHI, with a reduction of almost 50% after 1 week of therapy, Marshall and colleagues[28]

Table 3
Effects of zolpidem versus placebo on polysomnography

	Placebo (n = 16)	Zolpidem (n = 16)	P value
AHI, no/h	4.8 ± 1.4	2.7 ± 0.47	NS
AHI NREM, no/h	4.2 ± 6.4	2.2 ± 2 40	NS
AHI REM, no/h	7.1 ±11.1	5.6 ± 8.03	NS
AHI supine, no/h^2	7.3 ± 2.2	2.8 ± 1.1	NS
TST supine, %	61.3 ± 8.3	55.9 ± 8.0	NS
ODI no/h	1.46 ± 0.53	0.81 ± 0.29	NS
Lowest SaO$_2$, %	91.4 ± 0.6	91.0 ± 0.7	NS

Abbreviations: AHI, apnea hypopnea index; ODI, oxygen desaturation index; SaO$_2$, saturation oxygen; TST, total sleep time.
Data from Berry RB, Patel PB. Effect of zolpidem on the efficacy of continuous positive airway pressure as treatment for obstructive sleep apnea. Sleep 2006;29(8):1052–6.

**Percentage of Patients with Less Than 2 Hours
CPAP Usage Catagorized by Modified FAAS Scores**

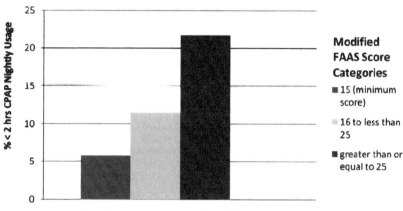

Fig. 2. Percentage of individuals who used CPAP for less than 2 hours nightly categorized by their score on a modified Fear and Avoidance Scale (FAAS). More than 20% of patients who scored ≥25 used CPAP for less than 2 hours, whereas only 5% of those with a minimum score of 15 used CPAP less than 2 hours. (*From* Chasens ER. Claustrophobia and adherence to CPAP treatment. West J Nurs Res 2005;27:307–21; with permission.)

did not show significant benefit with this medication. However, both studies agree that mirtazapine is not indicated as a treatment for sleep apnea. At any rate, further studies are needed to assess the role of sleep aids in long-term hypnotic use and CPAP therapy.

HEATED HUMIDIFICATION

Nasal symptoms (including nasal dryness, irritation, rhinorrhea, congestion, and sneezing), dry mouth, and dry throat are factors that may affect adherence to CPAP therapy.[30,31] Unidirectional airflow during CPAP therapy leads to a decrease in relative humidity of inspired air and in turn to drying of the nasal and oral passages, especially if nasal congestion leads to mouth leaks.[22,32,33] Mouth leaks lead to increased nasal airway blood flow and in turn to increased nasal airway resistance.[32] Richards and colleagues[34] illustrated this effect by measuring nasal resistance with posterior rhinomanometry. Test subjects deliberately produced a mouth leak during nasal CPAP use. This event was noted to cause increased nasal resistance (baseline mean of 2.21 cm H_2O/L/s to a maximum mean of 7.52 cm H_2O/L/s).

Martins de Araujo and colleagues[22] showed that significant mouth leaks are associated with decreased relative humidity in the nose. In their study, heated humidification significantly increased relative humidity. When compared with CPAP alone, added heated humidification raised the relative humidity from 60% ± 14% to 81% ± 14% with the mouth closed and from 43% ± 12% to 64% ± 8% with the mouth open.[22] When comparing spontaneous breathing without CPAP to CPAP use and to heated humidification added to CPAP, the levels of relative humidity were 80% ± 2% versus 63% ± 9% versus 82% ± 12%, respectively.[22] This finding indicates that the use of heated humidification more closely mimics the relative humidification found during spontaneous breathing. However, this was only true when the mouth was closed (**Fig. 3**).[22]

Because of this observation, addition of a face mask, which eliminated mouth leaks, showed comparable relative humidity regardless of the mouth being closed or opened (82% ± 9% vs 84% ± 8%, respectively).[22] However, it was also noted that changing to a full face mask did not necessarily improve compliance because the problems caused by the mask counteracted the benefit of eliminating mouth leaks.[22]

Two types of humidification are available: heated and cold passover. Richards and colleagues[34] compared the effects of a cold passover humidifier, which was noted to cause little change in nasal resistance (maximum mean, 8.27 cm H_2O/L/s), versus a hot water bath humidifier, which was shown to attenuate the manufactured increase in nasal resistance (maximum mean, 4.02 cm H_2O/L/s). In a separate study, Massie and colleagues[32] found no difference in compliance between cold passover and no humidification (**Table 4**). These studies show that compliance improved with use of heated humidity.

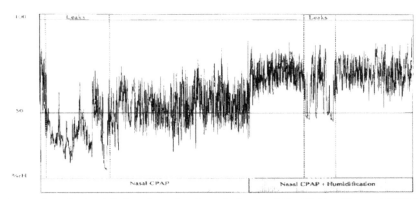

Fig. 3. Typical recording obtained during sleep showing relative humidity (%rH) with nasal CPAP (nCPAP) alone during the first part of the night (*left part of trace*) followed by nCPAP with heated humidification (*right part of trace*) during the second part of the night. The period of mouth leaks in each condition are indicated by vertical broken lines. (*From* Martins de Araujo MT. Heated humidification or face mask to prevent upper airway dryness during continuous positive airway pressure therapy. Chest 2000;117:142–7; with permission.)

Unfortunately, although current data show conflicting results regarding the effect of heated humidification on CPAP compliance **(Table 5)**,[32,33,35,36] most studies agree that heated humidification significantly improves nasal symptoms.[22,32,33,35] Mador and colleagues[33] found that heated humidification did not improve compliance, show greater improvement in sleepiness, or improve quality of life, but was associated with "fewer symptoms attributable to the upper airway."

Another study examined the effects of heated humidity on compliance when used with automatic positive airway pressure (APAP), defined as a CPAP machine that titrates the pressure based on an algorithmic estimate of airway obstruction. This study showed no benefit for heated humidification, with compliance at 7 days not significantly different between the APAP group with heated humidification and the APAP group without (4.9 ± 2.6 vs 5.2 ± 2.3 hours per night). The compliance at 30 days was also similar between the groups (5.3 ± 2.4 vs 5.2 ± 2.3 hours per night).[37] The investigators recommended that heated humidity only be used when patients are symptomatic with nasal complaints. However, this study highlights the fact that subjects' use of the assigned heated humidifier could not be measured objectively, and whether the humidifier was set to an optimal setting each night could not be established.[37]

Although some experts believe that heated humidity should be reserved for patients who complain of nasal symptoms, common practice

Table 4
Differences in outcome measures among CPAP use with heated humidity, CPAP use with cold passover humidity, and CPAP use without humidity

Outcome Measure	Heated Humidity	Cold Passover Humidity	Without Humidity
Use, h per night	5.52 ± 2.1[a]	5.15 ± 1.9	4.93 ± 2.2
Epworth sleepiness scale	6.2 ± 3.8[b]	7.2 ± 4.8[b]	6.7 ± 3.9[b]
Feeling on awakening	74.0 ± 15.95[c]	68.9 ± 23.4	62.0 ± 23.4
Satisfaction with CPAP	73.9 ± 19.1[c]	72.9 ± 22.6[d]	62.3 ± 27.6
No. adverse side effects (global score)	4.9 ± 3.3	6.2 ± 3.8	6.5 ± 4.9

[a] $P = .008$ versus without humidity.
[b] Results are significantly different from baseline ($P<.0001$).
[c] $P = .02$ versus without humidity.
[d] $P = .05$ versus without humidity.
Data from Massie CA. Effect of heated humidification on nasal symptoms and compliance in sleep apnea patients using continuous positive airway pressure. Chest 1999;116:403–8.

Table 5
CPAP compliance with and without heated humidification: a comparison of published studies

Study	Compliance without Heated Humidification	Compliance with Heated Humidification	Statistically Significant
Mador et al[33]	1 mo: 4.3 ± 2.4 3 mo: 4.8 ± 2.3 12 mo: 4.8 ± 2.4	1 mo: 4.3 ± 2.0 3 mo: 4.3 ± 2.0 12 mo: 4.2 ± 2.3	No No No
Massle et al[32]	3 wk: 4.93 ± 2.2	3 wk: 5.52 ± 2.1	Yes
Rakotonanahary et al[36]	3 mo: 3.51 ± 2.53	3 mo: 5.38 ± 2.26	Yes
Ryan et al[35]	4 wk: 5.21 ± 1.66	4 wk: 5.21 ± 1.84	No

in many areas is to prescribe a heated humidifier for each patient who needs CPAP therapy. Sleep providers must educate patients on the proper use of the heated humidifier, its function, and how it can improve the experience with CPAP. Anecdotally, the use of a heated humidifier can sometimes be difficult for patients, because this adjunct to therapy requires daily rinsing, regular cleaning using diluted acetic acid (white vinegar), and use of distilled water because tap or drinking water have minerals that can deposit onto the machine. Equipment damage may also result from water leaking to the wrong part of the unit, although some newer CPAP units have been redesigned to prevent this. Despite conflicting observations, humidification and general knowledge of CPAP may empower patients to adhere to CPAP therapy.

SUPPLEMENTAL OXYGEN

For patients who do not tolerate CPAP therapy and are nonsurgical candidates, supplemental oxygen has been proposed as an alternate therapy.[38] A task force from the American Academy of Sleep Medicine reviewed supplemental oxygen as an option for treating OSA. At the time of the task force, only four randomized controlled trials of supplemental oxygen as a treatment of OSA had been performed.[36,39–41] Conflicting results were reported on the effects of oxygen therapy for apneas and hypopneas associated with OSA. However, one consistent finding was that supplemental oxygen reduced the severity of hypoxemia.[38]

Transtracheal oxygen is a method of delivering oxygen through a small catheter inserted during a minor surgical procedure that is typically used to treat patients with chronic hypoxemia.[42] This technique is thought to deliver oxygen to the larynx, which acts as a reservoir to improve the efficiency of oxygen delivery.[43]

Two studies by Chauncey and Aldrich[39] and Farney and colleagues[40] examined the effect of transtracheal oxygen as an alternative treatment for OSA. In a small study of only four patients, Chauncey and Aldrich[39] showed that transtracheal oxygen delivery (TTOD) improved mean RDI in patients with moderate to severe OSA. Mean RDI was 54.3, 19.6, and 10.6 at baseline, after intervention with oxygen trough nasal cannula, and after intervention with TTOD, respectively. This improvement in RDI was associated with an improvement in the overall nocturnal oxygen saturation with TTOD (51% at baseline vs 43% with nasal cannula vs 87% with TTOD). These numbers show that when compared with nasal cannula oxygen delivery, TTOD improved RDI to a greater degree. Furthermore, in contrast to TTOD, no improvement in nocturnal hypoxemia or in daytime symptoms was noted with nasal cannula.[39] However, care must be taken in interpreting the data from this study, because the sample size was very small.

Farney and colleagues[40] showed that TTOD increased the low oxygen saturation (70.4% vs 89.7%) and significantly reduced the AHI (64.6 vs 26.2). This finding was in comparison to oxygen delivered through nasal cannula, which was shown to improve nocturnal desaturation (86.2%), but did not significantly reduce the AHI (59.0). The study also showed that nasal CPAP was most effective in reducing the AHI (13.9), but did not completely resolve the oxygen saturation nadir (80%).[40]

The studies were performed in patients with moderate to severe sleep apnea. Phillips and colleagues[44] studied the effects of 4 liters of oxygen delivered through nasal cannula in patients with mild sleep apnea. Again, oxygen was shown to improve oxygen saturation nadir (95.9% ± 0.3% vs 88.7% ± 2.8%) but not AHI (16.8 ± 3.2 vs 20.5 ± 4.8) when compared with baseline. The investigators also noted that nasal oxygen did not improve daytime sleepiness as measured

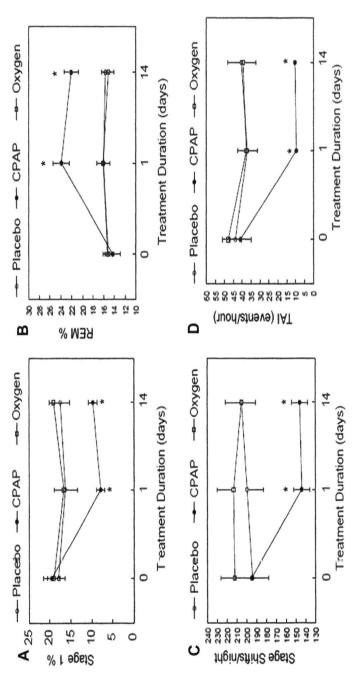

Fig. 4. Time plots of the effectiveness of CPAP (*closed circles*), supplemental oxygen (*open squares*), and placebo-CPAP (*opened circles*) on correcting sleep architecture sleep-quality variables. Values represent mean ± standard error of the mean. (*A*) Percentage of stage 1 sleep (stage 1%) is improved to near normal by CPAP. (*B*) Percentage of stage rapid eye movement sleep (REM%) is improved to within normal limits by CPAP. (*C*) Number of stage shifts per night is significantly reduced by CPAP. (*D*) Total arousal index (TAI) improved to within normal limits with CPAP. Supplemental oxygen at 3 L/min had no effects on sleep architecture. The effects of CPAP were apparent during the first night of therapy. Asterisk denotes statistically significant change from placebo-CPAP. (*From* Loredo JS. Effect of continuous positive airway pressure versus supplemental oxygen on sleep quality in obstructive sleep apnea: a placebo-CPAP – controlled study. Sleep 2006;29(4):564–71; with permission.)

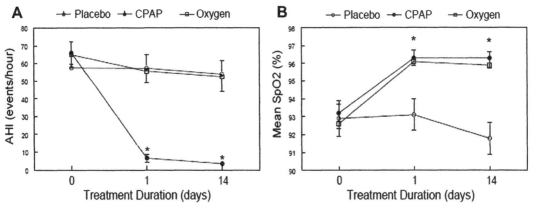

Fig. 5. Time plots of the effectiveness of CPAP (*closed circles*), supplemental oxygen (*open squares*), and placebo-CPAP (*opened circles*) on correcting respiratory sleep-quality variables. Values represent mean ± standard error of the mean. (*A*) CPAP improved to within normal AHI limits. (*B*) CPAP and supplemental oxygen at 3 L/min improved to within normal mean oxyhemoglobin saturation (SpO2) limits. The effects of CPAP and oxygen were apparent during the first night of therapy. Asterisk denotes statistically significant change from placebo-CPAP. (*From* Loredo JS. Effect of continuous positive airway pressure versus supplemental oxygen on sleep quality in obstructive sleep apnea: a placebo-CPAP-controlled study. Sleep 2006;29(4):564–71; with permission.)

in a mean sleep latency (MSL) test (baseline, 11.9 ± 1.6 minutes vs with nasal oxygen, 10.8 ± 1.6 minutes). In comparison, CPAP showed the best overall improvement in AHI (3.0 ± 0.9), improvement in oxygen saturation nadir (93.7% ± 0.9%), and best overall improvement in daytime sleepiness (15.1 ± 2.1 minutes).

A more recent study by Loredo and colleagues[45] examined the effect of oxygen delivered through a placebo-CPAP setup. In contrast to TTOD or nasal cannula, oxygen was delivered at 3 L/min using an oxygen concentrator combined with nontherapeutic CPAP (<1 cm H_2O at the mask). Supplemental oxygen given through this method corrected mean nocturnal oxygen saturation but did not significantly affect AHI, number of shifts in sleep stages, percent of REM sleep, percent of stage 1 sleep, or total arousals per hour of sleep (**Figs. 4** and **5**).

Other studies have examined the effects of oxygen on the adverse consequences of untreated sleep apnea. For instance, hypertension has been linked to sleep apnea. Norman and colleagues[46] compared the effects on blood pressure for CPAP and oxygen delivered through nasal cannula and showed a decrease in the daytime mean of diastolic blood pressure and systolic and diastolic blood pressure during nighttime measurements. However, a significant reduction in daytime systolic blood pressure was not appreciated. The effect of oxygen versus CPAP on cognitive deficits was also studied. Although neither intervention improved overall cognitive behavior in a 2-week treatment period, CPAP was shown to be helpful in terms of speed of information processing,

vigilance, and sustained attention/alertness. Supplemental oxygen did not have a significant effect.[47]

Care must be taken in prescribing oxygen in patients experiencing hypoventilation. A study by Masa and colleagues[48] showed that in patients with hypoventilation secondary to obesity, oxygen during sleep as the only treatment increased Pco_2 compared with Pco_2 daytime (52 ± 11 vs 42 ± 3). This finding is compared with noninvasive positive pressure ventilation (NIPPV), which did not cause a significantly decrease in Pco_2 between wake and sleep (40 ± 3 vs 44 ± 2).

In patients with obesity hypoventilation syndrome, treatment is recommended to consist of NIPPV (CPAP or bilevel device) with or without supplemental oxygen to keep oxygen saturation greater than 90%, because supplemental oxygen alone is likely inadequate.[49] In a recent study, Samolski and colleagues[50] showed that in patients with severe chronic obstructive pulmonary disease, adding 1 L of oxygen over the daytime prescription needed to keep the oxygen saturation greater than 90% resulted in increased hypercapnia and decreased pH. However, these patients did not have sleep apnea.

MISCELLANEOUS

Other adjunctive measures to CPAP are beyond the scope of this article, but may include weight loss through diet, exercise, and perhaps bariatric surgery[51]; nasal and pharyngeal surgeries for sleep apnea, such as uvulopharyngoplasty (UPPP), repair of a deviated nasal septum, tongue

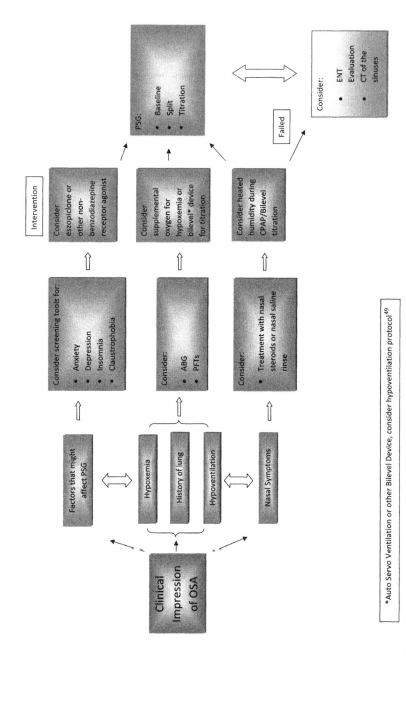

Fig. 6. A proposed algorithm to preempt CPAP intolerance for patients with clinical impression of OSA. ABG, arterial blood gas; ENT, Ear, Nose, Throat Physician; PFT, pulmonary function test; PSG, polysomnography.

*Auto Servo Ventilation or other Bilevel Device, consider hypoventilation protocol[49] base reduction, inferior turbinate reduction, and other surgeries of the upper airway[52]; mandibular advancement devices; jaw and chin straps[53,54]; and positional therapy.

SUMMARY

CPAP therapy has many adjunctive measures for controlling OSA. Sedatives and hypnotics may have a role in improving adherence to CPAP use, but long-term studies of the effectiveness of these medications are pending. Although evidence showing that heated humidification improves adherence is conflicting, it does have a role in improving nasal symptoms related to CPAP use. Oxygen clearly has a role in improving oxygen saturation nadir in patients with sleep-disordered breathing. It can also be helpful as a supplement to CPAP or bilevel devices for patients experiencing hypoventilation. The authors have proposed a simple algorithm for evaluating patients with a clinical impression of OSA (**Fig. 6**). In the end, the goal of health care providers is to improve the quality of life in patients with OSA and prevent the adverse consequences of untreated disease. For patients who agree to CPAP therapy, health care providers must work together with individual patients to tailor their care to improve adherence and, consequently, treatment of OSA.

REFERENCES

1. Ballard RD, Gay PC, Strollo PJ. Interventions to improve compliance in sleep apnea patients previously non-compliant with continuous positive airway pressure. J Clin Sleep Med 2007;3(7):706–12.
2. Punjabi NM, Sorkin JD, Katzel LI, et al. Sleep-disordered breathing and insulin resistance in middle-aged and overweight men. Am J Respir Crit Care Med 2002;165:677–82.
3. Aguiar M, Valença J, Felizardo M, et al. Obstructive sleep apnoea syndrome as a cause of road traffic accidents. Rev Port Pneumol 2009;15(3):419–31.
4. Loube DI, Gay PC, Strohl KP, et al. Indications for positive airway pressure treatment of adult obstructive sleep apnea patients: a consensus statement. Chest 1999;115:863–6.
5. Hanly P, Powles P. Hypnotics should never be used in patients with sleep apnea. J Psychosom Res 1993;37(Suppl 1):59–65.
6. Robinson RW, Zwillich CW. The effect of drugs on breathing during sleep. Clin Chest Med 1985;6(4):603–14.
7. Mendelson WB, Garnett D, Gillin JC. Flurazepam-induced sleep apnea syndrome in a patient with insomnia and mild sleep related respiratory changes. J Nerv Ment Dis 1981;169:261–4.
8. Guilleminault C, Silvestri R, Mondini Mondini S, et al. Aging and sleep apnea: action of benzodiazepine, acetazolamide, alcohol, and sleep deprivation in a healthy elderly group. J Gerontol 1984;39:655–61.
9. Dolly FR, Block AJ. Effect of flurazepam on sleep-disordered breathing and nocturnal oxygen desaturation in asymptomatic subjects. Am J Med 1982;73(2):239–43.
10. Berry RB, Kouchi K, Bower J, et al. Triazolam in patients with obstructive sleep apnea. Am J Respir Crit Care Med 1995;151(2):450–4.
11. Cirignotta F, Mondini S, Zucconi M, et al. Effect of brotizolam on sleep-disordered breathing in heavy snorers with obstructive apnea. Curr Ther Res 1992;51:360–6.
12. Ancoli-Israel S, Kripke DF, Zorick F, et al. Effects of a single dose of flurazepam on the sleep of healthy volunteers. Arzneimittelforschung 1984;34(1):99–100.
13. Sateia MJ, Hauri P, Kripke D, et al. Clinical safety of flurazepam and midazolam during 14-day use in chronic insomniacs. J Clin Psychopharmacol 1990;10(Suppl 4):28S–31S.
14. Berry RB, Patel PB. Effect of zolpidem on the efficacy of continuous positive airway pressure as treatment for obstructive sleep apnea. Sleep 2006;29(8):1052–6.
15. Nunes JL, Faria M, Winck JC. Apnea/hypopnea index and benzodiazepine use in patients with arterial hypertension and excessive weight. Int J Cardiol 2007;114:216–8.
16. Collen J, Lettieri C, Kelly W, et al. Clinical and polysomnographic predictors of short-term positive airway pressure compliance. Chest 2009;135(3):704–6.
17. Lettieri CJ, Collen JF, Eliasson AH, et al. Sedative use during continuous positive airway pressure titration improves subsequent compliance. Chest 2009;136:1263–8.
18. Lettieri CJ, Quast TN, Eliasson AH, et al. Eszopiclone improves overnight polysomnography and continuous positive airway pressure titration: a prospective, randomized, Placebo-Controlled Trial. Sleep 2008;31(9):1310–6.
19. Drake CL, Day R, Hudgel D, et al. Sleep during titration predicts continuous positive airway pressure compliance. Sleep 2003;26:308–11.
20. Bradshaw DA, Ruff GA, Murphy DP. An oral hypnotic does not improve continuous positive airway pressure compliance in men with obstructive sleep apnea. Chest 2006;130:1369–76.
21. Pelayo R. The role of hypnotics in continuous positive airway pressure compliance. Chest 2007;131(5):1616.
22. Martins de Araujo MT, Vieira SB, Vasquez EC, et al. Heated humidification or face mask to prevent upper airway dryness during continuous

positive airway pressure therapy. Chest 2000;117:142–7.

23. Chasens ER, Pack AI, Maislin G, et al. Claustrophobia and adherence to CPAP treatment. West J Nurs Res 2005;27:307–21.

24. Johnston M, Johnston DW, Wilkes H, et al. Cumulative scales for the measurement of agoraphobia. Br J Clin Psychol 1984;23:133–44.

25. Sadock BJ, Sadock VA. Benzodiazepines and drugs acting on the benzodiazepine receptor. Synopsis of psychiatry. 10th edition. Philadelphia: Lippincott, Williams and Wiklins, 2007. p. 1018.

26. Kohler M, Bloch KE, Stradling JR. Pharmacological approaches to the treatment of obstructive sleep apnoea. Expert Opin Investig Drugs 2009;18(5):647–56.

27. Carley DW, Olopade C, Ruigt GS, et al. Efficacy of mirtazapine in obstructive sleep apnea syndrome. Sleep 2007;30(1):35–41.

28. Marshall NS, Yee BJ, Desai AV, et al. Two randomized placebo-controlled trials to evaluate the efficacy and tolerability of mirtazapine for the treatment of obstructive sleep apnea. Sleep 2008; 31(6):824–31.

29. Sériès F, Workshop Participants. Can improving sleep influence sleep-disordered breathing? Drugs 2009;69(Suppl 2):77–91.

30. Engleman HM, Martin SE, Douglas NJ. Compliance with CPAP therapy in patients with sleep apnoea/hypopnea syndrome. Thorax 1994;49:263–6.

31. Pepin JL, Legar P, Veale D, et al. Side effects of nasal continuous positive airway pressure in sleep apnea syndrome. Chest 1995;107:375–81.

32. Massie CA, Hart RW, Peralez K, et al. Effects of humidification on nasal symptoms and compliance in sleep apnea patients using continuous positive airway pressure. Chest 1999;116:403–8.

33. Mador MJ, Krauza M, Pervez A, et al. Effect of heated humidification on compliance and quality of life in patients with sleep apnea using nasal continuous positive airway pressure. Chest 2005;128:2151–8.

34. Richards GN, Cistulli PA, Ungar RG, et al. Mouth leak with nasal continuous positive airway pressure increases nasal airway resistance. Am J Respir Crit Care Med 1996;154(1):182–6.

35. Ryan S, Doherty LS, Nolan GM, et al. Effects of heated humidification and topical steroids on compliance, nasal symptoms and quality of life in patients with obstructive sleep apnea syndrome using nasal continuous positive airway pressure. J Clin Sleep Med 2009;5(5):422–6.

36. Rakotonanahary D, Pelletier-Fleury N, Gagnadoux F, et al. Predictive factors for the need for additional humidification during nasal continuous positive airway pressure therapy. Chest 2001;119:460–5.

37. Salgado SM, Boleo-Tome JP, Canhao CM, et al. Impact of heated humidification with automatic positive airway pressure in obstructive sleep apnea therapy. J Bras Pneumol 2007;34(9):690–4.

38. Veasey SC, Guilleminault C, Strohl KP, et al. Medical therapy for obstructive sleep apnea: a review by the Medical Therapy for Obstructive Sleep Apnea Task Force of the Standards of Practice Committee of the American Academy of Sleep Medicine. Sleep 2006;29(8):1036–44.

39. Chauncey JB, Aldrich MS. Preliminary findings in the treatment of obstructive sleep apnea with transtracheal oxygen. Sleep 1990;13(2):167–74.

40. Farney RJ, Walker JM, Elmer JC, et al. Transtracheal oxygen, nasal CPAP and nasal oxygen in five patients with obstructive sleep apnea. Chest 1992;101:1228–35.

41. Landsberg R, Friedman M, Ascher-Landsberg J. Treatment of hypoxemia in obstructive sleep apnea. Am J Rhinol 2001;15:311–3.

42. Branditz FK, Kem KB, Campbell SC. Continuous transtracheal oxygen delivery during cardiopulmonary resuscitation. An alternative method to ventilation in a canine model. Chest 1989;95:441–8.

43. Kampelmacher MJ, Deenstra M, van Kesteren RG, et al. Transtracheal oxygen therapy: an effective and safe alternative to nasal oxygen administration. Eur Respir J 1997;10:828–33.

44. Phillips BA, Schmitt FA, Berry DTR, et al. Treatment of obstructive sleep apnea: a preliminary report comparing nasal CPAP to nasal oxygen in patients with mild OSA. Chest 1990;98(2):325–30.

45. Loredo JS, Ancoli-Israel S, Kim EJ, et al. Effect of continuous positive airway pressure versus supplemental oxygen on sleep quality in obstructive sleep apnea: a placebo-CPAP-controlled study. Sleep 2006;29(4):564–71.

46. Norman D, Loredo JS, Nelesen RA, et al. Effects of continuous positive airway pressure versus supplemental oxygen on 24-hour ambulatory blood pressure. Hypertension 2006;47:840–5.

47. Lim WJ, Bardwell WA, Loredo JS, et al. Neuropsychological effects of 2-week continuous positive airway pressure treatment and supplemental oxygen in patients with obstructive sleep apnea: a randomized placebo-controlled study. Sleep 2007;3(4):380–6.

48. Masa JF, Celli BR, Riesco JA, et al. Noninvasive positive pressure ventilation and not oxygen may prevent overt ventilatory failure in patients with chest wall diseases. Chest 1997;112:207–13.

49. Mokhlesi B, Tulaimat A. Recent advances in obesity hypoventilation syndrome. Chest 2007; 132:1322–36.

50. Samolski D, Tarrega J, Anton A, et al. Sleep hypoventilation due to increased nocturnal oxygen flow

in hypercapnic COPD patients. Respirology 2010; 15:283–8.

51. Greenburg DL, Lettieri CJ, Eliasson AH. Effects of surgical weight loss on measures of obstructive sleep apnea: a meta-analysis. Am J Med 2009; 122:535–42.

52. Lin HC, Friedman M, Chang HW, et al. The efficacy of multilevel surgery of the upper airway in adults with obstructive sleep apnea/hypopnea syndrome. Laryngoscope 2008;118:902–8.

53. Vorona RD, Ware JC, Sinacori JT, et al. Treatment of severe obstructive sleep apnea syndrome with a chinstrap. J Clin Sleep Med 2007;3(7):729–30.

54. Estrellita VJ, Phillips B. Evaluation of the "chin-up" strip [abstract]. Chest 1998;114:383S.

CPAP Effect on Cardiovascular Disease

Adrian Velasquez, MD[a],*, Shilpa Rahangdale, MD[b],
Atul Malhotra, MD[b]

KEYWORDS

- CPAP • OSA • Cardiovascular disease
- Cardiovascular outcomes

Obstructive sleep apnea (OSA) has well established neurocognitive and cardiovascular sequelae. Historically, the evidence for these relationships was primarily based on associations. Recently, interventional studies have provided evidence that treatment of OSA benefits the cardiovascular system in addition to its other neurocognitive effects. Although definitive data are still lacking regarding cardiovascular outcome benefits from the treatment of apnea, this article reviews rapidly evolving evidence of improvements in intermediate markers.

EFFECTS OF CONTINUOUS POSITIVE AIRWAY PRESSURE ON HYPERTENSION

The relationship between OSA and hypertension is supported by several clinic- and population-based studies, as well as experimental data from a canine OSA model. Hla and colleagues[1] were one of the earliest to demonstrate an independent association between OSA and hypertension from a community-based sample. They showed that use of continuous positive airway pressure (CPAP) for 3 weeks resulted in a decrease in blood pressure (BP) during the night, the persistence of lower BP after the treatment was terminated, and a decreasing trend in the BP after the therapy.[1] Lavie and colleagues[2] found that OSA was associated with hypertension independent of age, body mass index (BMI), and sex in a large clinic-based cohort (n = 2677). Peppard and colleagues[3] found

a similar relationship between OSA and hypertension in a prospective, population-based cohort of 709 subjects. They found a dose-response relationship between the presence and severity of OSA at baseline and the presence of incident hypertension 4 years later, independent of known confounding variables. These data show strong evidence of an important link between OSA and hypertension, but evidence remained elusive that OSA played a causative role in the development of hypertension, given the undefined role of common risk factors such as obesity. Evidence of a direct pathophysiologic link between the 2 diseases was derived from a canine model by Brooks and colleagues.[4] In tracheostomized dogs, the upper airways were reversibly obstructed with a device on detection of sleep by biotelemetry. Dogs with sleep fragmentation induced by acoustic arousals on detection of sleep were used as controls. Although night-time BP was elevated in OSA and sleep fragmentation controls, only the OSA group had sustained daytime hypertension, which resolved after cessation of OSA. Combined with the increased prevalence and incidence of hypertension in those with OSA, this model provides strong evidence that OSA is causally linked to hypertension.

Several interventional trials have suggested that CPAP therapy may be beneficial in the treatment of hypertension. Faccenda and colleagues[5] conducted a randomized, placebo-controlled trial investigating the effect of CPAP therapy on

a Department of Internal Medicine, Caritas Carney Hospital, Tufts University School of Medicine, 2100 Dorchester Avenue, Dorchester, MA 02124, USA
b Sleep Division, Brigham and Women's Hospital, 75 Francis Street, Boston, MA 02115, USA
* Corresponding author.
E-mail address: adrianvelasquezmd@gmail.com

Sleep Med Clin 5 (2010) 383–392
doi:10.1016/j.jsmc.2010.05.009
1556-407X/10/$ – see front matter © 2010 Elsevier Inc. All rights reserved.

24-hour BP in sleep clinic patients with OSA. Sixty-eight patients with an apnea-hypopnea index (AHI) of 15 events per hour or more were randomized to receive CPAP ($\geq$3.5 hours per night) or placebo capsule for one month; patients were switched to the alternative treatment for the second month. At the end of each month, 24-hour ambulatory BP data were collected. The investigators found that the use of CPAP resulted in no significant change in systolic BP but a statistically significant 1.5 mm Hg (P = .04) reduction in diastolic BP from 2 to 10 AM. The small absolute value of change is probably related to a floor effect, because enrolled subjects did not have hypertension and were not on antihypertensive therapy, excluding those with the most severe disease. Thus, one could argue that it is difficult to lower BP when the initial values are within the normal range. OSA patients with greater hypoxia (4% oxygen desaturation index of >20 events per hour, n = 14) had the largest response to CPAP therapy. In this subgroup of patients, CPAP resulted in a statistically significant decrease in systolic, diastolic, and mean arterial pressures (4.0-mm Hg decrease in systolic pressures and 5.0-mm Hg, in diastolic pressures).

CPAP therapy has been noted to have a greater effect in certain patient populations with higher baseline BP levels and untreated hypertension, in patients specifically noted to have nocturnal hypertension, and those with resistant hypertension.[6–9] Specifically, patients with resistant hypertension have been noted to have higher prevalence of OSA, with one study noting an 83% prevalence of OSA.[10] Logan and colleagues[6] conducted an interventional study of CPAP in patients who remained hypertensive despite optimal medical therapy and were found to have OSA. Refractory hypertension was defined as daytime clinic BP of 140 mm Hg systolic or greater or 90 mm Hg diastolic or greater.[11] Patients were treated with CPAP for 2 months; 24-hour BP was recorded before study initiation and at study completion. Of 19 patients with refractory hypertension, 16 were found to have OSA (84%); 11 agreed to participate in the study. After 2 months of CPAP therapy, statistically significant 24-hour systolic and diastolic BP reduction of 10.5 mm Hg and 5.7 mm Hg, respectively, was noted. Furthermore, nocturnal systolic BP was reduced by 14.4 mm Hg and daytime systolic BP, by 9.3 mm Hg, both with P<.05. Nocturnal diastolic BP was reduced by 7.8 mm Hg with statistical significance, although daytime diastolic BP reduction of 5.1 mm Hg did not attain statistical significance. These data are consistent with a marked effect of CPAP on BP in patients with refractory hypertension, although the lack of a control group

precludes assessment of the effects of natural history alone on BP in this cohort. These results suggest that patients with refractory hypertension may exhibit a significantly greater response to CPAP therapy than normotensive patients. Further randomized trials are required to draw more definitive conclusions.

The effectiveness of CPAP therapy in patients with mild OSA (AHI <15/h) remains an area of uncertainty. A small randomized controlled trial (RCT) by Barnes and colleagues[12] was conducted to evaluate presence and extent of cardiopulmonary treatment response to CPAP versus oral placebo in patients with mild (AHI 5–30/h) OSA. Patients exhibiting signs of severe disease, excessive desaturation during sleep, and those with clinically significant comorbidities were excluded from the study. Twenty-eight patients completed the entire protocol. The patients were randomized to receive CPAP or placebo tablet for 8 weeks after which they were switched to the alternative arm for another 8 weeks. Before the start of the trial and at the end of each 8-week period, patients' 24-hour BP was recorded. Of 24 patients, 7 (29%) were found to be hypertensive at baseline. Of these, 4 were found to be normotensive after CPAP therapy and 2 were found to be normotensive after CPAP and placebo. However, there were no statistically significant differences found in the 24-hour BP data after an 8-week treatment period compared with baseline. There was also no difference in BP outcomes between the 2 treatment arms. Furthermore, there was no benefit of CPAP over placebo in quality of life data analysis, and positive placebo effects were present in most neuropsychiatric and behavioral endpoints examined. These results bring into question the validity of some of the previously observed benefits from CPAP therapy in patients with mild OSA. Use of CPAP in these patients may be counterproductive to normalization of BP, given that some studies describe an association between placebo CPAP and increase in BP probably secondary to discomfort and anxiety associated with CPAP apparatus use.[13]

In summary, although some authors have reported that CPAP and sham CPAP (which may not be an ideal placebo) were associated with similar declines in daytime BP, most data point to a beneficial effect of CPAP on hypertension.[14] A meta-analysis of 18 RCTs involving 818 patients for a duration of at least 2 weeks demonstrated a 2.46 mm Hg reduction in BP with the use of CPAP[7] (Fig. 1). Even small average changes in BP associated with CPAP may be of clinical significance and carry significant health benefits. Earlier studies have shown that a 5-mm Hg decrease in

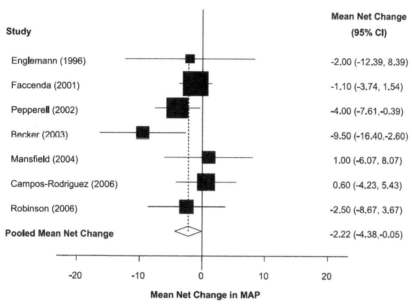

Fig. 1. CPAP treatment of OSA has been shown to lower blood pressure. (*Adapted from* Bazzano LA, Khan Z, Reynolds K, et al. Effect of nocturnal nasal continuous positive airway pressure on blood pressure in obstructive sleep apnea. Hypertension 2007;50:417–23; with permission.)

diastolic BP leads to a 42% decrease in cerebrovascular accident and 14% decrease in coronary artery disease (CAD) within a 5-year period (these studies looked at antihypertensive pharmacotherapy in non-OSA patients).[15] Also, nocturnal surges in BP, which are common in untreated OSA, are probably a substrate for plaque rupture. Thus, the magnitude of the BP improvement during the daytime may be less critical than the potential decrease in cardiovascular risk given that BP itself is a surrogate outcome measure.

EFFECTS OF CPAP IN PATIENTS WITH AND WITHOUT CAD

Treatment of patients with concomitant OSA and CAD has been observed to improve clinical outcomes in prospective and retrospective observational studies. Peled and colleagues[16] observed an increased prevalence of OSA in patients with CAD and attenuated nocturnal ischemia after only one night of treatment. Nocturnal myocardial ischemic events were observed in 51 patients with OSA and CAD but not in the control group of 17 OSA subjects without CAD. Nocturnal ischemic events, defined by ST-segment changes, were associated with measures of sleep apnea severity, sleep quality, and traditional cardiovascular risk factors.[16] ST-segment changes occurred more frequently in those with greater oxygen desaturations, lower sleep efficiencies, older age, more

severe CAD, and higher combined nocturnal BP and heart rate.[16] The AHI did not predict the presence of nocturnal ischemia, suggesting that the global cardiovascular health of the patient was more important in determining risk of nocturnal ischemia.[16] Treatment with CPAP diminished the number of nocturnal ischemic events from 13 to 6 on the first night of treatment. The investigators attribute the incomplete response to CPAP therapy to residual respiratory events. Thus, it seems that CPAP in the short term improves electrocardiographic measures of ischemia.

The best available evidence that CPAP also improves long-term outcomes in those with CAD come from several prospective observational studies demonstrating improvements in combined end points of cardiovascular events. Milleron and colleagues[17] prospectively followed 54 patients with CAD and OSA over 5 years for clinical end points of cardiovascular death, acute coronary syndrome, hospitalization for heart failure, and need for revascularization. During the follow-up, there were fewer cardiovascular events in the 25 treated subjects versus the 29 untreated subjects (6 and 17, respectively).[17] Also, the time to the first event in the treated group was longer compared with the untreated group. These results suggest that treatment with CPAP diminished the harmful effects of OSA on CAD outcomes.

Treatment of even mild-to-moderate forms of OSA has been associated with decreased serious cardiovascular events in a prospective observational study by Buchner and colleagues.[18] Patients who received CPAP therapy had a 10-year event-free survival of 80.3% versus 51.8% (n = 364 vs 85, respectively, P = .001), thus achieving an absolute risk reduction of 28.5%. The number needed to treat to prevent one event per 10 years was 3.5, suggesting that CPAP is a valuable treatment modality. OSA treatment was an independent predictor for cardiovascular events even after adjusting for age, gender, cardiovascular risk factors, and comorbidities.[18]

A larger observational study by Marin and colleagues[19] suggested that CPAP is beneficial in severe OSA. A total of 1651 subjects were studied: healthy men (n = 264), simple snorers (n = 377), those with mild-to-moderate OSA (n = 403), those with untreated severe OSA (n = 235), and those with treated severe OSA (n = 372).[19] The rate of fatal and nonfatal cardiovascular events was elevated in men with severe OSA over a 10-year follow-up and greatly reduced in subjects with severe untreated OSA who underwent treatment with CPAP[19] (Fig. 2).

The improved outcomes in the CPAP cohorts in the studies mentioned may be due to healthy-user bias, because treatment was not administered in a randomized controlled fashion. Patients who are adherent with therapy (even placebo) have a better prognosis than those who are not.[20] Adherence to therapy is probably a marker of a good prognosis, based on identifying more motivated patients who are more educated and more likely to follow suggestions including diet, exercise, medication use, and so forth.[21] Thus, despite a large number of patients and long follow-up, the evidence regarding the long-term efficacy of CPAP in cardiovascular outcomes is still limited at present. Further answers may be forthcoming from the Randomized Intervention with CPAP in CAD and OSA (RICCADSA) trial currently under way, a randomized controlled trial with a 3-year follow-up of 4 groups[1]: sleepy OSA/CAD patients treated with CPAP,[2] nonsleepy OSA/CAD patients treated with CPAP,[3] nonsleepy OSA/CAD patients treated conservatively without CPAP,[4] and CAD patients without OSA treated conservatively.[22]

Given that CPAP is associated with improved outcomes, some analysis of the factors contributing to adherence is worthwhile. Some findings may suggest that patients who are adherent to CPAP may be those with the most severe sleepiness, perhaps because of a greater relief of symptoms.[23] In contrast, Sampol, and colleagues[20] found that the absence of sleepiness did not affect adherence to CPAP treatment. Among patients with CAD, long-term adherence (at 12 months) to CPAP treatment was not affected by the lack of sleepiness.[20] The investigators emphasized the need for apnea therapy, even in the absence of sleepiness, because cardiovascular risk increases in untreated patients with OSA. The lack of the symptoms of sleepiness should not necessarily deter physicians from offering CPAP therapy, especially if the major concern is nonadherence. Further research in this area is needed.

EFFECTS OF CPAP ON ARRHYTHMIAS

Cardiac arrhythmias are commonly noted in those with OSA during polysomnography or Holter monitoring.[24] Bradyarrhythmias, tachyarrhythmias, sinus pauses, and AF have been associated with OSA.[25] Although the precise mechanisms by which OSA results in arrhythmogenesis are unclear, altered vagal tone, sympathetic surges, hypoxia, hypercarbia, and changes in transmural pressure associated with OSA are hypothesized to play a role. Bradyarrhythmias and pauses, for example, may result from hypervagotonia caused

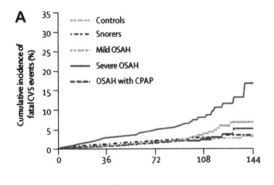

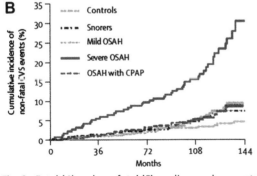

Fig. 2. Fatal (A) and nonfatal (B) cardiovascular events were elevated in untreated OSA subjects compared with other groups. (Adapted from Marin JM, Carrizo SJ, Vicente E, et al. Long-term cardiovascular outcomes in men with obstructive sleep apnoea-hypopnoea with or without treatment with continuous positive airway pressure: an observational study. Lancet 2005;365(9464):1046–53; with permission.)

by negative intrathoracic pressure and apnea.[26,27] Tachyarrhythmias, meanwhile, may result from intermittent postapneic arousal and the associated sympathetic surges. Also, hypoxemia and hypercapnia may act to disturb electrical stability of the heart, and inspiration against an obstructed airway with associated decrease in intrathoracic pressure may lead to episodic elevations in transmural pressure across the ventricles and, thus, may act to distort cardiac anatomy. All these adverse effects on the heart have the potential for being directly arrhythmogenic. Atrial stretch secondary to increase in transmural pressure, for example, may predispose to AF via stimulation of atrial stretch-responsive channels.[26]

The absolute rates of serious arrhythmias in milder forms of sleep-disordered breathing in a community based sample enrolled in the Sleep Heart Health Study (SHHS) were low. Monahan and colleagues[27] noted AF or nonsustained ventricular tachycardia in 2% of subjects (n = 2816 patients). Most subjects had an AHI less than 30 events per hour, and only 247 patients had an AHI greater than 30 events per hour. However, among those with severe OSA enrolled in the SHHS, cardiac arrhythmias were much more common when compared with controls (AHI>30 events per hour vs AHI<5 events per hour).[28] Mehra and colleagues[28] found an increased prevalence of AF (4.8% vs 0.9%), nonsustained ventricular tachycardia (5.3% vs 1.2%), and complex ventricular ectopy (25% vs 14.5%) in patients with OSA versus controls. These associations between rhythm disturbances and OSA persisted despite adjustment for potential confounders, such as cardiovascular risk factors and manifestations. Similarly, an 18% rate of serious arrhythmias on Holter monitoring was noted in moderate-to-severe OSA patients by Harbison and colleagues.[29] Cardiac pauses and bradycardias were also noted to be more frequent (47%) in those with moderate-to-severe OSA.[30]

Treatment of OSA has been shown to reduce or eliminate these rhythm disturbances in uncontrolled studies. An early study in 1977 by Tilkian and colleagues[31] found that the following arrhythmias improved after treatment of OSA with tracheostomy: bradycardia, asystole, second-degree atrioventricular block and ventricular tachycardia. CPAP treatment of OSA has also been found to be effective in eliminating cardiac rhythm disturbances. Harbison and colleagues[29] found that 8 of 45 patients with OSA (18%) had pathologically significant rhythm disturbances, such as ventricular tachycardia or fibrillation, ventricular ectopy, nonsinus supraventricular tachycardia, cardiac

pauses greater than 2 seconds, and second- or third-degree atrioventricular block. The most commonly noted disturbances were recurring sinus pauses, lasting as long as 10 seconds. After 2 to 3 days of CPAP therapy, 7 out of 8 patients had complete resolution of arrhythmias noted before CPAP use.

Simantirakis and colleagues[30] presented further compelling data on acute and long-term beneficial impact of CPAP on bradycardias and sinus pauses in OSA patients. They evaluated 23 patients with OSA (without underlying primary cardiac pathology) before, during, and after 16 months of CPAP therapy. Before initiation of CPAP, 47% of patients were noted to have rhythm disturbances (mostly severe bradycardic events and sinus pauses with a few supraventricular tachycardias). After 8 weeks of CPAP therapy, bradycardic events and sinus pauses were ameliorated in 6 of 11 patients. After 14 months of therapy, none of the patients were noted to have bradycardias or pauses, and 9 out of 11 patients remained absolutely free of any detectable cardiac arrhythmias. Based on these data, CPAP can be considered a potentially effective long-term treatment option for bradycardia and sinus pauses in patients with OSA.

Again, nonrandomized observational data suggest that treatment with CPAP may reduce recurrence of AF after cardioversion. Among patients with untreated OSA, Kanagala and colleagues[26] found an 82% recurrence of AF at 12 months compared with 42% in the treated group (P = .013) and 53% in the group without known OSA (P = .009; **Fig. 3**). Fifty-eight percent of OSA patients without recurrence were treated

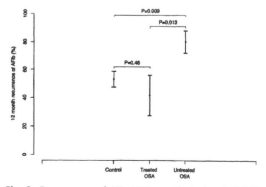

Fig. 3. Recurrence of AF at 12 months in treated OSA patients (42%) was comparable to those without OSA (53%) and much lower than those with untreated OSA (82%). (*From* Kanagala R, Murali NS, Friedman PA, et al. Obstructive sleep apnea and the recurrence of atrial fibrillation. Circulation 2003;107:2589–94; with permission.)

appropriately with CPAP, whereas only 19% of patients with recurrence were on appropriate OSA therapy (P = .013). Based on such findings, the authors propose that patients with AF should be screened for OSA and, if present, be treated.

EFFECTS OF CPAP ON PLATELET FUNCTION

Inappropriate platelet activation and aggregation has been proposed to be a mechanism linking OSA and cardiovascular morbidity and mortality. The nocturnal hypoxia, hemodynamic changes, and sleep fragmentation associated with OSA lead to stimulation of sympathetic nervous system activity and increased catecholamine levels in patients with OSA.[31] Elevated circulating epinephrine and norepinephrine act on alpha-2-adrenergic receptors on platelets resulting in platelet activation in vitro and in vivo.[32] Thus, repeated obstructive respiratory events can bring about a hypercoaguable state, predisposing to thrombosis and significantly increasing the risk of cardiovascular death.

Bokinsky and colleagues[33] published one of the earliest studies exploring spontaneous platelet activation and aggregation during OSA and the effects of CPAP on these 2 indices. Six subjects with OSA and 5 controls were observed before the study, hourly during the diagnostic polysomnographic night, on awakening, and on standing upright. For those with OSA, these measurements were repeated while on CPAP treatment. The investigators found a significant increase in spontaneous platelet activation during the night in patients with OSA and, to a much lesser degree, in controls. Differences between groups were negligible after assumption of the upright posture. Also, they noted a reduction in degree of spontaneous platelet activation and aggregation during the course of the night when CPAP was used. This study used an indwelling catheter, and although there were differences between groups, the indwelling catheter was associated with higher than usual platelet activation. Geiser and colleagues[31] confirmed the link between OSA and platelet activation (12 patients with OSA, 6 controls) by measuring platelet activation markers at 4 AM and 7 AM with a fresh blood draw, thus minimizing the activation caused by an indwelling catheter. After 2 nights of CPAP therapy, platelet activation was reduced without reaching statistical significance.[31]

CPAP improves platelet function within 1 to 2 nights, and such improvements are sustained even 6 months after initiating treatment.[32,34] Sanner and colleagues[32] evaluated in vitro nocturnal platelet aggregability in 15 healthy controls and before and after 6 months of CPAP therapy in 17 patients with OSA. Patients with OSA had slightly increased aggregability during the night (whereas controls had a decrease in aggregability); this aggregability almost normalized after treatment with CPAP, approaching the values seen in controls. Although in vitro platelet aggregation may not necessarily correlate with in vivo changes in platelet function, the findings of this study carry significant clinical implications, because in vitro platelet aggregability, specifically, is strongly associated with myocardial infarction, CAD, and other cardiovascular morbidities.[35]

Hui and colleagues[34] compared platelet activation in a larger group of 42 patients with OSA to 23 controls and re-examined OSA patients after 3 months of CPAP therapy. At baseline, OSA patients were found to have a significantly greater platelet activation compared with controls (15.1 vs 10.9, respectively, P = .05). Also, platelet activation positively correlated with the severity of OSA (AHI and log SaO_2 [oxygen saturation] <90%) and arousal index and total sleep time. In patients with OSA, platelet activation decreased after one night of CPAP treatment from 15.1 to 12.2 (P<.001) and decreased further after 3 months of CPAP therapy to 9.8 (P = .005), values similar to those of control subjects.

Results of published literature support the idea that untreated OSA contributes to alterations in platelet function and suggest that CPAP therapy may have a cardioprotective benefit by reducing platelet activation. Further research is necessary to characterize the role of platelet activation in specific subgroups of OSA patients and to investigate whether antiplatelet therapy might be useful in this group of patients.

IMPROVEMENT IN VASCULAR INFLAMMATION (C-REACTIVE PROTEIN, INTERLEUKIN-6) AND ENDOTHELIAL FUNCTION

Inflammatory processes and endothelial dysfunction also seem to play a role in cardiovascular morbidity associated with OSA. Fragmented sleep, sleep deprivation, and multiple nocturnal episodes of hypoxemia may be to blame for systemic inflammation and its associated risk of cardiovascular events. This hypothesis is supported by multiple works of research reporting that normal individuals experiencing hypoxia of high altitude have an increase in serum markers of inflammation, such as C-reactive protein (CRP) and interleukin 6 (IL-6); also, sleep deprivation alone was shown to induce an increase in cytokines responsible for regulating synthesis of CRP.[36]

Shamsuzzaman and colleagues[36] studied 22 otherwise healthy patients newly diagnosed with OSA and 20 controls to determine whether patients with OSA have increased plasma levels of CRP. The major findings of this work were that (1) OSA is, in fact, associated with elevated levels of CRP (0.81mg/dl in patients with OSA vs 0.28mg/dl in controls, $P<.008$) and (2) CRP levels positively correlate with AHI. Kokturk and colleagues[37] conducted an analogous study examining CRP levels in patients with OSA and cardiovascular disease, patients with OSA without cardiovascular disease, and patients without OSA but with cardiovascular disease (controls). CRP levels were significantly higher in patients with OSA and cardiovascular disease; no statistically significant difference was noted in CRP levels of patients with only OSA or only cardiovascular disease. Reclassifying the patients into 2 groups— those with OSA and those without—revealed that CRP levels were significantly elevated in patients with OSA compared with those without (3.36mg/dl vs 1.16mg/dl, respectively; $P<.05$). The investigators also reported that CRP levels correlated positively with AHI in patients with OSA, confirming the findings reported by Shamsuzzaman and colleagues.[36]

Possible pathogenetic mechanisms of CRP leading to cardiovascular dysfunction have been described. There are data to suggest that CRP may be directly involved in development of atherosclerotic lesions: atheromatous plaques contain CRP; increased levels of CRP in the blood are associated with vascular dysfunction; CRP acts on vascular endothelium to stimulate release of inflammatory mediators; and finally, CRP opsonizes low-density lipoprotein, which is then taken up by macrophages in atherosclerotic plaques.[37]

At this point in time, there is limited evidence supporting the hypothesis that OSA therapy can effectively reduce plasma CRP levels. Two interventional studies, one using surgical treatment and another using CPAP, reported significant reduction of plasma CRP after the intervention.[38,39] Friedman and colleagues[38] measured CRP levels pre- and postoperatively in 34 patients with OSA undergoing surgical treatment with uvulopalatopharyngoplasty. Mean CRP level was 0.33mg/dl preoperatively and decreased to 0.16mg/dl two months after the surgery ($P = .003$), and all patients achieved a reduction in AHI and improvement in OSA-associated symptoms. These findings suggest that treatment of OSA can be helpful in reducing plasma CRP levels

and decreasing risk of cardiovascular morbidity in patients with OSA. In their study, Ishida and colleagues[39] looked at whether CPAP therapy can be just as effective in treating OSA and reducing CRP in patients with OSA, avoiding the more invasive therapeutic option of surgery. Fifty-five patients newly diagnosed with OSA were assessed before and after 6 months of CPAP treatment. CRP levels were reduced significantly with CPAP therapy (0.23mg/dl before therapy vs 0.16mg/dl after therapy; $P<.05$) in patients with good compliance with CPAP (>4h/d, >5d/wk). The greatest reduction in CRP was noted in patients who had the most elevated plasma CRP levels before commencement of CPAP therapy (≥ 0.2mg/dl). In this patient subgroup, mean CRP at the beginning of the study was 0.48mg/dl, and after 6 months of CPAP, the CRP level decreased to 0.29mg/dl ($P<.05$).

IL-6 and CRP are acute-phase reactants that have been associated with cardiovascular outcomes. Yokoe and colleagues[40] showed the effect of CPAP treatment on CRP and IL-6. Of 44 subjects enrolled in the study, 30 had OSA syndrome and 14 were controlled obese subjects. Only 2 people had diabetes mellitus, one in each group. Measurement of the CRP and IL-6 was done at 5 AM before initiation of CPAP. Levels were much higher in men who were obese and had severe OSA, nocturnal hypoxia, and daytime sleepiness. Following one month of therapy, a significant decrease in the levels of CRP and IL-6 were observed. The observed improvement in these markers of cardiovascular risk is consistent with a decreased risk of major cardiovascular events; however, hard outcome data are lacking. Given the epidemiologic and mechanistic evidence supporting the significant role of CRP in cardiovascular pathology, these markers of systemic inflammation may explain the association between OSA, its treatment, and cardiovascular morbidity.

Impaired endothelial function, as a marker for atherosclerosis, has been linked with increased cardiovascular events. Flow-mediated dilation (FMD) has been one of the most commonly used methods to evaluate endothelial function. Bayram and colleagues[41] performed a prospective, controlled, and observational study assessing endothelial function in men with OSA but without hypertension after 6 months of treatment with CPAP. Forty-six men, 29 with OSA and 17 without, were enrolled. Baseline values of dilation, FMD, and endothelium-independent nitroglycerin (NTG)-induced dilation were measured with Doppler ultrasonography before the treatment. Those 2 variables were measured again after 6 months of treatment with CPAP. FMD was noted to be lower in patients with OSA. There was no difference in NTG-induced dilation in both groups. After CPAP therapy, FMD values were noted to increase significantly in the OSA group. A similar study about endothelial function with the use of FMD and NTG-induced dilation by Ip and colleagues[42] showed that patients with moderate-to-severe OSA have endothelial dysfunction that was noted to improve with CPAP treatment.

A prospective cohort study by Jelic and colleagues[43] evaluated endothelial function by assessing inflammation, oxidative stress, and repair capacity of the endothelium in patients with OSA. The purpose was to determine whether endothelial dysfunction occurs in vivo and whether improvement or reversal would be noted after treatment with CPAP. Aside from FMD, indicators of oxidative stress (nitrotyrosine) and proteins that control basal endothelial nitric oxide (NO) production (endothelial NO synthase [eNOS] and its phosphorylated form) and inflammation (inducible NOS and cyclooxygenase-2) were measured. Compared with controls, patients with OSA have reduced expression of eNOS and phosphorylated eNOS, and increased expression of nitrotyrosine, inducible NOS, and cyclooxygenase-2. After a 4-week treatment with CPAP, there was a reversal of the noted changes in OSA patients

These 3 studies established the improvement in endothelial function, which one might predict would reduce the number of cardiovascular events, and further emphasized the benefits of CPAP therapy with regard to cardiovascular outcomes and diseases.

EFFECTS OF CPAP ON VISCERAL FAT

Although increased visceral adiposity has been linked with OSA and generally thought to be one factor that can lead to the development of OSA, Chin and colleagues[44] showed that CPAP treatment of OSA actually decreased visceral fat after 6 months of therapy. These subjects had an average BMI close to 30 kg/m2 and were counseled to lose weight when they began CPAP therapy. Visceral fat decreased regardless of whether total body weight decreased. Follow-up studies by Vgontzas and colleagues[45] and Trenell and colleagues[46] included a more obese population treated with CPAP for 3 months. Visceral adiposity was reduced only in patients who used CPAP regularly (≥ 4 hours per night). These were, however, small observational studies, and further work is needed to define the role of CPAP

therapy in modulating visceral adiposity and with it, hopefully, metabolism.

SUMMARY

CPAP treatment for OSA has been shown in multiple observational trials to improve cardiovascular morbidity and mortality, including a reduction in BP, coronary ischemia and cardiac arrhythmias. These studies are supported by data showing that CPAP treatment decreases vascular inflammation, improves endothelial function, and also seems to improve visceral adiposity. The evidence suggests that it may be beneficial to treat moderate-to-severe OSA patients with coexistent CAD, certain arrhythmias, and hypertension with CPAP. Although some randomized controlled trials have been performed to determine CPAP treatment effect on hypertension outcomes, further RCTs are needed to determine the efficacy of CPAP treatment in other cardiovascular disorders.

REFERENCES

1. Hla KM, Young T, Bidwell T, et al. Sleep apnea and hypertension: a population-based study. Ann Intern Med 1994;120:382–8.
2. Lavie P, Herer P, Hoffstein V. Obstructive sleep apnea syndrome as a risk factor for hypertension: population study. BMJ 2000;320:479–82.
3. Peppard P, Young T, Palta M, et al. Prospective study of the association between sleep-disordered breathing and hypertension. N Engl J Med 2000; 342(19):1378–84.
4. Brooks D, Horner R, Kozar L, et al. Obstructive sleep apnea as a cause of systemic hypertension, evidence from a canine model. J Clin Invest 1997; 9(1):106–9.
5. Faccenda JF, Mackay TW, Boon NA, et al. Randomized placebo-controlled trial of continuous positive airway pressure on blood pressure in the sleep apnea-hypopnea syndrome. Am J Respir Crit Care Med 2001;163:344–8.
6. Logan AG, Tkacova R, Perlikowski SM, et al. Refractory hypertension and sleep apnoea: effect of CPAP on blood pressure and baroreflex. Eur Respir J 2003;21:241–7.
7. Bazzano LA, Khan Z, Reynolds K, et al. Effect of nocturnal nasal continuous positive airway pressure on blood pressure in obstructive sleep apnea. Hypertension 2007;50:417–23.
8. Baguet JP, Barone-Rochette G, Pépin JL. Hypertension and obstructive sleep apnoea syndrome: current perspectives. J Hum Hypertens 2009;23: 431–43.

9. Martínez-García MA, Gómez-Aldaraví R, Soler-Cataluña JJ, et al. Positive effect of CPAP treatment on the control of difficult-to-treat hypertension. Eur Respir J 2007;29:951–7.

10. Logan AG, Perlikowski SM, Mente A. High prevalence of obstructive apnea in drug resistant hypertension. J Hypertension 2001;19:2271–7.

11. Gifford RW Jr. Resistant hypertension. Introduction and definitions. Hypertension 1988;11(Suppl II):65–6.

12. Barnes M, Houston D, Worsnop CJ, et al. A randomized controlled trial of continuous positive airway pressure in mild obstructive sleep apnea. Am J Respir Crit Care Med 2002;165:773–80.

13. Pepperell JC, Ramdassing-Dow S, Crosthwaite N, et al. Ambulatory blood pressure after therapeutic and subtherapeutic nasal continuous positive airway pressure for obstructive sleep apnoea: a randomised parallel trial. Lancet 2002;3359:204–10.

14. Becker HF, Jerrentrup A, Ploch T, et al. Effect of nasal continuous positive airway pressure treatment on blood pressure in patients with obstructive sleep apnea. Circulation 2003;107:68–73.

15. Collins R, Peto R, MacMahon S, et al. Blood pressure, stroke, and coronary heart disease. 2. Short-term reductions in blood pressure: overview of randomized drug trial in their epidemiological context. Lancet 1990;335:827–38.

16. Peled N, Abinader EG, Pillar G, et al. Nocturnal ischemic events in patients with obstructive sleep apnea syndrome and ischemic heart disease. Effects of continuous positive air pressure treatment. J Am Coll Cardiol 1999;34:1744–9.

17. Milleron O, Pilliere R, Foucher A, et al. Benefits of obstructive sleep apnoea treatment in coronary artery disease: a long-term follow-up study. Eur Heart J 2004;25:728–34.

18. Buchner NJ, Sanner BM, Borgel J, et al. Continuous positive airway pressure treatment of mild to moderate obstructive sleep apnea reduces cardiovascular risk. Am J Respir Crit Care Med 2007; 176:1274–80.

19. Marin JM, Carrizo SJ, Vicente E, et al. Long-term cardiovascular outcomes in men with obstructive sleep apnoea-hypopnoea with or without treatment with continuous positive airway pressure: an observational study. Lancet 2005;365(9464): 1046–53.

20. Sampol G, Rodes G, Romero O, et al. Adherence to nCPAP in patients with coronary artery disease and sleep apnea without sleepiness. Respir Med 2007; 101(3):461–6.

21. Platt A, Kuna S, Asch D. Adherence to sleep apnea therapy and use and lipid-lowering drugs: a study of the healthy-user effect. Chest 2010;137(1):102–8.

22. Peker YK, Glantz H, Thunstrom E, et al. Rationale and design of the randomized intervention with CPAP in coronary artery disease and sleep apnoea–RICCADSA trial. Scand Cardiovasc J 2009;43:24–31.

23. McArdle N, Devereux G, Heidarnejad H, et al. Long-term use of CPAP therapy for sleep apnea/hypopnea syndrome. Am J Respir Crit Care Med 1999; 159(4 Pt 1):1108–14.

24. Alonso-Fernandez A, Garcia-Rio F, Racionero MA, et al. Cardiac rhythm disturbances and ST-segment depression episodes in patients with obstructive sleep apnea hypopnoa syndrome and its mechanisms. Chest 2005;127:15–22.

25. Schweitzer P. Cardiac arrhythmias in obstructive sleep apnea. Vnitr Lek 2008;54(10):1006–9.

26. Kanagala R, Murali NS, Friedman PA, et al. Obstructive sleep apnea and the recurrence of atrial fibrillation. Circulation 2003;107:2589–94.

27. Monahan K, Storfer-Isser A, Redline S, et al. Triggering of nocturnal arrhythmias by sleep-disordered breathing events. J Am Coll Cardiol 2009;54:1797–804.

28. Mehra R, Benjamin EJ, Shahar E, et al. Association of nocturnal arrhythmias with sleep-disordered breathing: the Sleep Heart Health Study. Am J Respir Crit Care Med 2006;173:910–6.

29. Harbison J, O'Reilly P, McNicholas WT. Cardiac rhythm disturbances in the obstructive sleep apnea syndrome: effects of nasal continuous positive airway pressure therapy. Chest 2000; 118:591–5.

30. Simantirakis EN, Schizab SI, Marketoua ME, et al. Severe bradyarrhythmias in patients with sleep apnoea: the effect of continuous positive airway pressure treatment: a long-term evaluation using an insertable loop recorder. Eur Heart J 2004;25: 1070–6.

31. Geiser T, Buck F, Meyer BJ, et al. In vivo platelet activation is increased during sleep in patients with obstructive sleep apnea syndrome. Respiration 2002;69:229–34.

32. Sanner BM, Konermann M, Tepel M, et al. Platelet function in patients with obstructive sleep apnoea syndrome. Eur Respir J 2000;16:648–52.

33. Bokinsky G, Miller M, Ault K, et al. Spontaneous platelet activation and aggregation during obstructive sleep apnea and its response to therapy with nasal continuous positive airway pressure. A preliminary investigation. Chest 1995;108:625–30.

34. Hui DS, Ko FW, Fok JP, et al. The effects of nasal CPAP on platelet activation in obstructive sleep apnea. Chest 2004;125:1768–75.

35. Thaulow E, Erikssen J, Sandvik L, et al. Blood platelet count and function are related to total and cardiovascular death in apparently healthy men. Circulation 1991;84:613–7.

36. Shamsuzzaman AS, Winnicki M, Lanfranchi P, et al. Elevated C-reactive protein in patients with obstructive sleep apnea. Circulation 2002;105:2462–4.

37. Kokturk O, Ciftci TU, Mollarecep E, et al. Elevated C-reactive protein levels and increased cardiovascular risk in patients with obstructive sleep apnea syndrome. Int Heart J 2005;46:801–9.

38. Friedman M, Bliznikas D, Vidyasagar R, et al. Reduction of C-reactive protein with surgical treatment of obstructive sleep apnea hypopnea syndrome. Otolaryngol Head Neck Surg 2006;135: 900–5.

39. Ishida K, Kato M, Kato Y, et al. Appropriate use of nasal con tenuous positive airway pressure decreases elevated C-reactive protein in patients with obstructive sleep apnea. Chest 2009;136(1): 125–9.

40. Yokoe T, Minoguchi K, Matsuo H, et al. Elevated levels of C-reactive protein and interleukin-6 in patients with obstructive sleep apnea syndrome are decreased by nasal continuous positive airway pressure. Circulation 2003; 107(8):1129–34.

41. Bayram NA, Ciftci B, Keles T, et al. Endothelial function in normotensive men with obstructive sleep apnea before and 6 months after CPAP treatment. Sleep 2009;32(10):1257–63.

42. Ip M, Tse H, Lam B, et al. Endothelial function in obstructive sleep apnea and response to treatment. Am J Respir Crit Care Med 2004;169:348–53.

43. Jelic S, Padeletti M, Kawut S, et al. Inflammation, oxidative stress, and repair capacity of the vascular endothelium in obstructive sleep apnea. Circulation 2008;117:2270–8.

44. Chin K, Shimizu K, Nakamura T, et al. Changes in intra-abdominal visceral fat and serum leptin levels in patients with obstructive sleep apnea syndrome following nasal continuous positive airway pressure therapy. Circulation 1999;100:706–12.

45. Vgontzas A, Zoumakis E, Bixler E, et al. Selective effects of CPAP on sleep apnea-associated manifestations. Eur J Clin Invest 2008;38(8):585–95.

46. Trenell MI, Ward JA, Yee BJ, et al. Influence of constant positive airway pressure therapy on lipid storage, muscle metabolism and insulin action in obese patients with severe obstructive sleep apnoea syndrome. Diabetes Obes Metab 2007;9:679–87.

Positive Airway Pressure in Congestive Heart Failure

Kirk Kee, MBBS[a], Scott A. Sands, BSc, BE[b], Bradley A. Edwards, PhD[b,c], Philip J. Berger, PhD[b], Matthew T. Naughton, MD[a,d,*]

KEYWORDS

• Heart failure • Positive airway pressure • Sleep apnea

Congestive heart failure (CHF) is an increasingly prevalent condition, which is estimated to affect 23 million people worldwide.[1] Despite significant recent advances in the medical management of this condition with an incidence reaching 12% in those older than 64 years,[2] it remains one of the leading causes of morbidity and mortality in the western world. Rates of hospitalization for CHF increased fourfold between 1971 and 1999,[3] corresponding with an aging population and greater survival for acute coronary syndromes, valvular disease, and other related conditions. Heart failure (HF) is now the leading cause of hospitalization in developed countries.

Positive airway pressure (PAP) delivered noninvasively via a mask (noninvasive ventilation [NIV]) has become increasingly used as adjunctive therapy in the acute and chronic settings for CHF. The provision of PAP by means of a face mask avoids the complications of intubation and the need for paralysis, sedation, associated instrumentation, and tracheostomy. Modern PAP flow generators are lightweight, simple to use, and accessible in hospital ward and outpatient settings. Similarly, today's masks are more comfortable, better fitting, and well tolerated. To understand how PAP works, one needs to look at the pathophysiology of CHF and explore how the various forms of NIV affect CHF.

CHF

CHF is defined by the inability of the heart to pump sufficient oxygenated blood to meet the metabolic needs of the body. Failure of the heart results in a complex clinical syndrome, which includes dyspnea (at rest and on exertion), fatigue, peripheral edema, orthopnea, tachypnea, tachycardia, and cardiomegaly. Although CHF may result from valvular disease or disturbances in cardiac rhythm or rate, it is most commonly the result of failure of the cardiac muscle pump.

Cardiac muscle pump failure, or cardiomyopathy, is generally divided into 2 types: systolic and diastolic dysfunction. Systolic dysfunction is defined by impaired left ventricular contractility and is usually the result of ischemic heart disease, long-standing hypertension, or unknown causes (idiopathic). It is defined by a reduced left ventricular ejection fraction (LVEF <55%) or impaired left ventricular fractional shortening (<28%). Diastolic dysfunction, recently renamed as HF with normal systolic function (HFNSF), is now recognized as being a significant cause of CHF.[4] It has been estimated that 13% to 74% of patients with CHF have normal systolic function,[5] with estimates varying widely depending on diagnostic criteria. The prevalence of HFNSF increases with age, at 15% in those younger than 50 years, rising to 50% in

[a] Department of Allergy, Immunology and Respiratory Medicine Alfred Hospital, Melbourne, Australia
[b] Ritchie Centre for Baby Health Research, Clayton, Victoria, Australia
[c] Brigham and Women's Hospital, Division of Sleep Medicine, Sleep Disorders Program and Harvard Medical School, Boston, MA, USA
[d] Faculty of Medicine, Monash University, Clayton, Victoria, Australia
* Corresponding author. Faculty of Medicine, Monash University, PO Box 315, Prahran 3181, Victoria, Australia.
E-mail address: m.naughton@alfred.org.au

Sleep Med Clin 5 (2010) 393–405
doi:10.1016/j.jsmc.2010.05.011
1556-407X/10/$ – see front matter © 2010 Elsevier Inc. All rights reserved.

those older than 70 years.[6] HFNSF is commonly due to "stiff" ventricular walls, which can result from hypoxia, tachycardia,[7] and hypertension. Less common causes include pericarditis, constrictive pericarditis, and myocardial infiltrative disorders (eg, amyloid, hemochromatosis), thus highlighting the need for an accurate diagnosis (eg, via echocardiography).

The end result of CHF of either cause is an inadequate cardiac output and fluid accumulation through activation of several neurohumoral pathways, including the sympathetic and renin-angiotensin systems. As a result, there is an increase in the pulmonary capillary wedge pressure and consequent leakage of fluid into the interstitium, then along the interlobular septa toward the peribronchovascular space and, eventually, into the hila. Fluid—up to 25% of the total extra body fluid in patients with CHF—also accumulates in the pleural space.[8] There is a resultant reduction in lung volumes and airflow obstruction from bronchial edema. With CHF, respiratory muscle weakness occurs[9] and the work of breathing increases, using a greater proportion of an already reduced cardiac output.

PAP IN HF

PAP in CHF is increasingly used in the acute and chronic settings. Although the evidence base for acute PAP in CHF is strong, the evidence for long-term PAP is more controversial. Acute PAP is used in the context of acute cardiogenic pulmonary edema, whereas long-term PAP has predominantly been used to manage sleep-disordered breathing (SDB) in those with heart failure.

Acute Cardiogenic Pulmonary Edema

Acute cardiogenic pulmonary edema (APO) is a common complication of CHF. As the left ventricle fails, pulmonary venous pressure increases, followed by pulmonary capillary pressure. Once hydrostatic pressure across the pulmonary capillary wall exceeds the osmotic pressure of the plasma proteins, fluid begins to accumulate in the interstitium. Once this fluid buildup exceeds lymphatic drainage, it moves into the alveoli, resulting in alveolar flooding and collapse especially in dependent areas of the lung. Such areas are unable to provide gas exchange and create areas of effective shunt,[10] leading to increased alveolar-arterial gradient and respiratory failure.

Several trials and meta-analyses have demonstrated that PAP decreases the need for intubation and improves respiratory parameters in acute respiratory failure secondary to APO when compared with medical therapy alone.[11–14] PAP is now standard treatment for severe APO and is usually initiated in the ambulance or emergency department.

The proposed acute mechanisms for the efficacy of PAP include[15–20]

1. Increased lung volume and increased oxygen availability
2. Reduced pulmonary atelectasis caused by edema
3. Increased intrathoracic pressure and reduced systolic left ventricular transmural pressure, resulting in reduced left ventricular afterload and mitral regurgitation and increasing cardiac output
4. Bronchodilatation
5. Assistance to inspiratory muscles when inspiratory PAP is greater than expiratory PAP.

The 2 modes of PAP most studied in APO are continuous (fixed) positive airway pressure (CPAP) and bilevel positive airway pressure (BPAP) at pressures of 4 to 25 cm H_2O. CPAP delivers a constant level of PAP irrespective of the respiratory cycle, whereas BPAP delivers a low level of pressure during expiration and a higher level during inspiration (usual difference>4 cm H_2O). In APO, CPAP and BPAP have been shown to reduce intubation rate and improve physiologic parameters, such as dyspnea, hypercapnia, acidosis, and heart rate.[11,13] Two meta-analyses concluded that CPAP results in mortality reduction,[11,14] although a recent large, multicentered trial suggested otherwise.[21] However, the overall intubation rate in this trial was low (<3%) and the population was elderly (mean age 77 years), suggesting that the patient cohort in the multicentered study was different to that examined in other trials. Also, the mean duration of PAP was less than 3 hours, and CHF was a clinical diagnosis (ie, without objective confirmation via echocardiography or brain natriuretic peptide [BNP] testing) and incorporated all causes of heart failure (pump, valvular, rate, and rhythm). Early concerns regarding an increased risk of acute myocardial infarction[14,22] with BPAP have been revoked with larger trials.[21,23] There is also good evidence that PAP can be used in the emergency department without needing intensive care or high-dependency units.[24] Direct comparison of CPAP and BPAP have generally not revealed any significant difference in efficacy between the 2 modalities, although there is some evidence that BPAP may relieve hypercapnia more quickly.

There is a high level of evidence that PAP (either CPAP or BPAP) should be standard therapy in cardiogenic APO resulting in respiratory failure. This therapy can be initiated in the emergency department and usually results in significant improvements in morbidity and mortality with minimal adverse events. The choice of CPAP versus BPAP can be dictated by local experience and preference, although BPAP may have some additional benefit to those with hypercapnic acidosis.

SDB

SDB includes obstructive (OSA) and central sleep apnea (CSA). By convention, the severity of CSA and OSA is commonly assessed by the apnea-hypopnea index (AHI). The prevalence of SDB in patients with CHF is more than tenfold that seen in the general community. Two large studies, one in Canada (n = 450)[25] and the other in Germany (n = 203),[26] have reported SDB (AHI >15) in 60 to 70% of CHF patients. In contrast, the incidence of SDB in the general population has been reported to be 6% to 17% (AHI >15 and >5, respectively).[27] In the general community, OSA is the predominant form of SDB, with CSA making up about 1% of cases. In CHF populations, CSA is far more common; in the 2 studies mentioned, OSA occurred in 38% to 43% of patients and CSA occurred in 28% to 38%.[25,26,28]

OSA

OSA occurs because of recurrent collapse of the pharyngeal airway following loss of muscle tone during sleep. Patients with OSA are at a 2.4-fold elevated risk of self-reported CHF,[29] which may occur as a result of OSA-related hypertension[30] and the impact of OSA on left ventricular function.[31,32] CHF may also augment a tendency toward OSA by increasing upper airway edema leading to a narrowing of the airway lumen, a factor especially important in the supine position.[33]

Most data suggest that an anatomically small pharyngeal airway[34–36] is a key factor in the development of upper airway obstruction, with pharyngeal dilator muscles compensating for the anatomic deficiency while awake, but not during sleep. However, measures of upper airway anatomy account for only a small percentage of the variability in apnea severity. Thus, other processes must influence apnea pathogenesis. As such, several variables have been recently revealed to interactively contribute to the development of OSA,[37,38] including dysfunction of the reflex response of the upper airway dilator muscles,[39] ease of triggering arousal from sleep by obstructed breathing efforts (ie, arousal threshold), and instability in

ventilatory control (ie, high loop gain).[40–43] Considerable evidence exists that a proportion of patients with CHF exhibit hypersensitive ventilatory responses to hypoxia, hypercapnia, and exercise,[44–46] particularly those with poor prognosis.[44,46] In those with OSA, the removal of upper airway obstruction with CPAP often reveals an underlying central instability in the form of CSA,[47] suggesting that upper airway obstruction is not the sole mechanism contributing to the condition. This observation and the finding that patients with CHF typically shift from obstructive to central apneas overnight[48] suggest that the 2 conditions have considerable overlap in pathophysiology.

The adverse physiologic effects of OSA are thought to be the consequence of

1. Recurrent arousal from sleep
2. Asphyxia and intermittent hypoxia
3. Negative intrathoracic pressure swings
4. Inflammatory endothelial injury due to formation of oxygen radicals
5. Direct vibrational trauma.

Intrathoracic pressure swings, asphyxia resulting in hypoxemia and hypercapnia, and apnea terminating in arousals result in a sympathetic surges, which may occur up to 800 times per night.[49,50] This increase in sympathetic activity results in tachycardia and increased blood pressure, an effect which is sustained in wakefulness. Intermittent hypoxia results in polycythemia[51,52] and inflammation,[53] which contribute to a hypercoagulable state. Also, intermittent hypoxia increases the sensitivity of the peripheral chemoreceptors[54,55]; markers of inflammation and hypercoagulability[56] and increased peripheral chemosensitivity[44] are strong predictors of mortality in patients with heart failure. The negative intrathoracic swings also result in increased left ventricular afterload and increased venous return with elevating right ventricular preload. The acute changes in cardiac parameters seen in OSA have been shown to be far more pronounced in those with CHF than in healthy subjects. In the general community, OSA is linked to systemic hypertension and type 2 diabetes.[57] Hypoxemia and tachycardia impair myocardial relaxation (diastolic dysfunction) and contractility (systolic dysfunction) and cause myocardial ischemia, premature atherosclerosis,[58] and greater cardiovascular morbidity and mortality.[59,60]

Randomized controlled trials have demonstrated that treatment of OSA in CHF with CPAP lowers sympathetic nervous system activity,[61,62] blood pressure, and heart rate,[63–65] reduces nocturnal ventricular arrhythmia,[65] and improves left ventricular function.[62–65] The results of these trials have been summarized in **Table 1**. To date, there have been no randomized trials demonstrating any improvement in mortality with CPAP use. However, a nonrandomized, prospective, observational study has demonstrated significantly better survival in CHF patients without SDB or treated OSA compared with those with untreated OSA (AHI >15).[66] Another observational study that divided patients with CHF and OSA into compliant (CPAP use>the 50th percentile) and noncompliant (CPAP use < the 50th percentile) demonstrated a significant difference in death or hospitalization after 25.3 ± 15.3 months followup. The compliant patients had an event rate of 15.6% versus 48.5% in the noncompliant group.[67] Both these studies suggest that effective treatment of OSA in patients with CHF results in improved outcomes.

CSA

CSA, often called periodic breathing or Cheyne-Stokes respiration (CSR), is rare in the general population, whereas it affects 28% to 38% of those with advanced CHF.[25,26,68] CSA is characterized by a crescendo-decrescendo pattern of ventilation followed by a central apnea and is associated with mild hypoxemia, modest hypocapnia, and an arousal at peak ventilation. Generally, CSA occurs more commonly in men than women with similar degrees of CHF. Typically, it has a periodicity of 45 to 90 seconds and occurs during non-rapid eye movement sleep stages 1 and 2 and is often triggered by an arousal or state change. Periodic breathing (ie, CSR with hypopneas rather than apneas) may occur during exercise or, occasionally, when awake. The predominant mechanism underlying CSA in patients with CHF is an unstable negative-feedback controlling ventilation during sleep.[69,70]

The negative-feedback system controlling ventilation normally maintains a constant partial pressure of arterial carbon dioxide ($PaCO_2$) and oxygen (PaO_2). Ventilatory command is modulated by chemoreceptor inputs from medullary neurons that respond to CO_2 or H^+ and from the carotid bodies, which are sensitive to PaO_2 and $PaCO_2$. The stability of this feedback loop has been quantified using an engineering criterion,[71] which states that if the gain of the feedback loop (*loop gain*) is greater than 1, the system is unstable and periodic oscillations in breathing will occur as a consequence (ie, CSA). If *loop gain* is less than 1, the feedback loop controlling ventilation is stable, and oscillations, if they develop, will gradually be attenuated. Detailed descriptions of *loop gain* have been given previously.[40,41,71–74]

Mathematical analyses of the control system[70–72,75] have revealed 4 major factors that contribute to the instability of breathing, as summarized by the relationship:

$$\text{Loop gain} = G \frac{PaCO_2 - PICO_2}{V_L} T \qquad (1)$$

where G is the chemosensitivity, defined as the strength of the ventilatory output in response to a given change in $PaCO_2$; $PaCO_2$ and $PICO_2$ are the arterial and inspired partial pressures of CO_2, respectively; V_L is lung volume (functional residual capacity); and T represents the combined effect of circulatory delay and the damping of oscillations between the lungs and the chemoreceptors. That is, CSA is favored by a hypersensitive chemoreceptor response, a low lung gas store, a delay in sensory information, and a large arterial-inspired CO_2 gradient promoting large changes in $PaCO_2$ for any fluctuation in ventilation.

There is considerable evidence that each factor contributes to the pathogenesis of CSA. Patients with CHF have a characteristically prolonged circulatory delay (T) as a consequence of low cardiac output. Indeed, CHF patients with CSA have been observed to have lower LVEF than patients without CSA.[76] Despite providing a background of instability, evidence suggests that prolonged circulatory delay alone is not sufficient to manifest CSA. Rather, enhanced chemosensitivity (G) has been revealed as the critical feature of CSA in patients with CHF.[45,70,77,78] In a study at the authors' laboratory, Solin and colleagues[45] demonstrated that the AHI in CHF-CSA is strongly associated with the single-breath hypercapnic ventilatory response, a measure of the peripheral response to CO_2. Furthermore, the investigators confirmed that decreased PaO_2 is an important contributor to CSA,[79] presumably via its action to increase G, the carotid body sensitivity to CO_2. Such findings, in combination with the observation that the lung-ear circulation delay is equal to the delay between the nadir CO_2 level and apnea during CSA,[80] strongly point to the dynamically-active carotid bodies as the chemoreceptors primarily responsible for CSA.

In a recent report, Francis and associates[70] demonstrated the power of *loop gain* in predicting the occurrence of unstable breathing. By measuring each of the factors in the *loop gain* equation (chemosensitivity, circulatory delay, lung volume, and $PaCO_2$), they were able to predict the occurrence of periodic breathing in patients with CHF during wakefulness with 100% sensitivity and 90% specificity (**Fig. 1**). As in the

Table 1
Randomized trials of PAP support in HF patients with OSA or CSA measuring cardiovascular outcomes

Study	Treatment	Follow-up (Months)	Baseline			Outcomes							
			N	AHI (eph)	LVEF (%)	AHI	BPsys	HR	SNA	LVEF	ExC	QOL	Death/ HTX
OSA													
Kaneko et al[63]	CPAP	1	24	41	27	↓↓↓	↓↓	→	na	↑↑	na	na	na
Usui et al[130]	CPAP	1	17	40	30	↓↓↓	↓↓	→	→	↑	na	na	na
Ryan et al[65]	CPAP	1	18	42	30	↓↓↓	↓↓	→	na	↑↑	na	na	na
Mansfield et al[62]	CPAP	3	40	26	36	↓↓↓	↔	na	→	↑	↔	↑	na
Smith et al[131]	APAP	1.5	26	36	29	na	na	na	na	↔	↔	(↑)	na
CSA													
Naughton et al[105]	CPAP	3	29	39	20	↓↓	na	na	→	↑↑	na	↑	na
Sin et al[108]	CPAP	3/26	29	39	20	↓↓↓	na	na	na	↑↑	na	na	(↓)
Bradley et al[106]	CPAP	26	258	40	24	↓↓	na	na	→	↑	↑	na	↔
Fietze et al[125]	BPAP	1.5	37	35	26	↓↓↓	na	↔	na	↑	na	↔	na
Pepperell et al[127]	ASV	1	30	20	35	na	na	na	→	↔	na	↔	na
Phillipe et al[128]	ASV	6	25	44	30	↓↓↓	na	na	na	(↑)	na	↑	na
Fietze et al[125]	ASV	1.5	37	32	25	↓↓↓	na	↔	na	↔	na	na	na
Kohnlein et al[123]	BPAP	0.5	16	27	24	↓↓	na	na	na	na	na	↑	na
Noda et al[122]	BPAP	3	21	28	33	↓↓	na	na	↓↓	↑↑↑	na	na	na

Abbreviations: APAP, Auto-titrating continuous positive airway pressure; ASV, adaptive pressure support servo-ventilation; BPsys, systolic arterial blood pressure; eph, events per hour; ExC, exercise capacity (6-minute–walk distance or peak oxygen uptake [VO2]); HR, heart rate; HTX, heart transplantation; na, not applicable; QoL, quality of life; SNA, sympathetic activity.

earlier study,[45] amongst the patients with CHF, chemosensitivity was the key factor contributing to periodic breathing, with no significant differences in the remaining factors within the patients with CHF.[70]

To assess whether an increase in chemosensitivity causes, rather than reflects, unstable breathing, Edwards and colleagues[73] augmented peripheral chemosensitivity with domperidone in a lamb model of periodic breathing. Following the administration of domperidone, peripheral chemosensitivity for O_2 and CO_2 increased by 35% and 70%, respectively, effects that were associated with an increased incidence and longer duration of periodic breathing. Also, domperidone was associated with greater swings in ventilation, shorter ventilatory duration, and longer apneas, features that the investigators demonstrated using mathematical modeling to indicate increased *loop gain*.[73] Thus, increasing peripheral chemosensitivity elevates *loop gain* and promotes unstable breathing.

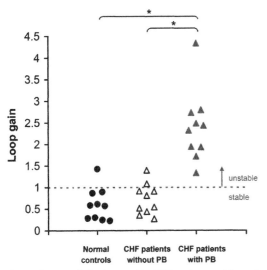

Fig. 1. *Loop gain* is elevated in CHF patients with periodic breathing (mean ± s.e. = 2.4 ± 0.3), but not in those without periodic breathing (0.7 ± 0.4) or control subjects without heart failure (0.6 ± 0.4). *Loop gain* was calculated from the *growth factor* data reported[70] by correcting for the period of the oscillation, t (min), using the relationship: *loop gain* = (*growth factor*)$^{t/2}$. This relationship can be derived by recognizing that the *growth factor* represents the expected increase in oscillatory amplitude after 1 minute, whereas *loop gain* represents the same over a half cycle (t/2). *P<.0001, student's *t*-test. s.e., standard error. (*Data from* Francis DP, Willson K, Davies LC, et al. Quantitative general theory for periodic breathing in chronic heart failure and its clinical implications. Circulation. 2000;102(18):2214–21).

Treatments that reduce chemosensitivity have been partially successful in reducing the severity of CSA in CHF. Studies have demonstrated that supplemental oxygen use in CHF can reduce chemosensitivity and AHI.[81–83] Similarly, the carbonic anhydrase inhibitor and diuretic acetazolamide has been found to reduce the severity of CSA.[84] Although its stabilizing actions may be multifactorial, acetazolamide is considered to reduce peripheral chemosensitivity and elevate central respiratory drive.[85,86] Acetazolamide increases the difference between resting $PaCO_2$ (eupnea) and the apneic threshold.[87] In essence, this increase in difference must represent a reduced chemosensitivity[87,88]; therefore, acetazolamide is likely to ameliorate CSA via a reduction in loop gain. Studies in cats demonstrated that even at low doses, acetazolamide administration reduces the hypoxic response and attenuates the increase in peripheral CO_2 sensitivity caused by hypoxia.[86,89] As such, treatments targeted toward reducing peripheral chemosensitivity may be particularly beneficial when combined with CPAP, because their effects on stabilization of breathing are expected to be multiplicative (Equation 1).

In addition to increased chemosensitivity, indirect evidence suggests that reduced lung volume plays an important role in the pathogenesis of CSA. Patients with CHF have a reduction in lung volumes[90,91] attributed to cardiomegaly, pleural effusions, respiratory muscle weakness, and pulmonary interstitial edema, which may vary to differing degrees with sleeping position and sleep state between patients. Krachman and colleagues[92] found that AHI in CHF-CSA patients was strongly associated with the rate of arterial oxygen desaturation during apnea, a factor strongly influenced by lung volume.[93–98] From their laboratory, Szollosi and colleagues[99] found that the lateral sleeping position strongly attenuated the AHI by 50% to 71% compared with the supine position, depending on sleep state. The lateral position attenuated the AHI-associated desaturation (4.7% vs 3.0%) with no difference in event duration. This change in desaturation and the known elevation in lung volume in the lateral position[100] are indirect evidence that lung volume might be of major importance in the pathogenesis of CSA. Whether the lateral position affects other factors, including cardiac output or chemosensitivity, in CHF patients is currently unknown.

There is substantial evidence that pulmonary congestion and interstitial edema may affect the stability of respiratory control. Szollosi and colleagues[79] observed that reduced pulmonary diffusing capacity measured with carbon monoxide (DLCO) in CSA patients was associated with increased severity of CSA as reflected by AHI. Earlier, it was found that elevated pulmonary capillary wedge pressure (PCWP) was associated with hypocapnia (an indication of elevated chemosensitivity[70]) and CSA frequency and severity.[101] Theoretical modeling would suggest that impaired pulmonary gas exchange may promote further hypoxemia during apnea and the delayed recovery from hypoxemia following apnea,[102] which could thereby augment the reflex increase in ventilation and promote ongoing cycles of apnea and hyperventilation. Alternatively, elevated pulmonary interstitial pressure secondary to edema stimulates pulmonary J receptors[103,104] that modulate ventilation,[103] perhaps by elevating chemosensitivity. Indeed, elevated peripheral and central chemosensitivity are associated with increased PCWP in CHF-CSA patients.[45] As such, the association between AHI and reduced DLCO and elevated PCWP may reflect this relationship. However, the mechanism by which pulmonary edema and dynamic chemosensitivity are related is yet to be established.

TREATMENT OF CSA

Apart from optimizing management of the underlying CHF, the best treatment of CSA specifically in CHF remains under debate. Although it is possible to suppress CSA with CPAP,[105,106] whether this translates into a mortality benefit remains unproven. **Table 1** summarizes the various trials that have looked at the use of PAP in CSA. The multicentered Canadian Continuous Positive Airway Pressure (CANPAP) trial was the largest randomized controlled trial that assessed the effect of CPAP on cardiac transplant-free survival in 258 patients who had CSA and CHF. Following a mean of 2.2 years, no significant difference in transplant-free survival, hospitalization, or quality of life was detected between the 2 groups.[106] However, significant improvements were observed in LVEF, plasma catecholamines, overnight oxygen levels, and AHI plus 6-minute walk distance with CPAP treatment.[106] Previous studies with smaller sample sizes had shown improvements in LVEF with CPAP when AHI was reduced to less than 15 events per hour (eph).[19,105,107,108] In the CANPAP trial, the mean AHI in the treatment arm was reduced to 19 eph, suggesting that many patients' CSA was not adequately controlled. Post hoc analysis of the CANPAP data, which divided the treatment arm into CSA-suppressed (AHI <15 eph at 3 months) and CSA-nonsuppressed groups, demonstrated improvements in LVEF (mean 25.6%–29.2%) and

transplant-free survival (approximately 95% vs approximately 50%, respectively) in the CSA-suppressed group compared with the CSA-nonsuppressed group.[109] Whether this is evidence for a benefit in suppressing CSA with CPAP remains to be proven. Alternative explanations include CSA-"suppressibility" being a marker for better prognosis or that some other unmeasured prognostic factor distinguished the 2 groups.

Compliance with CPAP may have been a factor that influenced the results of the CANPAP trial. The average compliance rates at 1 year were 3.6 hours per night.[106] Numerous studies have shown that compliance significantly affects the effectiveness of CPAP, with a cutoff of more than 4 hours per night being particularly advantageous.[67,110,111] Although these studies looked predominantly at CPAP in OSA, it is likely that CPAP compliance in CSA is equally important.

MECHANISMS OF ACTION OF CPAP IN CSA-CHF

The effectiveness of CPAP on breathing stability has long been attributed to the stabilization of the upper airway by its action of splinting the airway open. However, recent evidence indicates that, in addition to impact on the upper airway, PAP has stabilizing effects that result from lung inflation. Such effects are considered to result from increasing O_2 and CO_2 stores and damping oscillations in blood gases, which would otherwise increase *loop gain* and precipitate unstable breathing. The *loop gain* relationship (see Equation 1) predicts that an increase in lung volume due to CPAP would reduce *loop gain* and therefore provide for a more stable control system. The authors tested this hypothesis in their lamb model of periodic breathing, whereby with the upper airway bypassed, a CPAP-induced increase in lung volume was observed to strongly attenuate the duration and severity of periodic breathing induced following hyperventilation.[97] Such an effect was not attributable to changes in oxygenation in their controlled experiment. They also found that CPAP did not alter the cycle duration of periodic breathing; given that cycle duration is strongly related to circulatory delay/ejection fraction,[112,113] it is unlikely that cardiac output varied with CPAP in their study. Consistent with their observation of a lung inflation effect of CPAP, negative extrathoracic pressure applied to preterm infants to increase lung volume has been found to ameliorate periodic breathing.[114]

A common feature of studies examining the efficacy of different therapies for patients with CHF is that only some patients respond. Thus, CPAP has been found to be effective in reducing AHI to less than 15 eph only in approximately 50% of patients with HF.[106,109,115] No adequate explanation has yet been advanced to account for the uncertainty of treatment outcome. The authors suggest that the patients whose CSA does not resolve with treatment are those with the most unstable respiratory control or the highest *loop gain*. The potential for any particular therapy to be effective may be predicted using Equation 1. For example, if CPAP of approximately 10 cm H_2O increased functional residual capacity by approximately 1 L, or by approximately 50%, according to Equation 1, *loop gain* should reduce by 33%. Thus, PAP may only be effective at stabilizing breathing in patients who are bordering on stable breathing (*loop gain* <1.5).

Another unexplained phenomenon is that CPAP continues to provide benefit for CSA in patients with CHF over a 12-week period,[116] with patients exhibiting a baseline AHI of 41 ± 19 eph without CPAP, 22 ± 13 eph on initial CPAP implementation, and 13 ± 11 eph after 12 weeks on CPAP. Although the mechanisms underlying such long-term benefit are unknown, they may include an improvement in LVEF[108] or a reduction in chemosensitivity, perhaps occurring alongside either the reversal of sympathetic excitation[107,117,118] or a reversal of long-term sensitization of the peripheral chemoreflex via amelioration of intermittent hypoxia.[119,120] Indeed, the twofold elevation of chemosensitivity in patients with OSA versus healthy controls was found to be entirely normalized with one month of CPAP treatment.[121]

Alternative Modes of PAP Therapy

The equivocal findings from the CANPAP trial for CSA have led to a push for alternative methods of PAP. BPAP and adaptive pressure support servo-ventilation (ASV) provide varying levels of PAP in the hope of directly suppressing hypoventilation while providing the benefits of low-level CPAP.

BPAP provides a predetermined level of expiratory pressure with an increased level of inspiratory pressure. In small studies, BPAP has been shown to increase LVEF, reduce AHI and arousals, and decrease sympathetic outflow compared with medical therapy.[122,123] Similarly, small studies of BPAP in patients with CHF have shown positive results compared with CPAP and ASV. Three months of BPAP increased LVEF by 8.5% compared with 0.5% for those treated with CPAP in a study of 24 patients with CHF and OSA.[124] In patients with CHF in whom CSA predominates, a 6-week comparison of BPAP with ASV demonstrated a significant reduction in

AHI in both groups. LVEF increased significantly in those in the BPAP group but not in the ASV group.[125] However, the limitations of both studies are their small sample size, their short duration, and their design, which did not include functional or mortality outcomes.

ASV adopts a more complex approach to that of BPAP and CPAP in that it measures and aims to maintain a patient's ventilation at 90% of the prior 3-minute moving average.[126] ASV is designed to eliminate obstructive apneas and hypopneas with a minimum level of expiratory PAP and to modulate the inspiratory PAP to eliminate central apneas and hypopneas. Thus, ASV provides a low level of expiratory PAP (approximately 5 cm H_2O) and an adaptive level of inspiratory PAP (≥ 4 cm H_2O). Inspiratory PAP adapts to ventilatory effort; it increases as inspiratory effort falls and reduces as inspiratory effort increases. Thus, during central apneas, ASV provides inspiratory support (5–8 cm H_2O) at 15 breaths per minute, sufficient to maintain ventilation at 90% of the prior 3-minute average. However, ASV during sleep causes an acute 1 to 2 mm Hg rise in pCO_2 levels, possibly by increasing slow-wave and rapid-eye movement sleep and reducing arousals.[126] This may result in stabilization of ventilation.

Small medium-term studies demonstrate that ASV is more effective at reducing AHI compared with placebo[127] and CPAP.[128] A study comparing ASV with BPAP found that they were equally effective in reducing AHI.[125] Compliance data compared with CPAP is conflicting, with one study showing increased ASV use after 12 months[128] and another showing increased CPAP use after 12 months.[129] In terms of clinical benefits, improved cardiopulmonary exercise testing workload, maximal oxygen uptake (VO_2 max), LVEF, and N-terminal (NT)-proBNP levels have been demonstrated in an uncontrolled trial of 6 months of ASV.[129]

BPAP and ASV are promising new methods of delivering PAP to patients with CHF; however, solid, long-term data regarding mortality and morbidity benefits are lacking. The SERVE-HF and other similar large-scale, multicentered, randomized trials of ASV are expected to be completed between 2012 and 2015. Until then, routine use of either modality for the treatment of CSA cannot be recommended.

SUMMARY

The role of PAP in CHF is an evolving science. Although there has been considerable progress in the underlying science and the use of this treatment in the clinical setting, the picture is far from complete. It is known that the use of PAP in the treatment of APO due to left ventricular pump failure is safe and effective. It is also known that the medium- to long-term use of PAP in the ambulatory setting can improve respiratory, cardiac, and sleep physiology; however, definite mortality benefit is yet to be proven. Achieving this may require adapting the methods by which PAP is provided so that effectiveness and compliance are increased. The reasons for the lack of response to CPAP treatment in 50% of patients with CSA are unclear, as are the reasons that CPAP seems to yield further benefit following immediate use. As such, greater understanding of the underlying mechanisms behind the effects of PAP on the heart and lungs and, indeed, its influence on control of breathing (*loop gain*) is required. This may allow PAP to be implemented in a manner that specifically targets the required reduction in *loop gain* to ameliorate the disordered breathing of CHF and associated hypoxia, arousals, and sympathoexcitation, thus leading to better treatment outcomes.

REFERENCES

1. Schocken DD, Benjamin EJ, Fonarow GC, et al. Prevention of heart failure: a scientific statement from the American Heart Association Councils on Epidemiology and Prevention, Clinical Cardiology, Cardiovascular Nursing, and High Blood Pressure Research; Quality of Care and Outcomes Research Interdisciplinary Working Group; and Functional Genomics and Translational Biology Interdisciplinary Working Group. Circulation 2008;117(19): 2544–65.

2. Ho KK, Pinsky JL, Kannel WB, et al. The epidemiology of heart failure: the Framingham study. J Am Coll Cardiol 1993;22(4 Suppl A):6A–13A.

3. McCullough PA, Philbin EF, Spertus JA, et al. Confirmation of a heart failure epidemic: findings from the Resource Utilization Among Congestive Heart Failure (REACH) study. J Am Coll Cardiol 2002;39(1):60–9.

4. Maeder MT, Kaye DM. Heart failure with normal left ventricular ejection fraction. J Am Coll Cardiol 2009;53(11):905–18.

5. Vasan RS, Benjamin EJ, Levy D. Prevalence, clinical features and prognosis of diastolic heart failure: an epidemiologic perspective. J Am Coll Cardiol 1995;26(7):1565–74.

6. Zile MR, Brutsaert DL. New concepts in diastolic dysfunction and diastolic heart failure: part I: diagnosis, prognosis, and measurements of diastolic function. Circulation 2002;105(11):1387–93.

7. Serizawa T, Vogel WM, Apstein CS, et al. Comparison of acute alterations in left ventricular relaxation and diastolic chamber stiffness induced by hypoxia and ischemia. Role of myocardial oxygen supply-demand imbalance. J Clin Invest 1981; 68(1):91–102.

8. Gehlbach BK, Geppert E. The pulmonary manifestations of left heart failure. Chest 2004; 125(2):669–82.

9. Hamilton AL, Killian KJ, Summers E, et al. Muscle strength, symptom intensity, and exercise capacity in patients with cardiorespiratory disorders. Am J Respir Crit Care Med 1995;152(6 Pt 1):2021–31.

10. Schumacker PT. Pulmonary edema, shunt and blood flow distribution. Problems, progress and perspectives. Intensive Care Med 1993;19(4): 183–4.

11. Masip J, Roque M, Sanchez B, et al. Noninvasive ventilation in acute cardiogenic pulmonary edema: systematic review and meta-analysis. JAMA 2005; 294(24):3124–30.

12. Petersen JW, Felker GM. Inflammatory biomarkers in heart failure. Congest Heart Fail 2006;12(6): 324–8.

13. Winck JC, Azevedo LF, Costa-Pereira A, et al. Efficacy and safety of non-invasive ventilation in the treatment of acute cardiogenic pulmonary edema–a systematic review and meta-analysis. Crit Care 2006;10(2):R69.

14. Peter JV, Moran JL, Phillips-Hughes J, et al. Effect of non-invasive positive pressure ventilation (NIPPV) on mortality in patients with acute cardiogenic pulmonary oedema: a meta-analysis. Lancet 2006;367(9517):1155–63.

15. Gee MH, Williams DO. Effect of lung inflation on perivascular cuff fluid volume in isolated dog lung lobes. Microvasc Res 1979;17(2):192–201.

16. Pare PD, Warriner B, Baile EM, et al. Redistribution of pulmonary extravascular water with positive end-expiratory pressure in canine pulmonary edema. Am Rev Respir Dis 1983;127(5):590–3.

17. Fernandez Mondejar E, Vazquez Mata G, Cardenas A, et al. Ventilation with positive end-expiratory pressure reduces extravascular lung water and increases lymphatic flow in hydrostatic pulmonary edema. Crit Care Med 1996;24(9): 1562–7.

18. Naughton MT, Rahman MA, Hara K, et al. Effect of continuous positive airway pressure on intrathoracic and left ventricular transmural pressures in patients with congestive heart failure. Circulation 1995;91(6):1725–31.

19. Tkacova R, Liu PP, Naughton MT, et al. Effect of continuous positive airway pressure on mitral regurgitant fraction and atrial natriuretic peptide in patients with heart failure. J Am Coll Cardiol 1997;30(3):739–45.

20. Bradley TD, Holloway RM, McLaughlin PR, et al. Cardiac output response to continuous positive airway pressure in congestive heart failure. Am Rev Respir Dis 1992;145(2 Pt 1):377–82.

21. Gray A, Goodacre S, Newby DE, et al. Noninvasive ventilation in acute cardiogenic pulmonary edema. N Engl J Med 2008;359(2):142–51.

22. Mehta S, Jay GD, Woolard RH, et al. Randomized, prospective trial of bilevel versus continuous positive airway pressure in acute pulmonary edema. Crit Care Med 1997;25(4):620–8.

23. Bellone A, Monari A, Cortellaro F, et al. Myocardial infarction rate in acute pulmonary edema: noninvasive pressure support ventilation versus continuous positive airway pressure. Crit Care Med 2004; 32(9):1860–5.

24. Collins SP, Mielniczuk LM, Whittingham HA, et al. The use of noninvasive ventilation in emergency department patients with acute cardiogenic pulmonary edema: a systematic review. Ann Emerg Med 2006;48(3):260–9, 269.e1–4.

25. Sin DD, Fitzgerald F, Parker JD, et al. Risk factors for central and obstructive sleep apnea in 450 men and women with congestive heart failure. Am J Respir Crit Care Med 1999;160(4):1101–6.

26. Schulz R, Blau A, Borgel J, et al. Sleep apnoea in heart failure. Eur Respir J 2007;29(6):1201–5.

27. Young T, Peppard PE, Taheri S. Excess weight and sleep-disordered breathing. J Appl Physiol 2005; 99(4):1592–9.

28. Javaheri S. Central sleep apnea in congestive heart failure: prevalence, mechanisms, impact, and therapeutic options. Semin Respir Crit Care Med 2005;26(1):44–55.

29. Shahar E, Whitney CW, Redline S, et al. Sleep-disordered breathing and cardiovascular disease: cross-sectional results of the Sleep Heart Health Study. Am J Respir Crit Care Med 2001;163(1): 19–25.

30. Carlson JT, Hedner JA, Ejnell H, et al. High prevalence of hypertension in sleep apnea patients independent of obesity. Am J Respir Crit Care Med 1994;150(1):72–7.

31. Hedner J, Ejnell H, Caidahl K. Left ventricular hypertrophy independent of hypertension in patients with obstructive sleep apnoea. J Hypertens 1990;8(10):941–6.

32. Usui K, Parker JD, Newton GE, et al. Left ventricular structural adaptations to obstructive sleep apnea in dilated cardiomyopathy. Am J Respir Crit Care Med 2006;173(10):1170–5.

33. Redolfi S, Yumino D, Ruttanaumpawan P, et al. Relationship between overnight rostral fluid shift and obstructive sleep apnea in nonobese men. Am J Respir Crit Care Med 2009;179(3):241–6.

34. Suratt PM, Dee P, Atkinson RL, et al. Fluoroscopic and computed tomographic features of the pharyngeal airway in obstructive sleep apnea. Am Rev Respir Dis 1983;127(4):487–92.

35. Haponik EF, Smith PL, Bohlman ME, et al. Computerized tomography in obstructive sleep apnea. Correlation of airway size with physiology during sleep and wakefulness. Am Rev Respir Dis 1983; 127(2):221–6.

36. Schwab RJ, Gupta KB, Gefter WB, et al. Upper airway and soft tissue anatomy in normal subjects and patients with sleep-disordered breathing. Significance of the lateral pharyngeal walls. Am J Respir Crit Care Med 1995;152(5 Pt 1):1673–89.

37. Eckert DJ, Malhotra A, Jordan AS. Mechanisms of apnea. Prog Cardiovasc Dis 2009;51(4):313–23.

38. Eckert DJ, Malhotra A. Pathophysiology of adult obstructive sleep apnea. Proc Am Thorac Soc 2008;5(2):144–53.

39. Mezzanotte WS, Tangel DJ, White DP. Influence of sleep onset on upper-airway muscle activity in apnea patients versus normal controls. Am J Respir Crit Care Med 1996;153(6 Pt 1):1880–7.

40. Wellman A, Jordan AS, Malhotra A, et al. Ventilatory control and airway anatomy in obstructive sleep apnea. Am J Respir Crit Care Med 2004;170(11): 1225–32.

41. Wellman A, Malhotra A, Jordan AS, et al. Effect of oxygen in obstructive sleep apnea: role of loop gain. Respir Physiol Neurobiol 2008;162(2):144–51.

42. Onal E, Lopata M. Periodic breathing and the pathogenesis of occlusive sleep apneas. Am Rev Respir Dis 1982;126(4):676–80.

43. Younes M. Role of respiratory control mechanisms in the pathogenesis of obstructive sleep disorders. J Appl Physiol 2008;105(5):1389–405.

44. Ponikowski P, Chua TP, Anker SD, et al. Peripheral chemoreceptor hypersensitivity: an ominous sign in patients with chronic heart failure. Circulation 2001;104(5):544–9.

45. Solin P, Roebuck T, Johns DP, et al. Peripheral and central ventilatory responses in central sleep apnea with and without congestive heart failure. Am J Respir Crit Care Med 2000; 162(6):2194–200.

46. Chua TP, Ponikowski P, Harrington D, et al. Clinical correlates and prognostic significance of the ventilatory response to exercise in chronic heart failure. J Am Coll Cardiol 1997;29(7):1585–90.

47. Lehman S, Antic NA, Thompson C, et al. Central sleep apnea on commencement of continuous positive airway pressure in patients with a primary diagnosis of obstructive sleep apnea-hypopnea. J Clin Sleep Med 2007;3(5):462–6.

48. Tkacova R, Niroumand M, Lorenzi-Filho G, et al. Overnight shift from obstructive to central apneas in patients with heart failure: role of PCO2 and circulatory delay. Circulation 2001;103(2):238–43.

49. Somers VK, Dyken ME, Clary MP, et al. Sympathetic neural mechanisms in obstructive sleep apnea. J Clin Invest 1995;96(4):1897–904.

50. Tkacova R, Rankin F, Fitzgerald FS, et al. Effects of continuous positive airway pressure on obstructive sleep apnea and left ventricular afterload in patients with heart failure. Circulation 1998; 98(21):2269–75.

51. Moore-Gillon JC, Cameron IR. Right ventricular hypertrophy and polycythaemia in rats after intermittent exposure to hypoxia. Clin Sci (Lond) 1985; 69(5):595–9.

52. Moore-Gillon JC, Treacher DF, Gaminara EJ, et al. Intermittent hypoxia in patients with unexplained polycythaemia. BMJ 1986;293(6547):588–90.

53. Garvey JF, Taylor CT, McNicholas WT. Cardiovascular disease in obstructive sleep apnoea syndrome: the role of intermittent hypoxia and inflammation. Eur Respir J 2009;33(5):1195–205.

54. Lusina SJ, Kennedy PM, Inglis JT, et al. Long-term intermittent hypoxia increases sympathetic activity and chemosensitivity during acute hypoxia in humans. J Physiol 2006;575(Pt 3):961–70.

55. Koehle MS, Sheel AW, Milsom WK, et al. Two patterns of daily hypoxic exposure and their effects on measures of chemosensitivity in humans. J Appl Physiol 2007;103(6):1973–8.

56. Marcucci R, Gori AM, Giannotti F, et al. Markers of hypercoagulability and inflammation predict mortality in patients with heart failure. J Thromb Haemost 2006;4(5):1017–22.

57. Aronsohn RH, MJ, Ando S, et al. Impact of untreated obstructive sleep apnea on glucose control magnitude and time course of hemodynamic responses to Mueller maneuvers in type 2 diabetes patients with congestive heart failure. Am J Respir Crit Care Med 1998;85(4):1476–84.

58. Drager LF, Bortolotto LA, Figueiredo AC, et al. Effects of continuous positive airway pressure on early signs of atherosclerosis in obstructive sleep apnea. Am J Respir Crit Care Med 2007;176(7): 706–12.

59. Marin JM, Carrizo SJ, Vicente E, et al. Long-term cardiovascular outcomes in men with obstructive sleep apnoea-hypopnoea with or without treatment with continuous positive airway pressure: an observational study. Lancet 2005;365(9464): 1046–53.

60. Punjabi NM, Caffo BS, Goodwin JL, et al. Sleep-disordered breathing and mortality: a prospective cohort study. PLoS Med 2009;6(8):e1000132.

61. Gilman MP, Floras JS, Usui K, et al. Continuous positive airway pressure increases heart rate variability in heart failure patients with obstructive sleep apnea. Clin Sci (Lond) 2008;114(3):243–9.

62. Mansfield DR, Gollogly NC, Kaye DM, et al. Controlled trial of continuous positive airway pressure in obstructive sleep apnea and heart failure. Am J Respir Crit Care Med 2004;169(3): 361–6.

63. Kaneko Y, Floras JS, Usui K, et al. Cardiovascular effects of continuous positive airway pressure in patients with heart failure and obstructive sleep apnea. N Engl J Med 2003;348(13):1233–41.

64. Usui K, Bradley TD, Spaak J, et al. Inhibition of awake sympathetic nerve activity of heart failure patients with obstructive sleep apnea by nocturnal continuous positive airway pressure. J Am Coll Cardiol 2005;45(12):2008–11.

65. Ryan CM, Usui K, Floras JS, et al. Effect of continuous positive airway pressure on ventricular ectopy in heart failure patients with obstructive sleep apnoea. Thorax 2005;60(9):781–5.

66. Wang H, Parker JD, Newton GE, et al. Influence of obstructive sleep apnea on mortality in patients with heart failure. J Am Coll Cardiol 2007;49(15): 1625–31.

67. Kasai T, Narui K, Dohi T, et al. Prognosis of patients with heart failure and obstructive sleep apnea treated with continuous positive airway pressure. Chest 2008;133(3):690–6.

68. Javaheri S. Sleep disorders in systolic heart failure: a prospective study of 100 male patients. The final report. Int J Cardiol 2006;106(1):21–8.

69. Cherniack NS, Longobardo GS. Cheyne-Stokes breathing. An instability in physiologic control. N Engl J Med 1973;288(18):952–7.

70. Francis DP, Willson K, Davies LC, et al. Quantitative general theory for periodic breathing in chronic heart failure and its clinical implications. Circulation 2000;102(18):2214–21.

71. Khoo MC, Kronauer RE, Strohl KP, et al. Factors inducing periodic breathing in humans: a general model. J Appl Physiol 1982;53(3):644–59.

72. Wilkinson MH, Sia KL, Skuza EM, et al. Impact of changes in inspired oxygen and carbon dioxide on respiratory instability in the lamb. J Appl Physiol 2005;98(2):437–46.

73. Edwards BA, Sands SA, Skuza EM, et al. Increased peripheral chemosensitivity via dopaminergic manipulation promotes respiratory instability in lambs. Respir Physiol Neurobiol 2008;164(3):419–28.

74. Wellman A, Malhotra A, Fogel RB, et al. Respiratory system loop gain in normal men and women measured with proportional-assist ventilation. J Appl Physiol 2003;94(1):205–12.

75. Nugent ST, Finley JP. Periodic breathing in infants: a model study. IEEE Trans Biomed Eng 1987;34: 482–5.

76. Javaheri S, Parker TJ, Liming JD, et al. Sleep apnea in 81 ambulatory male patients with stable heart failure. Types and their prevalences, consequences, and presentations. Circulation 1998; 97(21):2154–9.

77. Topor ZL, Johannson L, Kasprzyk J, et al. Dynamic ventilatory response to CO(2) in congestive heart failure patients with and without central sleep apnea. J Appl Physiol 2001;91(1):408–16.

78. Javaheri S. A mechanism of central sleep apnea in patients with heart failure. N Engl J Med 1999; 341(13):949–54.

79. Szollosi I, Thompson BR, Krum H, et al. Impaired pulmonary diffusing capacity and hypoxia in heart failure correlates with central sleep apnea severity. Chest 2008;134:67–72.

80. Lorenzi-Filho G, Rankin F, Bics I, et al. Effects of inhaled carbon dioxide and oxygen on Cheyne-Stokes respiration in patients with heart failure. Am J Respir Crit Care Med 1999;159(5 Pt 1): 1490–8.

81. Franklin KA, Eriksson P, Sahlin C, et al. Reversal of central sleep apnea with oxygen. Chest 1997; 111(1):163–9.

82. Hanly PJ, Millar TW, Steljes DG, et al. The effect of oxygen on respiration and sleep in patients with congestive heart failure. Ann Intern Med 1989; 111(10):777–82.

83. Javaheri S, Ahmed M, Parker TJ, et al. Effects of nasal O2 on sleep-related disordered breathing in ambulatory patients with stable heart failure. Sleep 1999;22(8):1101–6.

84. Javaheri S. Acetazolamide improves central sleep apnea in heart failure: a double-blind, prospective study. Am J Respir Crit Care Med 2006;173(2): 234–7.

85. Bashir Y, Kann M, Stradling JR. The effect of acetazolamide on hypercapnic and eucapnic/poikilocapnic hypoxic ventilatory responses in normal subjects. Pulm Pharmacol 1990;3(3):151–4.

86. Teppema LJ, Dahan A. Low-dose acetazolamide reduces the hypoxic ventilatory response in the anesthetized cat. Respir Physiol Neurobiol 2004; 140(1):43–51.

87. Nakayama H, Smith CA, Rodman JR, et al. Effect of ventilatory drive on carbon dioxide sensitivity below eupnea during sleep. Am J Respir Crit Care Med 2002;165(9):1251–60.

88. Manisty CH, Willson K, Wensel R, et al. Development of respiratory control instability in heart failure: a novel approach to dissect the pathophysiological mechanisms. J Physiol 2006;577(Pt 1): 387–401.

89. Teppema LJ, Dahan A, Olievier CN. Low-dose acetazolamide reduces CO(2)-O(2) stimulus interaction within the peripheral chemoreceptors in the anaesthetised cat. J Physiol 2001;537(Pt 1): 221–9.

90. Naum CC, Sciurba FC, Rogers RM. Pulmonary function abnormalities in chronic severe cardiomyopathy preceding cardiac transplantation. Am Rev Respir Dis 1992;145(6):1334–8.

91. Torchio R, Gulotta C, Greco-Lucchina P, et al. Closing capacity and gas exchange in chronic heart failure. Chest 2006;129(5):1330–6.

92. Krachman SL, Crocetti J, Berger TJ, et al. Effects of nasal continuous positive airway pressure on oxygen body stores in patients with Cheyne-Stokes respiration and congestive heart failure. Chest 2003;123(1):59–66.

93. Sands SA, Edwards BA, Kelly VJ, et al. A model analysis of arterial oxygen desaturation during apnea in preterm infants. PLoS Comput Biol 2009;5(12):e1000588.

94. Findley LJ, Ries AL, Tisi GM, et al. Hypoxemia during apnea in normal subjects: mechanisms and impact of lung volume. J Appl Physiol 1983; 55(6):1777–83.

95. Poets CF, Rau GA, Neuber K, et al. Determinants of lung volume in spontaneously breathing preterm infants. Am J Respir Crit Care Med 1997;155(2): 649–53.

96. Series F, Cormier Y, La Forge J. Role of lung volumes in sleep apnoea-related oxygen desaturation. Eur Respir J 1989;2(1):26–30.

97. Edwards BA, Sands SA, Feeney C, et al. Continuous positive airway pressure reduces loop gain and resolves periodic central apneas in the lamb. Respir Physiol Neurobiol 2009;168(3):239–49.

98. Hurewitz AN, Sampson MG. Voluntary breath holding in the obese. J Appl Physiol 1987;62(6):2371–6.

99. Szollosi I, Roebuck T, Thompson B, et al. Lateral sleeping position reduces severity of central sleep apnea/Cheyne-Stokes respiration. Sleep 2006; 29(8):1045–51.

100. Hurewitz AN, Susskind H, Harold WH. Obesity alters regional ventilation in lateral decubitus position. J Appl Physiol 1985;59(3):774–83.

101. Solin P, Bergin P, Richardson M, et al. Influence of pulmonary capillary wedge pressure on central apnea in heart failure. Circulation 1999;99(12): 1574–9.

102. Sands SA, Kelly VJ, Edwards BA, et al. A dynamic model for assessing the impact of diffusing capacity on arterial oxygenation during apnea. Respir Physiol Neurobiol 2010;171(3):193–200.

103. Roberts AM, Bhattacharya J, Schultz HD, et al. Stimulation of pulmonary vagal afferent C-fibers by lung edema in dogs. Circ Res 1986;58(4):512–22.

104. Paintal AS. Mechanism of stimulation of type J pulmonary receptors. J Physiol 1969;203(3):511–32.

105. Naughton MT, Liu PP, Bernard DC, et al. Treatment of congestive heart failure and Cheyne-Stokes respiration during sleep by continuous positive airway pressure. Am J Respir Crit Care Med 1995;151(1):92–7.

106. Bradley TD, Logan AG, Kimoff RJ, et al. Continuous positive airway pressure for central sleep apnea and heart failure. N Engl J Med 2005;353(19):2025–33.

107. Naughton MT, Benard DC, Liu PP, et al. Effects of nasal CPAP on sympathetic activity in patients with heart failure and central sleep apnea. Am J Respir Crit Care Med 1995;152(2):473–9.

108. Sin DD, Logan AG, Fitzgerald FS, et al. Effects of continuous positive airway pressure on cardiovascular outcomes in heart failure patients with and without Cheyne-Stokes respiration. Circulation 2000;102(1):61–6.

109. Arzt M, Floras JS, Logan AG, et al. Suppression of central sleep apnea by continuous positive airway pressure and transplant-free survival in heart failure: a post hoc analysis of the Canadian Continuous Positive Airway Pressure for Patients with Central Sleep Apnea and Heart Failure Trial (CANPAP). Circulation 2007;115(25):3173–80.

110. Ishida K, Kato M, Kato Y, et al. Appropriate use of nasal continuous positive airway pressure decreases elevated C-reactive protein in patients with obstructive sleep apnea. Chest 2009;136:125–9.

111. Dorkova Z, Petrasova D, Molcanyiova A, et al. Effects of continuous positive airway pressure on cardiovascular risk profile in patients with severe obstructive sleep apnea and metabolic syndrome. Chest 2008;134(4):686–92.

112. Solin P, Roebuck T, Swieca J, et al. Effects of cardiac dysfunction on non-hypercapnic central sleep apnea. Chest 1998;113(1):104–10.

113. Hall MJ, Xie A, Rutherford R, et al. Cycle length of periodic breathing in patients with and without heart failure. Am J Respir Crit Care Med 1996; 154(2 Pt 1):376–81.

114. Thibeault DW, Wong MM, Auld PA. Thoracic gas volume changes in premature infants. Pediatrics 1967;40(3):403–11.

115. Javaheri S. Effects of continuous positive airway pressure on sleep apnea and ventricular irritability in patients with heart failure. Circulation 2000; 101(4):392–7.

116. Arzt M, Schulz M, Schroll S, et al. Time course of continuous positive airway pressure effects on central sleep apnoea in patients with chronic heart failure. J Sleep Res 2009;18(1):20–5.

117. Yamada K, Asanoi H, Ueno H, et al. Role of central sympathoexcitation in enhanced hypercapnic chemosensitivity in patients with heart failure. Am Heart J 2004;148(6):964–70.

118. Kaye DM, Mansfield D, Aggarwal A, et al. Acute effects of continuous positive airway pressure on cardiac sympathetic tone in congestive heart failure. Circulation 2001;103(19):2336–8.

119. Chowdhuri S, Shanidze I, Pierchala L, et al. Effect of episodic hypoxia on the susceptibility to hypocapnic central apnea during NREM sleep. J Appl Physiol 2010;108:369–77.

120. Lee DS, Badr MS, Mateika JH. Progressive augmentation and ventilatory long-term facilitation are enhanced in sleep apnoea patients and are mitigated by antioxidant administration. J Physiol 2009;587(Pt 22):5451–67.

121. Salloum A, Rowley JA, Mateika JH, et al. Increased propensity for central apnea in patients with obstructive sleep apnea: effect of nasal continuous positive airway pressure. Am J Respir Crit Care Med 2010;181(2):189–93.

122. Noda A, Izawa H, Asano H, et al. Beneficial effect of bilevel positive airway pressure on left ventricular function in ambulatory patients with idiopathic dilated cardiomyopathy and central sleep apnea-hypopnea: a preliminary study. Chest 2007; 131(6):1694–701.

123. Kohnlein T, Welte T, Tan LB, et al. Assisted ventilation for heart failure patients with Cheyne-Stokes respiration. Eur Respir J 2002;20(4):934–41.

124. Khayat RN, Abraham WT, Patt B, et al. Cardiac effects of continuous and bilevel positive airway pressure for patients with heart failure and obstructive sleep apnea: a pilot study. Chest 2008;134(6): 1162–8.

125. Fietze I, Blau A, Glos M, et al. Bi-level positive pressure ventilation and adaptive servo ventilation in patients with heart failure and Cheyne-Stokes respiration. Sleep Med 2008;9(6):652–9.

126. Teschler H, Dohring J, Wang YM, et al. Adaptive pressure support servo-ventilation: a novel treatment for Cheyne-Stokes respiration in heart failure. Am J Respir Crit Care Med 2001;164(4): 614–9.

127. Pepperell JC, Maskell NA, Jones DR, et al. A randomized controlled trial of adaptive ventilation for Cheyne-Stokes breathing in heart failure. Am J Respir Crit Care Med 2003;168(9): 1109–14.

128. Philippe C, Stoica-Herman M, Drouot X, et al. Compliance with and effectiveness of adaptive servoventilation versus continuous positive airway pressure in the treatment of Cheyne-Stokes respiration in heart failure over a six month period. Heart 2006;92(3):337–42.

129. Oldenburg O, Schmidt A, Lamp B, et al. Adaptive servoventilation improves cardiac function in patients with chronic heart failure and Cheyne-Stokes respiration. Eur J Heart Fail 2008;10(6):581–6.

130. Usui K, Bradley TD, Spaak J, et al. Inhibition of awake sympathetic nerve activity of heart failure patients with obstructive sleep anea by nocturnal continuous positive airway pressure. J Am Coll Cardiol 2005;45:2008–11.

131. Smith LA, Vennelle M, Gardner RS, et al. Auto-titrating continuous positive airway pressure therapy in patients with chronic heart failure and obstructive sleep apnoea: a randomized placebo-controlled trial. Eur Heart J 2007;28(10): 1221–7.

Positive Airway Pressure Treatment of Central Sleep Apnea with Emphasis on Heart Failure, Opioids, and Complex Sleep Apnea

S. Javaheri, MD[a,b,*]

KEYWORDS
• Central sleep apnea • Heart failure • Opioids
• Positive airway pressure treatment

Central sleep apnea (CSA) is due to temporary failure in the pontomedullary inspiratory pacemaker generating breathing rhythm. Consequently, there is no medullary inspiratory neural output through the phrenic and intercostals nerves innervating inspiratory thoracic pump muscles. This results in the loss of any ventilatory efforts, which, if it lasts 10 seconds or more, is defined a central apnea. Polygraphically, central apnea is recognized by the absence of naso-oral airflow and thoracoabdominal excursions. The absence of any breathing excursions, that is, presence of flat (not diminished) lines from naso-oral flow probes, and thoracoabdominal excursions are critical criteria for accurate recognition of central apnea. I follow these strict criteria to minimize cross-contamination with other obstructive disordered breathing events.

A central apnea index (CAI) of greater than or equal to 5 per hour of sleep is considered abnormal. Central hypopneas, however, have not been included in this threshold. This is in contrast to the index used in defining presence of polysomnographically (PSG) significant obstructive disordered breathing events, when hypopneas are included in the threshold. Therefore, the minimum number of central events (apneas plus hypopneas) required during sleep to represent a distinct disorder or syndrome (a condition associated with consequences [eg, insomnia, excessive daytime sleepiness, impaired quality of life, morbidity, or mortality]) is not known.

The reason for not including central hypopneas in the index relates to the difficulty in accurately and precisely differentiating central and obstructive hypopneas from each other. In particular, in PSGs with mixed pattern of breathing, observed in patients with systolic heart failure or those on opioids, concomitant presence of both forms of hypopnea poses a problem.

In patients with systolic heart failure, we have used arbitrary PSG criteria[1–3] to classify the disordered breathing into predominant central apnea or obstructive sleep apnea (OSA). But, what the minimum clinically significant central apnea-hypopnea index (AHI) should be remains to be defined. In our studies of patients with heart failure, arbitrarily, an AHI of 15 or more per hour has been used, but this does not mean that it is the appropriate threshold, as we have more

[a] College of Medicine, University of Cincinnati, Cincinnati, OH, USA
[b] Sleepcare Diagnostics, Cincinnati, OH, USA
* College of Medicine, University of Cincinnati, Cincinnati, OH.
E-mail address: Javaheri@snorenomore.com

Sleep Med Clin 5 (2010) 407–417
doi:10.1016/j.jsmc.2010.05.006
1556-407X/10/$ – see front matter © 2010 Elsevier Inc. All rights reserved.

recently reported that AHI values less than 15 are associated with excess mortality.[4]

Box 1 shows the various physiologic and pathologic conditions associated with CSA.[5] The mechanisms and description of CSA associated with various disorders are detailed elsewhere[1–3,6–11] and are not discussed in this article. The focus of this article is on three disorders: systolic heart failure, opioid-induced sleep apnea, and complex sleep apnea.

SYSTOLIC HEART FAILURE
Prevalence of Central Apnea in Systolic Heart Failure

Heart failure is a highly prevalent syndrome. It is estimated that at least 5 to 6 million Americans, approximately 2% of the population, and 10% of those above 65 years age have heart failure.[12] Because heart failure is highly prevalent and CSA is common in the setting of the failing heart, heart failure is the most common cause of CSA in general population.

It has been long recognized that periodic breathing in systolic heart failure is characterized by crescendo-decrescendo breathing arms. This is due to a long arterial circulation time, a pathophysiologic feature of systolic heart failure. We refer to this pattern of periodic breathing as Hunter-Cheyne-Stokes breathing because John Hunter, a British surgeon, described it 37 years before John Cheyne's description.[13,14]

Many early studies[1–3,15–26] of consecutive patients with stable heart failure and left ventricular systolic dysfunction show a high prevalence of sleep apnea. The disordered breathing events include central apnea and OSA, and they commonly occur together.

The largest and most systematic PSG study[18] involved 100 ambulatory male patients with stable, treated heart failure. In this study, 114 consecutive eligible subjects who were followed in a cardiology and a primary care clinic were asked to participate (88% recruitment) without regard to any symptom of sleep apnea. They spent 2 nights in the sleep laboratory, the first night for habituation. Using an AHI of 15 per hour or greater as the threshold for moderate to severe sleep apnea, we found that 49 subjects (49% of all patients) met this criterion with an average index of 44 per hour. The index included central and obstructive events.

In our studies, 10% of the patients were on β-blockers, and, because this family of drugs is part of contemporary therapy in the management of heart failure, the question arises if their use has decreased the prevalence of sleep apnea in heart failure.

Box 1
Central sleep apnea

1. Physiologic CSA
   - Sleep-onset
   - Postarousal/postsigh
   - Phasic rapid eye movement sleep

2. Hypocapnic (nonhypercapnic) CSA
   - Systolic heart failure
   - Idiopathic
   - Idiopathic pulmonary arterial hypertension
   - High altitude
   - Poststroke

3. Hypercapnic[a] CSA
   - Alveolar hypoventilation with normal pulmonary function

     Congenital central hypoventilation syndrome

     Primary chronic alveolar hypoventilation syndrome

   - Brainstem and spinal cord disorders

     Encephalitis; brain tumors and infarcts

     Cervical cordotomy

     Anterior cervical spinal artery syndrome

     Neurodegenerative disorders

     Amyotrophic lateral sclerosis

     Multiple sclerosis

     Chiari malformation

   - Muscular disorders

     Myotonic and Duchenne dystrophies

     Acid maltase deficiency

     Guillain-Barré syndrome

   - Opioids

4. CSA with endocrine disorders
   - Acromegaly
   - Hypothyrodism

5. CSA with OSA
   - A minor component of OSA
   - With CPAP therapy (complex sleep apnea)
   - Post-tracheotomy

6. CSA with upper airway disorders

[a] P_{CO_2}, however, may be at times normal.
Data from Javaheri S. Central sleep apnea. In: Lee-Chiong T, editor. Sleep Medicine Essentials. Hoboken (NJ): Wiley-Blackwell; 2009. p. 81–9.

Based on the results of recent studies,[27–30] in which up to 85% of the patients were receiving β-blockers (**Table 1**), I conclude that these drugs have had no significant impact on the high prevalence of sleep apnea in heart failure. **Table 1** shows the prevalence of sleep apnea and OSA in some of the largest studies using an AHI greater than or equal to 15 per hour. Combining the results of these studies, involving a total of 1250 consecutive patients and using an AHI of 15 greater than or equal to per hour of sleep as the threshold, 52% have moderate to severe sleep apnea, 31% have CSA, and 21% have OSA (**Fig. 1**).

Treatment of Central Sleep Apnea in Systolic Heart Failure

The various therapeutic options for CSA have been reviewed elsewhere.[1–3,31] These include positive airway pressure (PAP) devices, nocturnal oxygen,[32] theophylline,[33] acetazolamide,[34] and cardiac transplantation.[35]

This article discusses treatment with PAP devices. Several such devices, including continuous positive airway pressure (CPAP), bilevel pressure, and adaptive pressure support servo-ventilation, have been used to treat sleep apnea, both OSA and CSA, in systolic heart failure.

There is a major difference in the therapeutic effects of these devices when treating OSA and CSA, however. In contrast to treatment of OSA when application of nasal CPAP invariably results in virtual elimination of the disordered breathing events,[36] in CSA, response to therapy is not uniform, with some patients responding well and others not at all.[36]

There are many short-term studies (for review, see articles by Javaheri[1–3,37]) of CPAP to treat CSA in systolic heart failure showing differing results,[36,38–42] with several trials showing no effects. In our study,[36] first-night CPAP titration was effective in eliminating OSA in all, and CSA in 43%, of the patients in whom the average AHI decreased from 36 to 4 per hour. The remaining 57% were considered CPAP nonresponsive.

The question that I like to address is if long-term CPAP use will prove effective in these first night CPAP nonresponders. As discussed later, the answer is generally no. There is only one long-term randomized clinical trial, the multicenter Canadian study, which for obvious reasons (discussed later) failed to confirm a beneficial effect of CPAP on mortality. In that trial,[43] 130 patients were randomized to the control group and 128 to the CPAP arm. The baseline features were similar between the two randomized groups. The patients in the therapeutic arm were adapted to CPAP over 1 to 3 nights (without PSG to determine who had not responded to CPAP) and were discharged at CPAP level of approximately 8 to 10 cm H_2O. The idea was that with time, patients CSA would improve and first-night titration is not representative of long-term response (an erroneous assumption).

A second PSG was performed at 3 months in both groups.[43] In the CPAP arm, the mean AHI (I emphasize the mean, which represents AHI values of all individuals, some of whom might have not responded to CPAP) decreased by 50%, with improvement in desaturation, plasma norepinephrine level, and left ventricular ejection fraction (all mean values statistically significant). The mean values for these variables remained unchanged in the control group. In spite of these improvements in the surrogates of mortality, an interim analysis revealed worse transplantation-free survival (due to progressive heart failure and sudden death) of the CPAP-treated patients compared with the control group ($P = .02$). Although the survival curves diverged after approximately 3 years favoring the CPAP arm, the difference was not statistically significant ($P = .06$).

What was the reason for early excess mortality in the CPAP group? I speculated[44] that CPAP therapy could have resulted in excess early mortality for the following reasons: Those who died were heart failure patients with CSA whose periodic breathing was CPAP nonresponsive to begin with. (This assumption was based on the

Table 1
Worldwide prevalence of sleep apnea in systolic heart failure

Author, Country (y)	n	% of Patients with AHI ≥ 15/h	% of Patients on β-Blockers
Javaheri, USA (2006)	100	49	10
MacDonald, USA (2008)	108	61	82
Wang, Canada (2007)	287	47	80
Vazir, UK (2007)	55	53	78
Oldenburg, Germany (2007)	700	52	85

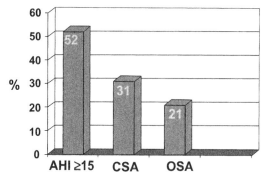

Fig. 1. Prevalence of sleep apnea (AHI ≥15/h) in 1250 consecutive patients with systolic heart failure. (*From* Javaheri S. Cardiovascular disorders. In: Kryger MH, editor. Atlas of clinical sleep medicine. Philadelphia: Saunders/Elsevier; 2010; with permission.)

results of the overnight study[36] showing 57% were CPAP nonresponsive). Furthermore, these patients were confronted with adverse hemodynamic effect of CPAP as a result of increased intrathoracic pressure. In particular, in heart failure patients whose ventricular function (according to the Frank-Starling curve) is preload dependent, any reduction in venous return by the increased intrathoracic pressure, with application of CPAP, could decrease right ventricular stroke volume and, consequently, the preload of the left ventricle, decreasing left ventricular stroke volume enhancing neurohormonal activation, and causing hypotension, diminished coronary blood flow, myocardial ischemia, and arrhythmias. Adverse effect of CPAP on blood pressure is further augmented during sleep when blood pressure normally decreases. In this context, we have reported that in patients with systolic heart failure, a low diastolic blood pressure (a major determinant of coronary blood flow), a low right ventricular ejection fraction, and presence of CSA were independent predictors of mortality.[4]

If the aforementioned assumptions[44] were correct, then, in the Canadian trial,[43] CPAP responders should have had improved survival compared with the untreated control group, and in turn, the control group should have had a better survival compared with CPAP nonresponders. Confirmation came from the post hoc analysis[45] of mortality in the Canadian trial (**Fig. 2**), showing that in those whose CSA responded to CPAP, transplantation-free survival was significantly improved when compared with the untreated control group. In addition, the mortality of CPAP nonresponders seemed the worst, although the number of patients was small for statistical significance.

In the Canadian trial at 3 months, 43% of heart failure patients with CSA were CPAP nonresponsive[44] compared with 57% in our study[36] of first-night use. Typically, CPAP-nonresponsive patients had more severe CSA than CPAP-nonresponsive patients.[36,44] For these patients, and those who are intolerant to CPAP, we recommend use of adaptive pressure support servoventilators devices. These devices act like a buffer ventilator, maintaining stable breathing (buffer PAP). These devices provide varying amounts of inspiratory support (on top of the expiratory pressure) during different phases of periodic breathing. The inspiratory support is variable and proportional; it is minimal (and could be zero in some devices) during the hyperpneic phase of periodic breathing (and when breathing is stable) and is maximal during periods of diminished breathing. In addition, the device initiates a breath on a timely basis aborting any impending apnea. In a newly Food and Drug Administration–approved device, BiPAP autoSV Advanced, the expiratory pressure changes automatically.[46]

There are many short-term studies[46–55] on treatment of CSA in congestive heart failure, generally with excellent results. In an acute (1-night) study of 14 subjects with systolic heart failure and CSA, one of these devices (VPAP Adapt SV, ResMed, San Diego, CA, USA) decreased AHI more than oxygen, CPAP and bilevel devices.[47] In a preliminary study of 10 patients with Hunter-Cheyne-Stokes breathing, another buffer PAP (BiPAP AutoSV Advanced, Monroeville, PA, USA) was effective in treatment of periodic breathing and was superior to CPAP.[46] Similar results were reported by Arzt and colleagues.[54]

In the only randomized, sham-controlled, double-blind, parallel trial of 1 month's duration,[48] VPAP Adapt device decreased AHI from 25 to 5 per hour; in addition, urinary metadrenaline and brain naturetic peptide decreased significantly, although left ventricular ejection fraction did not increase significantly.

I optimistically predict that systematic long-term studies with buffer PAP devices will prove effective in treatment of CSA, which should translate to improved survival of patients with heart failure. In the mean time, these devices are effective in treating CSA and OSA, and because these two forms of sleep disorders commonly occur together in the same patient, the distinction as to which kind of sleep apnea is predominant becomes academic.[55] For elimination of obstructive disordered breathing events, the expiratory pressure is increased using the same protocol as used during CPAP titration. The expiratory pressure is increased to eliminate obstructive apneas, hypopneas, flow limitation,

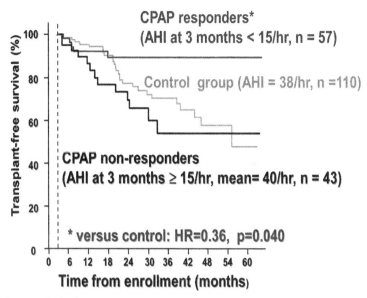

Fig. 2. Transplant-free survival of 210 patients with systolic heart failure and CSA. During the follow-up period, the occurrences of the primary endpoints were 9% in the CPAP responders, 23% in the control untreated group, and 30% in CPAP nonresponders. (*From* Javaheri S. Cardiovascular disorders. In: Kryger MH, editor. Atlas of clinical sleep medicine. Philadelphia: Saunders/Elsevier; 2010; with permission.)

and snoring. The algorithms for pressure increase differ between devices; similarly, the algorithm for pressure support differs among different devices and one needs to be familiar with the algorithm of the device used.

In conclusion, pressure support servoventilator devices are effective in treating sleep apnea in systolic heart failure and I recommend them for heart failure patients who are first-night CPAP nonresponders. In our laboratory, no heart failure patient is discharged with CPAP after overnight CPAP titration unless the AHI was effectively lowered below 15 per hour sleep the night before.

OPIOIDS
Prevalence of Sleep Apnea in Patients Taking Opioids

Ventilatory depression during wakefulness is a well-known effect of opioid drugs. With chronic use, however, daytime hypoventilation is generally mild, but sleep apnea is prevalent.[56–59] Two systematic studies have shown a high prevalence of sleep apnea in this population. In a case control study reported by Walker and associates,[58] 60 patients taking opioids for pain management were matched for age, gender, and body mass, with 60 patients not taking opioids. In patients on opioids, AHI was 44 per hour, which was significantly higher than the AHI in the control group

(30/h). The difference in the two indices was primarily due to an increase in the number of central apneas (13/h) in the opioid group.

In the second study, Webster and associates,[59] being aware of high prevalence of sleep apnea associated with opioids, routinely recommended PSG to 392 consecutive subjects in their pain clinic. Of the 140 subjects who underwent PSG in their institution, 75% had an AHI greater than or equal to 5 per hour, 50% had an AHI greater than or equal to 15 per hour, and 36% had severe sleep apnea with an index of AHI greater than or equal to 30 per hour. As found in other studies, opioid use was associated with a mixed pattern of disordered breathing events characterized by presence of central and obstructive events, although central apneas commonly predominate.

Recently there has been a marked acceleration in the use of opioids for the management of chronic pain. Therefore, with the reported high prevalence of sleep apnea associated with opioids, many patients suffer from sleep apnea. Many patients on opioids are also on benzodiazepines. This combination may be particularly fatal, and sleep apnea could contribute to excess unexplained mortality in this population. In this context, many patients on opioids are found dead in the morning or in bed during the day. Therefore, diagnosis and appropriate treatment of sleep apnea may improve survival of such patients.

Treatment of Opioid-Induced Sleep Apnea

Treatment of sleep apnea due to opioids with CPAP has proved difficult because of simultaneous presence of OSA and CSA, with the latter resistant to therapy.[60] This observation is somewhat similar to that in systolic heart failure (discussed previously). Also similar to that in systolic heart failure, a preliminary study[60] shows that new-generation pressure support servoventilator is effective in the treatment of OSA and CSA associated with use of opioids. Titration with appropriate adjustment of expiratory pressure and inspiratory support, however, is critical[60]; otherwise, residual disordered breathing events remain.

COMPLEX SLEEP APNEA
Prevalence of Complex Sleep Apnea

Few central apneas are often observed in PSGs of patients with OSA and are appropriately ignored because they are of no clinical significance. Some patients referred for evaluation of OSA, however, may develop CSA during initiation of CPAP therapy; others may have excess central apneas to begin with that persists or increases during initiation of CPAP therapy.[61] In others, central apneas go away with continued use of CPAP. The phenotype of the patients and the reasons for evolution of CSA are variable (discussed later).

Presence of CSA (CAI ≥ 5/h) on CPAP could be emergent (ie, was not present on diagnostic PSG) or considered persistent (ie, CSA was also present on diagnostic PSG). The term, *complex sleep apnea*, has been used to denote presence of CSA (CAI ≥ 5/h) along with other disordered breathing events on first-night CPAP titration (**Table 2**).[62]

Prevalence of complex sleep apnea varies from 5% to 20%,[61 66] although most recent studies[61,65,66] show a prevalence of approximately 5% to 6% (**Table 3**).

In our study,[61] which included 1286 patients referred for evaluation of OSA, the monthly incidence of CSA during initial CPAP titration (CPAP1) varied from 3% to 10% during a 1-year period, with an average of 6.5%. One aspect of this study had to do with determination of the natural history of CSA on CPAP. Of the 42 patients who had developed CPAP1-CSA, CSA was eliminated in most with long-term use of CPAP (average therapeutic time on CPAP/night = 5.6 h). Therefore, the

prevalence of CPAP-persistent CSA, CSA present after long-term use, was 1.5%. This decrease in the number of central apneas with continued use of CPAP is consistent with results of two tracheotomy studies and one CPAP study in which OSA patients underwent serial PSGs. In an early study, Guilleminault and colleagues[67] showed that OSA patients who underwent therapeutic tracheotomy initially had CSA, which decreased later on a repeat PSG. A similar observation was reported by Coccagna and colleagues.[68] In the serial CPAP study of Dernaika and colleagues,[63] most of the CSAs had resolved 9 weeks later in 12 of the 14 patients who had a repeat PSG, yielding an estimate of 1.5% for persistent CSA, the prevalence observed in our study.[61]

The reasons for a low prevalence of complex sleep apnea in the Cincinnati study,[61] compared with that in the Mayo study[62] and some other studies,[63,64] have to do with several issues, including the large number of patients enrolled in our study and separate full-night diagnostic and CPAP titration PSGs (not split-night study), followed by an additional third-night CPAP/PSG after long-term use of CPAP. In three studies[62–64] of high prevalence of complex sleep apnea, several patients were enrolled if they had CPAP-CSA during the second half of a split-night study. Half-night CPAP titration is not representative of the whole night, and, in addition, in a split-night study, placement of the mask and a rapidly escalating pressure for hasty titration during the second half of the night could be disruptive to sleep, resulting in arousals and transitions in sleep stages with consequent fluctuation in P_{CO_2}, which could promote instability of breathing. Consequences of disruptive sleep could account for most central apneas on the first night or even full night of CPAP titration, as in our study,[61] such patients had many arousals that contributed to instability of breathing, increasing the likelihood of central apneas; that CSA goes away in most patients with continued use of, and adaptation with, CPAP is consistent with this notion. In addition to disruptive sleep as a cause of CSA with CPAP, rapid titration, overtitration, or a combination thereof could potentially lead to oral leak, which, if long enough could polygraphically appear as a central apnea. Excess pressure, in particular, by increasing lung volume may activate lung stretch receptors, inhibiting central respiratory motor output. In this regard, we did find excessive numbers of central apneas at high CPAP levels in a few patients, but central apneas also occurred frequently at CPAP levels as low as 5 cm H_2O (**Fig. 3**).

Table 2
Distribution of central apneas across the night at various CPAP levels in a typical patient

	Complex Sleep Apnea				
CPAP (cm H_2O)	CA (#)	OA (#)	HYP (#)	AHI Index	Low SaO_2
6	0	0	1	50	91%
7	1	0	15	108	89%
8	4	0	26	72	86%
9	5	0	11	107	87%
10	3	0	6	98	85%
11	7	0	9	31	85%
12	8	0	3	12	81%
13	47	1	22	91	87%
14	57	0	7	113	86%
15	12	1	4	91	91%
16	7	0	0	40	93%

Note presence of central apneas, obstructive disordered breathing events, including obstructive apneas, and oxyhemoglobin desaturatuion across the night, from low to high pressures as CPAP level progressively increased.

Abbreviations: AHI, apnea-hypopnea index; CA, central apnea; HYP, hypopnea; OA, obstructive apnea; SaO_2, saturation measured by pulse oximetry.

There is at least one more reason for presence of complex sleep apnea[69] on the first night of CPAP exposure and its elimination with continued use of CPAP. It is conceivable that such patients have increased loop gain manifested in increased chemosensitivity above and below eupnea, similar to patients with systolic heart failure.[7] Increased loop gain predisposes patients to central apneas. Using proportional assist ventilation to assess loop gain during sleep, Younes and colleagues[70] showed that patients with severe OSA (AHI = 88/h), compared with those who mild to moderate OSA

(AHI = 27/h), had increased loop gain. This finding has important implications to CPAP-emergent and -persistent CSA. We found that one of the risk factors for long-term CPAP-persistent CSA was the severity of OSA (**Table 4**). In our study,[61] the baseline AHI of those with persistent CSA (after long-term use of CPAP) was 79 per hour compared with 39 per hour in those without CPAP-emergent CSA and 56 per hour (P = .02) compared with those who had CSA on the first-night exposure to CPAP but not with long-term (several weeks) use. The results of other studies

Table 3
Prevalence of complex sleep apnea

Author/Site (y)	n	Complex Sleep Apnea	PSG	AHI (n/h)	Follow-up PSG
Morgenthaler/ Rochester, USA (2006)	223	15%	Split	32	—
Derniaka/Oklahoma, USA (2006)	116	20%	Split	51	2%
Lehman/Adelaide, Australia (2007)	99	13%	Mixed	72	—
Javaheri/Cincinnati, USA (2009)	1286	6.5%	Full night	57	2%
Endo/Japan (2007)	1232	5.3%	Full night	59	—
Yaegashi/Japan (2009)	297	5.7%	Full night	56	—

In two studies in which CPAP had been used long-term, the prevalence of complex sleep apnea decreased to approximately 2%.

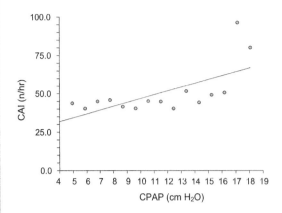

n   84 84 84 82 82 76 60 45 36 26 16 11 6   3   1

Fig. 3. Average CAI at various CPAP levels in 84 patients. Central apneas occurred at various CPAP levels, though increased much at very high pressures. (*From* Javaheri S, Smith J and Chung J. The prevalence and Natural history of complex sleep apnea. J Clin Sleep Med 2009;5:205–11; with permission.)

seem consistent with our observation (see **Table 4**) and that of Younes and colleagues.[70] I hypothesize that, due to severity of sleep apnea, these patients have such a heightened chemosensitivity (increased loop gain), which, after elimination of sleep apnea with CPAP, would take a long time to normalize. Anecdotally, in one of our patients who continued to have CSA on CPAP after few weeks (CPAP2), CSA was eliminated a few weeks later on a repeat PSG (S. Javaheri, MD, unpublished data). Salloum and colleagues[71] have shown that patients with OSA have increased CO_2 chemosensitivity below eupnea, a finding similar to patients with systolic heart failure[9] (discussed previously). In these patients, Pco_2 failed to increase on sleep onset, a finding similar to that in patients with systolic heart failure. In the latter patients, we have hypothesized[7] that the lack of rise in Pco_2 is due to concomitant presence

of left ventricular diastolic dysfunction; the same may apply to OSA patients, some of whom may suffer from diastolic dysfunction.

Treatment of Complex Sleep Apnea

Controlled randomized clinical trials to assist sleep physicians in making appropriate therapeutic decisions are lacking. Based on the aforementioned data, our approach to finding CSA (CAI ≥ 5/h) on the first night of CPAP titration is to call patients back for follow-up within few days to discuss the reasons for CSA and to take appropriate therapeutic steps. Because most commonly these central apneas are eliminated with continued use of CPAP, I assure patients and encourage adherence. I may lower the pressure if overtitration is suspected. Many patients with CSA on the first night of CPAP titration report oral leak, which is often noticed by a technician. Under such circumstances, the excess pressure forces the mouth open and, graphically, oral leak appears as a central apnea (this is a pseudo-CSA). At times, a night technician may use a chin strap (which frequently is ineffective) or switch from a nose mask to a naso-oral mask. In that case, during the follow-up, if I lower the air pressure, I may switch back to a nose mask or discontinue the use of chin strap. I assure patients that with continued use of CPAP, CSA will go away. There are some exceptions, however, such as CSA associated with opioids, systolic heart failure, and some cases of atrial fibrillation.

What should be done for the 2% to 3% of OSA patients with persistent CSA after long-term use of CPAP? If a patient is nonadherent to CPAP or continues to be symptomatic (eg, excessive daytime sleepiness), I recommend a titration with a pressure support servoventilator. The process of titration is critical in elimination of disordered breathing (discussed previously).

Table 4
Comparison of AHI in OSA patients with and without complex sleep apnea

	Without	With
Morgenthaler	21	32[a]
Dernaika	47	51
Lehman	53	72[a]
Javaheri	39	79[a]
Endo	49	59[a]
Yaegashi	49	56 (NR)

In study by the author, the apnea-hypopnea index of 79 belongs to patients who had persistent central apneas after longterm (several weeks) use of CPAP.
Abbreviation: NR, not reported.
[a] Statistically significant.

SUMMARY

There are many causes of CSA[5,10] (see **Box 1**). This article has briefly reviewed CSA associated with three specific conditions: systolic heart failure, opioids, and complex sleep apnea. In systolic heart failure, many patients have CSA to begin with. In almost half of these patients, CSAs are eliminated with initiation of CPAP therapy, and these patients survive long. In those heart failure patients who have CSA on the first night of CPAP titration, central apneas remain CPAP resistant (ie, they do not go away with continued use of CPAP). In this group of patients, continued use of CPAP contributes to poor survival and they must stop using CPAP. Preliminary studies show that these patients can be effectively treated with the new pressure support servoventilators. Randomized clinical trials are in progress.

The story of opioids is different from systolic heart failure in that in these individuals central apneas remain resistant to CPAP, not going away with continued use of CPAP. Therefore, our approach to treatment of disordered breathing events in patients on opioids is to proceed to the new-generation pressure support servoventilaton devices (without a trial of CPAP). Preliminary studies show that these devices are effective in improving opioid-associated disordered breathing events.

The approach to complex sleep apnea is different from that to systolic heart failure and to opioid-associated sleep apnea. Complex sleep apnea refers to the presence of central apneas along with hypopneas during initiation of CPAP therapy. Our experience is consistent with the notion that in most individuals, with continued use of CPAP, these apneas go away. Therefore, there is no need to switch to more expensive and perhaps deleterious therapeutic options. In a few of these patients, however, central apnea persists and is resistant to CPAP. In these individuals, if they continue to be symptomatic, intolerant to CPAP, or noncompliant with it, I recommend a trial of the new-generation pressure support servoventilator devices. Long-term trials are needed to determine whether or not the persistence of central apneas in otherwise asymptomatic patients needs any treatment if at all.

REFERENCES

1. Javaheri S. Heart failure. In: Kryger MH, Roth T, Dement WC, editors. Principles and practices of sleep medicine. 5th edition. Philadelphia: WB Saunders Company; 2010, in press.
2. Javaheri S. Sleep dysfunction in heart failure. Curr Treat Options Neurol 2008;10:323–35.
3. Javaheri S. Sleep-related breathing disorders in heart failure. In: Mann DL, editor. Heart failure, a companion to Braunwald's heart disease. Philadelphia: WB Saunders; 2010, in press.
4. Javaheri S, Shukla R, Zeigler H, et al. Central sleep apnea, right ventricular dysfunction and low diastolic blood pressure are predictors of mortality in systolic heart failure. J Am Coll Cardiol 2007;49: 2028–38.
5. Javaheri S. Central sleep apnea. In: Lee-Chiong T, editor. Sleep medicine essentials. Hoboken (NJ): Wiley-Blackwell; 2009. p. 81–9.
6. Skatrud JB, Dempsey JA. Interaction of sleep state and chemical stimuli in sustaining rhythmic ventilation. J Appl Physiol 1983;55:813–22.
7. Javaheri S, Dempsey J. Mechanisms of sleep apnea and periodic breathing in systolic heart failure. In: Lee-Chiong T, editor. Sleep medicine clinics: sleep and cardiovascular disease. Philadelphia: WB Saunders; 2007. p. 623–30. Guest editor: S Javaheri.
8. Nakayama H, Smith CA, Rodman JR, et al. Effect of ventilatory drive on CO_2 sensitivity below eupnea during sleep. Am J Respir Crit Care Med 2002; 165:1251–8.
9. Xie A, Skatrud JB, Puleo DS, et al. Apnea-hypopnea threshold for CO_2 in patients with congestive heart failure. Am J Respir Crit Care Med 2002;165: 1245–50.
10. Javaheri S. Central sleep apnea. In: Lee-Chiong T, editor. Sleep: a comprehensive handbook. New Jersey: Wiley-liss; 2006. p. 46–62.
11. Javaheri S. A mechanism of central sleep apnea in patients with heart failure. N Engl J Med 1999;341: 949–54.
12. Heart disease and stroke statistics—2009 update. Circulation 2009;119:e1–161.
13. Ward M. Periodic respiration. A short historical note. Ann R Coll Surg Engl 1973;52:330–4.
14. Cheyne J. A case of apoplexy, in which the fleshy part of the heart was converted into fat. Dublin Hospital Reports and Communications 1818;2:216–23.
15. Javaheri S, Parker TJ, Wexler L, et al. Occult sleep-disordered breathing in stable congestive heart failure. Ann Intern Med 1995;122:487–92 [erratum in: Ann Intern Med 1995;123:77].
16. Hanly PJ, Millar TW, Steljes DG, et al. Respiration and abnormal sleep in patients with congestive heart failure. Chest 1989;96:480–8.
17. Javaheri S, Parker TJ, Liming JD, et al. Sleep apnea in 81 ambulatory male patients with stable heart failure: types and their prevalences, consequences, and presentations. Circulation 1998;97:2154–9.
18. Javaheri S. Sleep disorders in 100 male patients with systolic heart failure. A prospective study. Int J Cardiol 2006;106:21–8.
19. Tremel F, Pépin J-L, Veale D, et al. High prevalence and persistence of sleep apnea in patients referred

for acute left ventricular failure and medically treated over 2 months. Eur Heart J 1999;20:1201–9.

20. Solin P, Bergin P, Richardson M, et al. Influence of pulmonary capillary wedge pressure on central apnea in heart failure. Circulation 1999;99:1574–9.

21. Sin DD, Fitzgerald F, Parker JD, et al. Risk factors for central and obstructive sleep apnea in 450 men and women with congestive heart failure. Am J Respir Crit Care Med 1999;160:1101–6.

22. Yasuma F, Nomura H, Hayashi H, et al. Breathing abnormalities during sleep in patients with chronic heart failure. Jap Circ J 1989;53:1506–10.

23. Lofaso F, Verschueren P, Rande JLD, et al. Prevalence of sleep-disordered breathing in patients on a heart transplant waiting list. Chest 1994;106:1689–94.

24. Ferrier K, Campbell A, Yee B, et al. Sleep-disordered breathing occurs frequently in stable outpatients with congestive heart failure. Chest 2005;128:2116–22.

25. Staniforth AD, Kinnear WJM, Starling R, et al. Nocturnal desaturation in patients with stable heart failure. Heart 1998;79:394–9.

26. Lanfranchi PA, Braghiroli A, Bosimini E, et al. Prognostic value of nocturnal Cheyne-Stokes respiration in chronic heart failure. Circulation 1999;99:1435–40.

27. Vazir A, Hastings PC, Dayer M, et al. A high prevalence of sleep disorder breathing in men with mild symptomatic chronic heart failure due to left ventricular systolic dysfunction. Eur J Heart Fail 2007;9:243–50.

28. Oldenburg O, Lamp B, Faber L, et al. Sleep disordered breathing in patients with symptomatic heart failure: a contemporary study of prevalence in and characteristics of 700 patients. Eur J Heart Fail 2007;9:251–7.

29. MacDonald M, Fang J, Pittman SD, et al. The current prevalence of sleep disordered breathing in congestive heart failure patients treated with beta-blockers. J Clin Sleep Med 2008;4:38–42.

30. Wang H, Parker JD, Newton GE, et al. Influence of obstructive sleep apnea on mortality in patients with heart failure. J Am Coll Cardiol 2007;49:1625–31.

31. Javaheri S. Treatment of obstructive and central sleep apnoea in heart failure: practical options. Eur Respir Rev 2007;16:183–8.

32. Javaheri S. Pembrey's dream: the time has come for a long-term trial of nocturnal supplemental nasal oxygen to treat central sleep apnea in congestive heart failure. Chest 2003;123:322–5.

33. Javaheri S, Parker TJ, Wexler L, et al. Effect of theophylline on sleep-disordered breathing in heart failure. N Engl J Med 1996;335:562–7.

34. Javaheri S. Acetazolamide improves central sleep apnea in heart failure: a double-blind prospective study. Am J Respir Crit Care Med 2006;173:234–7.

35. Javaheri S, Abraham WT, Brown C, et al. Prevalence of obstructive sleep apnea and periodic limb movement in 45 subjects with heart transplantation. Eur Heart J. 2004;25:260–6.

36. Javaheri S. Effects of continuous positive airway pressure on sleep apnea and ventricular irritability in patients with heart failure. Circulation 2000;101:392–7.

37. Javaheri S. Heart failure and sleep apnea: emphasis on practical therapeutic options. Clin Chest Med 2003;24:207–22 Chest Clinics of North America, W.B. Saunders, New York.

38. Naughton MT, Liu PP, Benard DC, et al. Treatment of congestive heart failure and Cheyne-Stokes respiration during sleep by continuous positive airway pressure. Am J Respir Crit Care Med 1995;151:92–7.

39. Sin DD, Logan AG, Fitzgerald FS, et al. Effects of continuous positive airway pressure on cardiovascular outcomes in heart failure patients with and without Cheyne-Stokes respiration. Circulation 2000;102:61–6.

40. Guilleminault C, Clerk A, Labanowski M, et al. Cardiac failure and benzodiazepines. Sleep 1993;16:524–8.

41. Davies RJ, Harrington KJ, Ormerod OJ, et al. Nasal continuous positive airway pressure in chronic heart failure with sleep- disordered breathing. Am Rev Respir Dis 1993;147:630–4.

42. Buckle P, Millar T, Kryger M. The effects of short-term nasal CPAP on Cheyne-Stokes respiration in congestive heart failure. Chest 1992;102:31–5.

43. Bradley T, Logan A, Kimoff J, et al. Continuous positive airway pressure for central sleep apnea and heart failure. N Engl J Med 2006;353:2025–33.

44. Javaheri S. CPAP should not be used for central sleep apnea in congestive heart failure patients. J Clin Sleep Med 2006;2:399–402.

45. Arzt M, Floras JS, Logan AG, et al. Suppression of central sleep apnea by continuous positive airway pressure and transplant-free survival in heart failure. A post-hoc analysis of the Canadian Continuous Positive Airway Pressure for patients with central sleep apnea and heart failure trial (CANPAP). Circulation 2007;115:3173–80.

46. Javaheri S, Khayat R, Goodwin J, et al. Complex central sleep apnea (COMP CSA) treatment with auto servoventilation. Chest 2009;136:43S.

47. Teschler H, Döhring J, Wang YM, et al. Adaptive pressure support servo-ventilation. Am J Respir Crit Care Med 2001;164:614–9.

48. Pepperell J, Maskell NA, Jones DR, et al. A randomized controlled trial of adaptive ventilation for Cheyne-Stokes breathing in heart failure. Am J Respir Crit Care Med 2003;168:1109–14.

49. Philippe C, Stoica-Herman M, Drouot X, et al. Compliance with and effectiveness of adaptive servoventilation versus continuous positive airway pressure in the treatment of Cheyne-Stokes respiration in heart failure over a six month period. Heart 2006;92:337–42.

50. Szollosi I, O'Driscoll DM, Dayer MJ, et al. Adaptive servo-ventilation and deadspace: effects on central sleep apnoea. J Sleep Res 2006;15:199–205.

51. Kasai T, Narui K, Dohi T, et al. First experience of using new adaptive servo-ventilation device for Cheyne-Stokes respiration with central sleep apnea among Japanese patients with congestive heart failure. Circ J 2006;70:1148–54.

52. Fietze I, Blau A, Glos M, et al. Bi-level positive pressure ventilation and adaptive servo ventilation in patients with heart failure and Cheyne-Stokes respiration. Sleep Med 2008;9:652–9.

53. Oldenburg O, Schmidt A, Lamp B, et al. Adaptive servoventilation improved cardiac function in patients with chronic heart failure and Cheyne-Stokes respiration. Eur J Heart Fail 2008;10:581–6.

54. Arzt M, Wensel R, Montalvan S, et al. Effects of dynamic bilevel positive airway pressure support on central sleep apnea in men with heart failure. Chest 2008;134:61–6.

55. Randerath W, Galetke W, Stieglitz S, et al. Adaptive servo-ventilation in patients with coexisting obstructive sleep apnoea/hypopnoea and Cheyne-Stokes respiration. Sleep Med 2008;9:823–30.

56. Teichtahl H, Prodromidis A, Miller B, et al. Sleep-disordered breathing in stable methadone programme patients: a pilot study. Addiction 2001;96:395–403.

57. Fareny RJ, Walker JM, Cloward RS. Sleep-disordered breathing associated with long-term opioid therapy. Chest 2003;123:632–9.

58. Walker M, Farney J, Rhondeau SM, et al. Chronic opioid use a risk factor for the development of central sleep apnea and ataxic breathing. J Clin Sleep Med 2007;3:455–61.

59. Webster L, Choi Y, Desai H, et al. Sleep disordered breathing and chronic opioid therapy. Pain Med 2008;9:425–32.

60. Javaheri S, Malik A, Smith J, et al. Adaptive pressure support servoventilation: a novel treatment for sleep apnea associated with use of opioids. J Clin Sleep Med 2008;4:305–10.

61. Javaheri S, Smith J, Chung J. The prevalence and natural history of complex sleep apnea. J Clin Sleep Med 2009;5:205–11.

62. Morgenthaler T, Kagramanov V, Hanak V, et al. Complex sleep apnea syndrome: is it a unique clinical syndrome? Sleep 2006;29:1203–8.

63. Dernaika T, Tawk M, Nazir S, et al. The significance and outcome of continuous positive airway pressure-related central sleep apnea during split-night sleep studies. Chest 2007;132:81–8.

64. Lehman S, Anic N, Thompson C, et al. Central sleep apnea on commencement of continuous positive airway pressure in patient with primary diagnosis of obstructive sleep apnea-hyperpnoea. J Clin Sleep Med 2007;3:462–6.

65. Endo Y, Suzuki M, Inoue Y, et al. Prevalence of complex sleep apnea among Japanese patients with sleep apnea syndrome. Tohoku J Exp Med 2008;215:349–54.

66. Yaegashi H, Fujimoto K, Abe H, et al. Characteristics of Japanese patients with complex sleep apnea syndrome: a retrospective comparison with obstructive sleep apnea syndrome. Intern Med 2009;48:427–32.

67. Guilleminault C, Simmons B, Motta J, et al. Obstructive sleep apnea syndrome and tracheostomy. Arch Intern Med 1981;141:985–8.

68. Coccagna G, Mantovani M, Brignani F, et al. Tracheostomy in hypersomnia with periodic breathing. Bull Physiopathol Respir (Nancy) 1972;8:1217–27.

69. Malhotra A, Bertisch S, Wellman A. Complex sleep apnea: it isn't really a disease. J Clin Sleep Med 2008;4:1–2.

70. Younes M, Ostrowski M, Thompson W, et al. Chemical control stability in patients with obstructive sleep apnea. Am J Respir Crit Care Med 2001;163:1181–90.

71. Salloum A, Rowley JA, Mateika JH, et al. Increased propensity for central sleep apnea in patients with obstructive sleep apnea; effect of continuous positive airway pressure. Am J Respir Crit Care Med 2010;181:189–93.

Adaptive Servo-Ventilation for Sleep Apnea: Technology, Titration Protocols, and Treatment Efficacy

Lee K. Brown, MD, BS (Electrical Engineering)[a,b,*]

KEYWORDS

- Sleep apnea • Hypoventilation • Ventilatory support
- Mechanical ventilation • Noninvasive ventilation

General Bogan: Mr Knapp here knows as much about electronic gear as anyone. He'd like to say something.

Gordon Knapp: The more complex an electronic system gets, the more accident prone it is. Sooner or later it breaks down.

Secretary Swenson: What breaks down?

Gordon Knapp: A transistor blows... a condenser burns out... sometimes they just get tired—like people.

Professor Groeteschele: Mr Knapp overlooks one factor, the machines are supervised by humans. Even if the machine fails a human can always correct the mistake.

Gordon Knapp: I wish you were right. The fact is, the machines work so fast... they are so intricate... the mistakes they make are so subtle... that very often a human being just can't know whether a machine is lying or telling the truth.

Fail-Safe (1964), Directed by Sidney Lumet. Based on the novel 'Fail-Safe' by Eugene Burdick and Harvey Wheeler.

It is important to remember that any feedback control system (and an adaptive servo-ventilator is surely such a system) must be furnished with a set of operating parameters and constraints. Because few control systems can be designed to account for every possible variation in the greater environment in which it operates, those responsible for designing the system must consider incorporating into the design the ability for the operator to adjust these parameters and constraints to account for such variations. This is particularly true for feedback control systems that interact with the human organism in disease, given that much harm can occur if the system fails to adequately maintain its controlled variable within physiologic bounds.[1]

Financial disclosures: L.K.B. recently completed terms on the boards of directors of the American Academy of Sleep Medicine, Associated Professional Sleep Societies LLC, and American Sleep Medicine Foundation. He currently receives no grant or commercial funding pertinent to the subject of this article but was the recipient of grant funding from ResMed Inc. between 2004 and 2005 for an investigation involving the AutoSet CS2.

[a] Division of Pulmonary, Critical Care, and Sleep Medicine, Department of Internal Medicine, University of New Mexico School of Medicine, MSC10 5550, 1 University of New Mexico, Albuquerque, NM 87131-0001, USA
[b] Program in Sleep Medicine, University of New Mexico Health Sciences Center, 1101 Medical Arts Avenue North East, Building 2, Albuquerque, NM 87102, USA
* Division of Pulmonary, Critical Care, and Sleep Medicine, Department of Internal Medicine, University of New Mexico School of Medicine, MSC10 5550, 1 University of New Mexico, Albuquerque, NM 87131-0001.
E-mail address: lkbrown@alum.mit.edu

Sleep Med Clin 5 (2010) 419–437
doi:10.1016/j.jsmc.2010.05.004

ADAPTIVE SERVO-VENTILATION AND RELATED DEVICES: HISTORICAL CONTEXT

The history of automating the control of mechanical ventilation in human disease dates back more than 30 years, with a report from Menn and colleagues[2] of a computerized decision support tool. In such systems, information concerning the clinical status of the patient is evaluated by the computer, which outputs recommended changes in ventilator settings that must be instituted by an intervening human operator. A variety of computerized decision support tools were subsequently described up through the early 1990s in relation to tasks such as weaning from mechanical ventilation,[3] determining ventilator settings (tidal volume, respiratory rate, and so forth) for standard ventilator modes,[4] and recommending settings for complex respiratory assist devices in the treatment of adult respiratory distress syndrome (ARDS)[5,6] and chronic obstructive pulmonary disease (COPD).[7] All of these methodologies interposed a human being—a clinician—between the decisions made by the computer and any actual changes in ventilator settings, much as a human being—a member of the military—was at first interposed between the receipt of a firing command and the actual firing of a missile, as in the prologue to *Fail-Safe*. Of importance is that clinician disagreement with a significant proportion (6%–10%) of expert system instructions was reported in the ARDS studies[5,6] and more than one-quarter of the time in the COPD study.[7]

Not long after the advent of computerized expert systems, reports also began appearing of the use of computers to control the process of weaning from mechanical ventilation without the interposition of a clinician. Initially, minute ventilation was measured and either the number of machine-initiated breaths or the level of pressure support (PS) was varied to achieve a minute ventilation target (mandatory minute volume, MMV).[8,9] Unfortunately, no evidence ever appeared suggesting that these strategies resulted in better clinical outcomes.[10] The description of the rapid shallow breathing index by Yang and Tobin[11] led some investigators to explore the use of this parameter to automatically determine changes in synchronized intermittent mandatory ventilation (SIMV) rate and PS, with improved outcomes as compared with a control group in terms of time to weaning and number of arterial blood gas draws, although subject numbers were low.[12] At approximately the same time, the concept of adaptive support ventilation (ASV) was introduced as a technique not just for weaning but also for initial and ongoing ventilator management in critically ill patients.[13] This technology, similar in concept to that of noninvasive adaptive servo-ventilation, also eliminated the human clinician from the control loop. Initial target minute ventilation was entered by the operator, following which a standard set of SIMV settings for a limited period of time were used to gather various pieces of data including properties such as anatomic dead space, total respiratory system compliance, and RC time constant. Thereafter, the controller varied respiratory rate and PS consistent with the target minute ventilation and the ongoing collection of gas exchange and mechanical parameters, as well as theoretical considerations pertaining to minimizing work of breathing. Over the ensuing years, descriptions of ever more sophisticated ASV systems have appeared that incorporated additional measured input variables (eg, oxyhemoglobin saturation, functional residual capacity) and controlled more aspects of the mechanical ventilator (eg, positive end-expiratory pressure, FIO_2, flow rates, I/E ratio).[14–19] However, serious difficulties remain in relinquishing control to the computer for ventilator management, in part related to problems designing systems that can accommodate a wide spectrum of respiratory pathophysiology (eg, obstructive airways disease) and a lack of randomized controlled trials.[20] Despite more than 30 years' research and development of computer-controlled invasive mechanical ventilation, approval to market such devices (let alone wide-scale deployment of them) has lagged.

Automated control of positive airway pressure devices for the treatment of sleep-disordered breathing in the home has not suffered the same fate, presumably because the apparatus is noninvasive and the patients are considerably less fragile clinically. Originally described in the mid-1990s,[21–23] autotitrating continuous positive airway pressure devices (auto-CPAP) were approved by the US Food and Drug Administration (FDA) in 1999. Unlike the situation pertaining to invasive ASV, several randomized controlled trials and one meta-analysis of smaller studies (all considered level 1 evidence after Sackett[24]) tend to support the efficacy of certain of these devices. Still, the latest American Academy of Sleep Medicine (AASM) guidelines state that auto-CPAP only "may" be used for out-of-laboratory CPAP titration, grading the recommendation at the "Option" level indicating uncertain clinical utility. Furthermore, the AASM recommendation limits their use only to patients having moderate to severe obstructive sleep apnea (OSA) who have no significant comorbidities.[25] Two additional factors complicate the status of auto-CPAP for widespread clinical use. First, the specific manner in which a given brand and model measures respiratory events, and the algorithm each uses to determine the extent and timing of pressure changes, are rarely or never published in detail due to proprietary concerns. Moreover, changes in these parameters may be made from time to time in production and not widely publicized, as has been demonstrated in bench tests of seemingly identical models over a 5-year span.[26] Second, wide variations have been shown to occur with respect to how different brands and models respond to standardized simulations of sleep-disordered breathing,[27–31] and can differ significantly in their determination of the optimum CPAP setting in any given patient.[32–38] Data such as these suggest that the performance of each individual make, model, and version of an autotitrating CPAP device should be the subject of more rigorous testing and reporting so as to facilitate more informed prescribing.[39] Alternatively, one group has suggested that the algorithms used by autotitrating CPAP be more standardized,[29] and another option would consist of prescribing only autotitrating CPAP generators that have performed well in randomized controlled trials. The latter strategy presupposes that manufacturers resist making substantive changes in the technology and algorithms employed as they market newer versions of their devices, no doubt an unrealistic assumption. Another option, sleep laboratory testing of the specific make, model, and version of the autotitrating CPAP device on the patient for whom it is prescribed, is clearly impractical given the volume involved, but may be the best choice in more difficult situations such as when complex sleep apnea syndromes are treated with ASV, as is further discussed herein.[40]

In 1999, Berthon-Jones applied for a United States patent (granted in 2003 and assigned to ResMed, Ltd, North Ride, Australia) covering most of the underlying technology for a bilevel PAP device that would vary the degree of PS to maintain a percentage of measured long-term spontaneous minute ventilation.[41] Teschler and colleagues[42] successfully employed a device derived from this patent (AutoSet CS, ResMed, Sydney, Australia) in a group of patients with Cheyne-Stokes respiration (CSR) and congestive heart failure (CHF) in 2001. The AutoSet CS used an algorithm that reportedly varied PS to achieve 90% of the measured long-term minute ventilation, but was housed in a modified Sullivan IV CPAP case, making it somewhat large and bulky. A more compact version (AutoSet CS2) was marketed in Europe some time later, and in 2006 a slightly modified version was marketed in the

United States (renamed the VPAP Adapt SV) following a successful clinical trial.[43] Meanwhile, Hill filed for a patent in 2001 (granted in 2004 and assigned to Respironics, Inc, Murrysville, PA) that embodied much of the technology that appeared in the Respironics BiPAP autoSV and later, the BiPAP autoSV Advanced.[44] The actual patent makes for interesting reading, as it incorporates peak inspiratory flow as the parameter used to determine the level of PS, which is perhaps not as intuitive as the recent average ventilation target used by ResMed but presumably avoids the issue of patent infringement. The Hill patent also described additional strategies for normalizing respiration, including an algorithm for automatically setting a backup respiratory rate, and a process for titrating expiratory positive airway pressure (EPAP; also termed end-expiratory pressure or EEP in some of the literature, but EPAP will be used exclusively hereafter) to aid in the elimination of CSR. The former technique seems to have been incorporated into both BiPAP autoSV models, while the latter does not yet seem to have been implemented commercially; as is described below, the Advanced model uses the older REMStar Auto algorithm aimed strictly at obstructive events. It is interesting that despite using a radically different target for the PS algorithm (peak inspiratory flow rather than minute ventilation), US FDA 510(k) marketing approval was sought on the basis that the BiPAP autoSV was substantially equivalent to the ResMed VPAP Adapt. According to the application, "…comprehensive bench testing was performed…including collecting waveform performance data, triggering data, alarms data, and overall event diction [sic?] and control data for comparison to the VPAP Adapt," and this view was sustained by the FDA in February of 2007.[45] Clearance of the ResMed VPAP Adapt SV was itself approved by the FDA on the basis of "substantial equivalence" with the VPAP III ST-A, an interesting glimpse into how little significance the FDA places on major changes in technology.[46] In 2006, the first published data on the clinical use of BiPAP autoSV appeared in the form of a small case series reporting the successful treatment of 4 patients with CSR and CHF.[47] Respironics also markets a generator that is not, strictly speaking, an ASV device. The BiPAP AVAPS (average volume assured pressure support) model uses an operator-set target tidal volume rather than an ongoing assessment of the patient's breathing pattern to determine the level of PS, and is therefore marketed as a noninvasive positive pressure ventilator. A similar device was reported to successfully treat patients with severe OSA,[48] and conceivably may have utility in managing central sleep apnea (CSA) and complex sleep apnea syndromes. However, no reports of such use are available, and therefore the BiPAP AVAPS is not discussed further here. A third company, Weinmann Medical Technology (Hamburg, Germany), also markets an ASV device that is available in most countries but not currently in the United States. The SOMNOvent CR adjusts EPAP, PS, and end-expiratory positive airway pressure (EEPAP) based on measurements of average minute ventilation, flattening of the inspiratory limb of the flow versus time waveform or absent flow, and snoring.[49] In addition, this device incorporates either a manual setting or automatic determination of a backup rate. The SOMNOvent CR is discussed here only in the context of the somewhat similar Bilevel autoSV Advanced flow generator that is currently available in the United States.

TECHNICAL AND CLINICAL ASPECTS OF THE AVAILABLE DEVICES

In general, specific technical information concerning the manner in which each device measures various input variables, and the algorithms by which they compute changes in EPAP, PS, and backup rate, are closely held by each manufacturer as being highly proprietary in nature. Sources of such information include equipment brochures, published scientific articles, and patents applied for or granted. The latter are not necessarily of great utility, as patent descriptions are frequently broad in nature in order to secure exclusive rights to as much of the art as possible; thus, a given device may not include every feature described in a patent, and the specific implementation of a given technique may not be discernible. In addition, any particular device may incorporate technology from earlier patents assigned to the manufacturer or technology that is licensed from the holders of other patents, making it excessively laborious to associate a given device with any specific patent. In the following descriptions, information that is more uncertain is identified; moreover, some details may change as each particular model is replaced by newer versions.

RESMED VPAP ADAPT SV
Flow Generator Characteristics

The VPAP Adapt SV flow generator differs from most other such devices in that the hose connecting the mask to the generator incorporates an additional small-bore tube for sampling pressure near the mask, and consequently other brands of PAP hoses cannot be used. The generator is available with or without an integral humidifier, with the basic unit weighing just under 4 kg (the empty humidifier adds about 0.5 kg). Sound pressure level is specified as less than 30 dBA. The device can record compliance data onto a plug-in memory module, and will sense whether the patient is wearing the interface allowing it to stop and start the blower automatically. A ramp feature is not available in the ASV mode. ResMed seems to encourage the use of only specific interfaces of their own manufacture, including several different nasal and full face masks (both hospital and outpatient types) but not nasal pillows. The algorithm accounts for the type of interface being used through manual entry of the ResMed product name and then a "learn" algorithm during which various calibrations are made with the interface off of the patient. The following alarms are available: high maximum pressure; high mean mask pressure; low mask pressure; insufficient PS; high leak; flow blocked. The flow generator is specified for working pressures between 4 and 25 cm H_2O, with EPAP adjustable from 4 to 15 cm H_2O. A further limit constrains maximum PS (inspiratory PAP [IPAP] minus EPAP) to 16 cm H_2O.[50] The manufacturer notes that the device's inherent inspiratory triggering sensitivity is also predicated on the assumption that only patients with "essentially normal lungs" will use the device.[51]

Respiratory Parameter Determination and Control Algorithm

A microcontroller (similar to the central processing unit integrated circuit in a personal computer) is the basis of operation for all ASV devices. The microcontroller receives digital representations of the various pressure and flow measurements, rapidly performs the necessary and often complex computations based on these inputs, and then outputs electrical signals that control various functions such as blower speed and the operation of valves that determine respiratory phase. The VPAP Adapt SV determines instantaneous respiratory airflow using techniques common to several previous generations of CPAP and bilevel PAP devices. The method described in the patent consists of first estimating instantaneous mask leak, then subtracting this from total mask airflow.[41] Instantaneous mask leak is computed by measuring instantaneous mask airflow and pressure, low-pass filtered to eliminate high-frequency noise; the conductance (inverse of resistance) of the sum of the leakage pathways is estimated by dividing instantaneous mask airflow by the square root of instantaneous mask pressure; mask leak is then derived from this conductance multiplied by the square root of the instantaneous mask pressure. Once respiratory airflow has been determined, the microprocessor "learns" the patient's recent average ventilation by continuously computing the absolute value of the 100-second low-pass filtered instantaneous respiratory airflow. Note that a low-pass filter, especially one with such a long time constant, is essentially computing the integral of the instantaneous respiratory airflow and therefore the result is proportional to average ventilation. In addition, the patent document specifies that the length of the time constant is chosen to exceed the typical lung-chemoreceptor delay time as well as the typical cycle time for CSR.[41] It is stated that a time constant of this magnitude is thought to better suppress periodic breathing without requiring an undue amount of time to converge on a steady-state degree of ventilation; shorter time constants could result in less stability and longer time constants could delay achieving an equilibrium condition.

A percentage of the recent average ventilation is then computed to be used as the target input in a regulatory control loop (also known as a negative feedback controller) The patent document specifies that 95% of the recent average ventilation is used, whereas published investigations and reviews that describe the ResMed device seem to consistently mention 90%[42,52,53] as does the manufacturer's informational material.[54] According to the patent, using too high a percentage of recent average ventilation results in positive feedback and drift in the steady-state level of ventilation, while too low a percentage does not allow for complete control of CSR. The other input to the regulatory control loop consists of the absolute value of the instantaneous respiratory airflow, and the controller itself (also implemented within the microprocessor) is constructed as an integral clipped controller. That is, an error term (the absolute value of instantaneous respiratory airflow minus the target value) is multiplied by a constant, integrated over a short interval (the patent seems to indicate a time span equivalent to a few breaths) and bounded so as not to fall below a minimum value and not to exceed a maximum value. An integral controller is chosen so as to ensure that variations in PS from the device are opposite in phase to the patient's own variations in ventilatory drive; that is, maximum PS occurs when the patient's ventilatory drive is at a minimum, and minimum ventilatory support occurs when the patient's own ventilatory drive has peaked. The manufacturer's published specifications indicate

that the controller PS limits are 3 to 16 cm H_2O, subject to the additional constraint that EPAP plus maximum PS cannot exceed 25 cm H_2O.[50] The patent states a typical value for the constant used by the integral controller as -0.3 cm H_2O per L/min per second,[41] and 2 published articles indicate that this is the actual value used in the algorithm for the predecessor AutoSet CS model.[42,53] Finally, the microprocessor uses the instantaneous respiratory airflow signal to judge respiratory phase and thus determine transitions between EPAP and IPAP (ie, when to supply PS). The patent offers 2 methods to identify phase: one is simply based on the sign of instantaneous respiratory airflow; the other uses the sign of the instantaneous respiratory airflow and its rate of change to determine "fuzzy" categories of respiratory phase. In addition, the 5-second low-pass filtered absolute value of instantaneous respiratory airflow is used to determine whether the patient is exhibiting a regular respiratory rate or requires a timed backup rate. The manufacturer's literature states that the device assesses the "instantaneous direction, magnitude, and rate of change of the patient's airflow," implying that the second, more complicated method is implemented in the marketed device.[55]

Settings and Titration

It should be apparent from the preceding discussion that there are a myriad of possible ways in which the algorithm could conceivably be adjusted. Some of these are listed in **Table 1**, which also highlights the fact that very few of these parameters can be altered by the clinician. In practice, only EPAP, minimum PS, and maximum PS can be changed, and these only within limited ranges. The manufacturer provides little guidance as to how best to perform a titration, but little is actually needed because the device is so fully automated.[56] After selecting an interface (as noted above, the manufacturer specifies a limited range of full facemasks and nasal masks of their own design) and verifying that the leak does not exceed 24 L/min, the mask type is entered into the "Settings" menu. With the mask not worn by the patient and in the clear, the "Learning circuit" mode is started and will stop automatically after about 20 seconds with the indication "Circuit learned successfully." The manufacturer recommends allowing the device to use the default settings as indicated in **Table 1**, although it is likely that the patient has already undergone conventional CPAP (and very possibly bilevel PAP) titration from which an informed choice of EPAP can be made. When a component of OSA is present,

Table 1
Parameters used by the VPAP adapt SV algorithm

Parameter	Range, if Operator Adjustable	Default Value
Low-pass filter time constant for computing recent average ventilation	n/a	100 s
Proportion of recent average ventilation used as controller target	n/a	90%
Time interval employed by integral controller	n/a	"Few breaths"
Gain of integral controller	n/a	-0.3 cm H_2O per L/min per s
Internal limits of integral controller	n/a	3–16 cm H_2O
Maximum pressure support (PS)	n/a	25 cm H_2O
Pressure waveform	n/a	Resembles a decaying exponential ("ocean wave")
Expiratory positive airway pressure (EPAP)	4–15 cm H_2O	5 cm H_2O
PS limits (IPAP − EPAP)	3–16 cm H_2O[a]	3–15 cm H_2O
Respiratory phase determination (used for EPAP/IPAP transitions and computation of patient's recent respiratory rate)	n/a	Fuzzy logic table using airflow magnitude, sign, rate of change, and 5 s low-pass filtered absolute value; and 20 s low-pass filtered phase rate of change
Backup respiratory rate	n/a	15 breaths/min or patient's own recent respiratory rate

[a] Device will not allow maximum PS − minimum PS of less than 5 cm H_2O and EPAP + PS of greater than 25 cm H_2O.
Data from Refs.[41,52,54]

the level of CPAP or EPAP necessary to suppress obstructive apneas should already be known and EPAP should be set to that value.[43] Another published approach calls for setting EPAP to the level that abolished all obstructive events (apneas, hypopneas, and snoring) during the previous CPAP or bilevel PAP titration,[57] but this should not be necessary if the minimum value of PS is manually titrated during the night to eliminate obstructive hypopneas and snoring.[58] If the patient is not known to have a component of obstructive sleep apnea but rather pure CSR or CSA, then the default setting of EPAP can be used (5 cm H_2O). Alternatively, some investigators recommend setting EPAP to the level of CPAP that resulted in "abolishing or significantly decreasing" CSR.[59] Finally, it is usually most effective to set the PS upper limit so as to permit automatic titration to the highest value of PS possible (within the constraints noted in **Table 1**) to fully suppress CSR or CSA. During the course of a titration in the laboratory, EPAP can be increased as necessary if obstructive apneas are observed. The increase in EPAP is indicated because both theory

and practice hold that a fully closed airway at end-expiration will not open during the subsequent inspiration in response to IPAP greater than EPAP, but an airway that is partially obstructed at end-expiration will open further when exposed to the higher pressure of IPAP. Essentially no other adjustments are possible during the course of the night, given the extent of automation built in to the device.

Efficacy

Unlike the situation with autotitrating CPAP devices, there are no published studies that have examined the behavior of the VPAP Adapt SV (or for that matter, either BiPAP AutoSV models) on the bench using breathing simulators. The FDA 510(k) approval covers a fairly broad indication for the clinical use of this ASV device: "non-invasive ventilatory support to treat adult patients with OSA and Respiratory Insufficiency caused by central and/or mixed apneas and periodic breathing."[46] Note that this indication does not include ventilatory support for hypercapnic respiratory failure, although several reports have appeared investigating efficacy in sleep-disordered breathing due to chronic opiate use, which may have included patients with hypercapnia.[60,61] There is no particular reason not to anticipate, however, that additional such indications may be forthcoming. At present, the literature supports the use of the VPAP Adapt SV in two specific settings: CSR/CSA and complex sleep apnea (CompSA). The definition of the latter condition varies, with some investigators restricting its use to the appearance of central apneas when patients with OSA receive CPAP[62]; the following discussion uses a broader definition encompassing any sleep apnea syndrome demonstrating both obstructive and central components.[63,64]

The initial patent suggests that the technology was initially viewed as a treatment for CSR.[41] This would, at first sight, seem to be counterintuitive because CSR/CSA (as usually associated with CHF, stroke, or when idiopathic) is a hyperventilatory phenomenon with arterial pCO_2 transitioning above and below the apneic threshold.[65] Previous strategies for treating CSR/CSA have concentrated on raising arterial pCO_2 safely above the apneic threshold either by reducing ventilatory drive (eg, oxygen administration),[66] ventilatory loading (one possible mechanism for CPAP),[67] rebreathing (another possible mechanism for CPAP but also achieved by adding dead space to a noninvasive breathing circuit),[68] administering CO_2 exogenously,[69] or effective treatment of any underlying CHF (another possible mechanism for CPAP).[70] An explanation of the putative mechanism for ASV's suppression of CSR/CSA appears in the patent[41]: ASV is thought to provide a component of ventilation that is anticyclic to the patient's own respiratory drive periodicity. That is, during the hyperventilatory phase of CSR/CSA, ASV provides a minimal amount of ventilatory support that is not sufficient to worsen hyperventilation, while during the hypoventilatory or apneic phase, ASV significantly augments ventilation. These effects are exactly opposite the periodicity of the patient's own respiratory drive and act to dampen the oscillations in respiratory drive that underlie CSR/CSA. An analogy that is not exact, but perhaps will serve, is the effect of shock absorbers in an automobile's suspension system that counters the tendency of the springs to cause the vehicle to bounce up and down once perturbed by a bump in the road. In addition, it is possible that some of the other mechanisms attributed to CPAP in CHF may similarly accompany ASV treatment.

The first report of VPAP Adapt SV (in fact, the predecessor Autoset CS) efficacy in CSR/CSA accompanying CHF was that of Teschler and colleagues.[42] Fourteen patients with stable, treated CHF and an oxyhemoglobin desaturation index (ODI) greater than 15 on overnight pulse oximetry were subjected to 5 nights of nocturnal polysomnography (NPSG). During the first (baseline) night they received no treatment, while the next 4 nights incorporated, in random order, treatment with oxygen, CPAP, bilevel PAP in spontaneous/timed mode, and ASV. The most profound improvement in apnea/hypopnea index (AHI; number of apneas and hypopneas per hour of sleep) occurred with ASV, falling from a mean ± standard error of the mean (SEM) of 44.5 ± 3.4 to 6.3 ± 0.9, accompanied by substantial improvements in sleep architecture. It is interesting that arterialized capillary pCO_2 measured in the morning after treatment was significantly higher after ASV than it was the morning after the baseline NPSG (mean ± SEM, 35.2 ± 0.8 vs 30.8 ± 0.8 mm Hg) in the 10 subjects with available data, and also higher than that measured in the evening before the ASV night (mean ± SEM of 31.6 ± 1.1 mm Hg) in 8 subjects, results that tend to support the contention that ASV does not worsen the hyperventilation of CSR/CSA. Several subsequent reports of case series documented the success of the same device (Autoset CS) in suppressing CSR/CSA in CHF[71,72] and idiopathic CSR/CSA,[73] in a total of 34 patients and with treatment lasting as long as 12 months. All 3 studies reported baseline mean AHI greater than 30, falling to a mean AHI of less than 10 with ASV. One study of CHF patients also demonstrated significant improvements in 6-minute walk test distance and left ventricular ejection fraction (LVEF)[72] while the other reported significant improvement in quality of life as measured by the Minnesota Living with Heart Failure questionnaire (MLHFQ).[71] Another study, again in patients with CHF, compared baseline polysomnography with 2 weeks of oxygen supplementation, then 2 weeks of no therapy, followed by 2 weeks of ASV (Autoset CS) in fixed order.[74] Mean ± standard deviation (SD) AHI for the 14 subjects fell modestly from 34.5 ± 6.1 at baseline to 27.8 ± 8.2 on oxygen, and further declined substantially to 6.5 ± 0.8 with ASV. In addition, 6-minute walking distance increased to the largest degree after 2 weeks of ASV therapy and LVEF increased significantly only after the use of ASV. Szollosi and colleagues[75] compared polysomnography on ASV (probably Autoset CS) or added dead space (500 mL) via a full face mask to baseline in 10 men with stable CHF and severe CSR/CSA. The one night of testing under each condition occurred in random order with each trial separated by 7 ± 1 days. Similar degrees of improvement in AHI occurred with both treatments, although both dropped mean AHI only to approximately 15. End-tidal pCO_2 was measured during wakefulness and on both modalities of treatment during eupneic sleep. An increase from wakefulness to sleep was only demonstrated during the nights with added dead space, although it is possible that the end-tidal values while on ASV might have been falsely reduced by dilution with PAP air flow. Sleep architecture was significantly disrupted during the dead space nights, an effect that the investigators attributed to arousals from elevated levels of arterial pCO_2. Kuzniar and colleagues,[57] in a study primarily aimed at demonstrating the utility of a multimodal titration night in the treatment of predominantly CSR/CSA, reported on the efficacy of a variety of treatments (oxygen, CPAP, bilevel PAP in spontaneous mode, bilevel PAP in spontaneous/timed mode, ASV) in a retrospective review of the experience at one institution. With success defined as attaining an AHI on treatment of less than 10 for at least 30 minutes, ASV (most likely VPAP Adapt SV, although the device used is not specified) resulted in suppression of sleep-disordered breathing in 36 of 46 patients (78%), oxygen alone was next best (12/23 or 52%), and bilevel PAP in spontaneous/timed mode with or without an oxygen bleed was almost as good as oxygen alone (6/13 or 46% and 21/41 or 51%, respectively), whereas CPAP with or without oxygen (10/35 or 29% and 3/106 or 3%) and lastly bilevel PAP in spontaneous mode with or without oxygen (0/3 and 0/25) were both much less effective.

To date, there have appeared 4 controlled prospective trials of ResMed ASV devices in patients with CSR/CSA and CHF.[59,76–78] Bitter and colleagues[76] recently reported on a prospective study of ASV (Autoset CS2) in 39 patients with diastolic CHF (normal LVEF) treated for a mean of 11.6 ± 3 months compared with 21 similar patients who declined or were unable to use ASV. On average, subjects in the treatment and control groups had severe CSR/CSA and most were men (approximately 85% of each group). Sleep-disordered breathing was essentially abolished with ASV treatment: AHI (mean $\pm$ SD) was 3.5 ± 1.7. Adherence averaged 5.3 ± 2.1 hours of use per night, with 4 hours of use demonstrated in $64.0 \pm 30.4\%$ of nights. Both treatment and control patients experienced similar improvements in New York Heart Association class and N-terminal pro–brain natriuretic peptide (NT-proBNP) levels, but treated subjects had significant increases in cardiopulmonary exercise parameters of cardiac function (oxygen consumption at anaerobic threshold, peak oxygen consumption, and O_2 pulse) that the control group did not share. Echocardiographic indices of diastolic function (left atrial dimension, Doppler mitral inflow velocity, ratio of peak early and peak atrial Doppler mitral inflow velocities, mean early diastolic lengthening velocity, and ratio of early mitral valve flow velocity and early diastolic lengthening velocities) all significantly improved on ASV treatment. One randomized controlled trial compared ASV (Autoset CS) with CPAP in 25 patients with severe CSR/CSA and stable systolic CHF.[59] Sleep-disordered breathing was more completely suppressed by ASV, with AHI less than 10 at 6 months in all subjects in that group, while AHI remained 20 or greater in 3 patients on CPAP. Adherence was better in the ASV patients and LVEF increased only in the ASV group, while quality of life (MLHFQ) was enhanced in both treated patients and controls but improved to a greater degree in the ASV group. A second randomized controlled trial contrasted bilevel PAP with ASV (Autoset CS) in 37 patients, once more in patients with systolic CHF and severe CSR/CSA.[77] After baseline NPSG, subjects were randomized to either bilevel PAP (spontaneous/timed mode) or ASV and underwent 2 nights of titration with the assigned device. Polysomnography was repeated after 6 weeks of treatment in the 30 patients who returned for reevaluation. Similar degrees of CSR/CSA suppression occurred with both treatments, although a small number of patients in each group failed to adequately respond to PAP therapy (3 on bilevel PAP, 2 on ASV). Although LVEF increased in both groups, the change was greater in the bilevel PAP group. A final randomized controlled trial differs from previous investigations in that indices of sleep-disordered breathing severity were not measured after treatment.[78] Pepperell and colleagues[78] enrolled 30 patients (29 men) with moderately severe CSR/CSA and systolic CHF who were then randomized to either therapeutic or subtherapeutic ASV (Autoset CS). Changes in sleepiness (Osler test), BNP, and urinary metadrenaline excretion were assessed at baseline and after 1 month of treatment. Machine-estimated AHI demonstrated resolution of CSR/CSA with ASV but not with subtherapeutic ASV; Osler test improved significantly in the ASV group, as did BNP and urinary catecholamine excretion, whereas subtherapeutic ASV failed to provide these salutary effects.

There is at present only one report of a randomized controlled trial of ResMed ASV in OSA or CompSA. Morgenthaler and colleagues[43] compared bilevel PAP with ASV (VPAP Adapt SV) in 21 patients (19 men) with a variety of sleep apnea syndromes: 6 had CSR/CSA, 6 had predominantly mixed apneas, and 9 had CompSA. The study subjects overall had severe disease (mean ± SD AHI of 51.9 ± 22.8) and 15 had poor response to CPAP. All subjects were randomized to receive bilevel PAP titration or ASV on the first night of the study and then crossed over to the other treatment for the second night. Both treatments were effective in suppressing sleep-disordered breathing, although control was more complete during the ASV night compared with the bilevel PAP night: mean ± SD AHI of 0.8 ± 2.4 versus 6.2 ± 7.6, P<.002. In a nonrandomized trial, Hastings and colleagues[79] compared 11 men with stable CHF receiving ASV (Autoset CS) for 6 months with 8 men who declined ASV and did not undergo specific treatment for their sleep-disordered breathing. On average, the ASV group had severe sleep-disordered breathing (mean ± SD AHI of 49 ± 35.1) with obstructive events predominating in 5 and central in 6 of the patients, whereas the control group had slightly more moderate disease (mean ± SD AHI of 28 ± 12.6); all of the control patients had predominantly CSA. Polysomnography at 6 months in the treated group revealed significant improvement in AHI (7.6 ± 14.6), although the high value of the reported SD likely indicates that AHI was not normalized in some patients (individual values were not tabulated). There were significant improvements in LVEF and quality of life by Short Form 36 questionnaire (SF-36) for the treated group but not the controls.

With respect to reports of case series, 3 published studies are available. Morrell and colleagues[80] studied the acute effects of ASV (Autoset CS) on cerebral vascular reactivity in 10 patients with systolic CHF and severe, predominantly obstructive, sleep apnea. Each subject underwent 2 nights of NPSG in fixed order, first without and then with ASV; compared with the control night, ASV treatment essentially abolished sleep-disordered breathing (control mean ± SD AHI, 48.1 ± 11.7; ASV mean ± SD AHI, 4.2 ± 0.9). However, ASV did not affect cerebrovascular reactivity as assessed by left middle cerebral artery Doppler flow velocity at varying levels of inhaled CO_2. Finally, Yao and Zhang[81] have published, in the Chinese literature but with an English abstract, a study of patients with OSA treated with CPAP who complained of residual sleepiness. Of 50 patients with moderate to severe OSA treated with CPAP, 26 were recruited who complained of residual sleepiness and 24 had no residual sleepiness. All received 1 month of treatment with an autotitrating CPAP device and then 1 week of treatment with ASV (Autoset CS2). Whereas no

difference in overall AHI or Epworth Sleepiness Scale was apparent between the 2 groups before treatment, the subjects with residual sleepiness had, on average, a higher central sleep apnea index (CSAI) that decreased on ASV treatment. In addition, sleepiness as assessed by the Epworth Sleepiness Scale score, and inflammatory state as reflected by tumor necrosis factor α both decreased in the patients with residual sleepiness when treated with ASV.

As mentioned previously, 2 published studies describe series of patients with sleep-disordered breathing due to chronic opiate use that were treated with the VPAP Adapt SV.[60,61] Javaheri and colleagues[60] reported on 5 middle-aged adults (4 men) medicated for 2 to 5 years with opiates for chronic pain syndromes; opiate dosages were the equivalent of between 120 and 450 mg of morphine (mean, 252 mg). All presented with snoring, unrestorative sleep, hypersomnia, and witnessed apneas. All exhibited severe sleep apnea on diagnostic polysomnography (mean ± SD AHI, 70 ± 19) with both OSA and a prominent central component (mean ± SD central apnea index, 26 ± 27). There is no mention in the article of any component of Biot's respiration or ataxic breathing, a finding that has reportedly been associated with opiate use.[61] Only modest improvement was demonstrated on best CPAP after titration during a second night of NPSG (mean ± SD AHI, 55 ± 25), whereas application of ASV on a third night resulted in much more significant improvement (mean ± SD AHI, 13 ± 13). Note that there is a discrepancy in the published article between the ASV AHI in the abstract and the value given in a table and parts of the text; the result given here is from the abstract and is consistent with the graph in the article's Table 4, while the SD is inferred from the table based on the listed hypopnea index. During the ASV night, mean ± SD EPAP was titrated to 7 ± 2 cm H_2O and maximum IPAP was set to 10 cm H_2O. Farney and colleagues,[61] in the same issue of the journal, reported their experience in treating 22 patients (9 men) aged 22 to 76 years also chronically medicated with opiates for pain syndromes (dosages not reported). In contrast to subjects in the previous cohort, these patients had a significant component of ataxic breathing that was judged as moderate or severe at baseline in more than 80%. The degree of sleep-disordered breathing was severe on diagnostic NPSG (mean ± SD AHI, 66.6 ± 37.3) and remained severe in the 18 patients who underwent CPAP titration (mean ± SD AHI, 70.1 ± 32.6). During the ASV night, EPAP was initially set to the default value of 5 cm H_2O, but apparently at some point in the series they began titrating EPAP to as high as 10 cm H_2O in an attempt to suppress sleep-disordered breathing. PS was set to a minimum of 3 cm H_2O and a maximum of 10 cm H_2O. In contrast to the results reported by Javaheri and colleagues, these 22 patients did not respond adequately to ASV (mean ± SD AHI, 54.2 ± 33.0) with only 4 subjects achieving an AHI of less than 20. The proportion of subjects with moderate or severe ataxic breathing remained above 80% while receiving ASV.

RESPIRONICS BIPAP AUTOSV AND BIPAP AUTOSV ADVANCED
Flow Generator Characteristics

The BiPAP autoSV and BiPAP autoSV Advanced flow generators use a standard, single-lumen hose to connect the mask to the generator.[82–86] The generators can be equipped with an optional integral humidifier, and weigh 1.8 kg. Sound pressure level is not specified. As with the ResMed flow generator, both devices can record compliance data onto a plug-in memory module, and will sense whether the patient is wearing the interface allowing it to stop and start the blower automatically (this feature must be enabled on setup). Unlike the ResMed, a ramp feature is available in the ASV mode. The Provider Manuals state that these devices are "intended for use with Respironics-approved patient circuits," but also allows for "masks and accessories...recommended by the health care professional or respiratory therapist."[83,86] There is an understandably strict warning that if there is no exhalation port on the interface itself, then an exhalation port must be inserted between the interface and the circuit tubing. There is no mention of any need to identify the type of mask when initializing the flow generator, and the device does not require a calibration process before starting treatment. However, because pressure is only measured at the proximal end of the circuit, fixed compensation for the resistance of the hose is employed that assumes standard 6-ft (183 cm) smooth-bored tubing. The Provider Manuals supply a graph that displays the expected pressure drop versus flow in the patient circuit if a Respironics bacteria filter or a filter and a Respironics humidifier are added to the circuit. Both models of flow generator are equipped with 2 sets of alarms, divided into "system" alerts and "patient" alerts. The system alarms include high and low pressure regulation (triggered when IPAP is 5 cm H_2O above or below the required pressure) and a low PS alarm (activates after 60 seconds of a low PS condition); the patient alarms alert when patient disconnect, low minute ventilation, or apnea are detected

according to parameters input at setup. Because pressure is not sampled at the interface, it is not possible to detect circuit obstructions reliably. Both flow generators are specified for working pressures between 4 and 30 cm H_2O for IPAP and 4 and 25 cm H_2O for EPAP, and consequently can provide a maximum PS (IPAP minus EPAP) of 26 cm H_2O. In addition, the autoSV devices allow for tailoring inspiratory pressure rise times within a range of 0.1 to 0.6 seconds in steps of 0.1 second. As with the ResMed device, intended application is in adult patients with OSA, CSR/CSA, or CompSA, and use in patients without spontaneous respiratory drive or with existing respiratory failure is contraindicated.

Respiratory Parameter Determination and Control Algorithm

With the exception of the autotitration of EPAP that is incorporated into the BiPAP autoSV Advanced but not its predecessor BiPAP autoSV, the internal operation of both devices appears to be similar. The following discussion applies to both unless otherwise specified. A microcontroller again serves as the component that performs all manipulations, calculations, and control functions that result in changes in blower speed and valve positions so as to control the values of, and alternate between, EPAP and IPAP. As with the ResMed device, an estimate of instantaneous patient air flow is the basis for the control algorithm. The patent does not describe the specific manner in which this is done,[44] although previous patents incorporated by reference (and also listed in the Provider Manual) specify 2 possible techniques.[87] The more simple method involves computing instantaneous air flow averaged over multiple breaths (this is essentially the low-pass filter technique as used in the ResMed device). This average air flow, derived as it is from a single-limb patient circuit, represents average leak because inspiratory and expiratory tidal volumes will cancel each other. Instantaneous air flow, when subtracted from this average flow, then represents an estimate of instantaneous patient air flow. The other method for estimating instantaneous patient air flow is similar to that used in the ResMed device. Rather than computing leak pathway conductance on an instantaneous basis, Respironics apparently computes this value averaged over an entire breath and then computes instantaneous mask leak air flow by multiplying this average conductance by the square root of the instantaneous circuit pressure. Subtracting this value from instantaneous system air flow then results in an estimate of instantaneous patient air flow.

Although this is conjecture, it is likely that the former method is used in controlling transitions between EPAP and IPAP as well as computing the patient's respiratory rate, while the latter technique is used in the pressure control algorithm.

The algorithm controlling the level of IPAP delivered in any given breath is complex, assuming that all aspects of the process described in the patent are actually implemented in the marketed device.[44] The underlying goal is to achieve a target peak flow (in contrast to the average ventilation target employed by ResMed) by comparing this value with the measured peak flow for a given breath. The value of IPAP for the next breath is then adjusted so as to reach that target, within the constraints of maximum and minimum IPAP as set by the provider. There are 3 parameters involved: a CSR shape index, CSR severity index, and a PS index. The latter index is perhaps easiest to understand, in that it is simply the percentage of breaths during the previous 2 to 3 minutes (or, alternatively, the previous 2 CSR cycles) that required a value of PS above a threshold level (typically 2 cm H_2O according to the patent). Both CSR indices are derived from an array of peak flows collected over the previous 2 to 5 minutes. The array of peak flows are, in effect, high-pass filtered to ensure that they vary above and below a zero flow point; 3 zero crossings are detected and used to identify 2 putative sequences of CSR. The peak flows are then compared with a standard template of peak flows (the patent describes using a triangle function, but presumably other functions could be employed) that models an extreme degree of CSR, and a coherence value computed (ranging from 0% to 100%) that is a measure of how closely the actual array of peak flows conforms to the template's model of severe CSR. Finally, the CSR severity index is computed as the ratio of the last minimum peak flow over the last maximum peak flow, or an average of these ratios over a set interval (time span not specified in the patent), converted to a percentage that ranges between 0% and 100%. A severity index of 50% or greater is considered "normal," meaning that peak flow during normal breathing may vary to that degree; values less than 50% indicate the presence of CSR, with a value of zero representing the occurrence of a central apnea. The actual computation that determines changes in IPAP for each breath incorporates 3 factors: (1) a target peak flow (2) that is continually adjusted using the 3 parameters described above, and (3) the difference between the previous breath's peak flow and the target peak flow multiplied by a constant ("gain") that is nominally 9 cm H_2O per L/s. In addition, the amount that IPAP changes with each breath is proportional to this difference value, so that large discrepancies between actual and target peak flow result in greater changes in IPAP then would result from small differences in this metric.

Two backup rate mechanisms are available, or the device can be set to spontaneous mode only. One mechanism allows for a provider-chosen backup respiratory rate between 4 and 30 breaths/min, while the other calculates the patient's customary respiratory rate (tidal volumes less than 100 mL are discarded) and adds a machine breath when too much time passes without a spontaneous breath. Respironics also employs several proprietary methods to determine cycling between EPAP and IPAP. Transitions from EPAP to IPAP occur when either an accumulated inspired volume of 6 mL is detected, or when expiratory air flow crosses a transformed flow waveform called the "shape signal." The latter is the patient's actual flow decreased by a constant 15 L/min and delayed by a constant 300 milliseconds. This method is said to allow trigger sensitivity to adjust to different values of leak and spontaneous breathing patterns. Transitions from IPAP to EPAP are also governed in 2 ways: during inspiration, when instantaneous patient air flow falls below a value proportional to instantaneous tidal volume; or when time in IPAP exceeds 3.0 seconds.[83]

The BiPAP autoSV Advanced adds 2 types of functionality to the previous model. The BiFlex mode allows for a brief reduction in pressure spanning the latter part of inspiration and the beginning of expiration. This feature may be set to values between "1" and "3," corresponding to progressively greater degrees of pressure relief and slightly different pressure versus time profiles, neither of which are described quantitatively. Presumably the setting is empirically determined and should be chosen so as to maximize patient comfort.[86] The other feature added in the Advanced model replicates the autotitrating CPAP function from previous generations of Respironics devices such as the REMStar Auto.[88] As implemented in the BiPAP autoSV Advanced, the additional algorithm allows for automatic adjustment of EPAP in response to evidence of upper airway obstruction. Discussions of autotitrating CPAP technology are reviewed elsewhere[89,90] and are not the subject of this review. Therefore, the details of the algorithm are not described in detail other than to note that Respironics literature[91] indicates that the device detects apneas and hypopneas based on reductions in flow during a moving window in time, analyzes the shape of the inspiratory limb of the flow signal to identify flow limitation, and senses snoring from characteristic vibrations superimposed on the flow signal. In addition, the algorithm prevents counterproductive increases in CPAP/EPAP when a central apnea is misidentified as an obstructive event by limiting the step up in CPAP/EPAP unless and until additional evidence of flow limitation appears.

Settings and Titration

The BiPAP autoSV uses even more internal parameters than its ResMed cousin, and the Advanced model adds a few additional user-selectable variables. **Tables 2** and **3** list some of these parameters, including those that can be altered by the clinician. After selecting an interface, the device is turned on and executes a self-check program. The Provider Manual does not indicate that the device starts with any default settings, and therefore the clinician should be careful to enter all settings anew at the beginning of a titration. Unlike the literature available from ResMed, Respironics provides a fairly clear titration protocol.[92] For patients with primarily OSA but an additional component of CSA (either treatment-emergent or coexisting), it is again likely that the patient has previously undergone a PAP titration. This allows for an informed choice of EPAP, which should be set to the level of CPAP or EPAP that suppressed obstructive apneas during the previous titration. If the patient is not known to have a component of OSA but rather pure CSR or CSA, Respironics recommends setting EPAP to 4 cm H_2O, although consideration could be given to using the value of CPAP that resulted in significant improvement of CSR in a previous CPAP titration as in the ResMed device.[59] In both clinical scenarios, Respironics recommends setting minimum IPAP to the same value as EPAP and maximum IPAP to 10 cm H_2O above EPAP, although it would not seem unreasonable to set maximum IPAP to a higher value depending on the clinician's judgment of how well the patient would tolerate higher pressures. This strategy may allow the automatic titration algorithm to more fully suppress CSR or CSA. Setting minimum IPAP to equal EPAP allows the device to revert to CPAP if it senses that ventilation is adequate and stable. The protocol calls for allowing the patient to sleep for 20 minutes at these settings so that breathing can stabilize. If obstructive apneas are observed, then EPAP, minimum IPAP and maximum IPAP are all raised together in 1 cm H_2O increments until these are suppressed. The reasoning behind increasing EPAP in this situation is the same as outlined previously with respect to the VPAP Adapt SV: to

convert a fully closed airway at end-expiration to one that is partially open, which can then be fully expanded by IPAP. If other evidence of obstruction is noted (hypopneas, respiratory effort related arousals, snoring) and the device is consistently choosing to deliver maximum IPAP, then the value of maximum IPAP should be increased in 2 cm H_2O increments. This same strategy can be considered if CSR/CSA persists, but if unsuccessful then a backup rate can be set to 2 breaths/min less than the spontaneous respiratory rate along with an inspiratory time of at least 1.2 seconds. If primarily central apneas persist, then the backup rate can be set to either 10 breaths/min or 2 breaths/min less than the spontaneous respiratory rate, and again inspiratory time should be at least 1.2 seconds. The Respironics protocol gives no advice as to when to use the automatic backup rate setting, but presumably the clinician can try this mode when CSA/CSR persists during the standard titration.

The Biflex setting on the BiPAP autoSV Advanced is simply chosen on the basis of patient comfort and tolerance. Respironics literature gives no specific guidance as to how to choose minimum and maximum EPAP when using the Advanced model, and there have been no published studies as of yet employing this device in the sleep laboratory. It would seem reasonable to use this flow generator in patients with CompSA when the patient is unable to tolerate the fixed level of EPAP capable of suppressing obstructive apneas in all body positions. It is also possible that the variable level of EPAP may be capable of more effectively suppressing the wide variety of respiratory events seen in CompSA. It would be wise to systematically assess this device's efficacy in treating any specific patient during formal polysomnography in the sleep laboratory. A satisfactory approach may be to set minimum EPAP to 4 cm H_2O and maximum EPAP to 2 cm H_2O above the level of CPAP or EPAP that suppressed obstructive apneas during a previous titration, and allow the flow generator to select the delivered EPAP within that range. Peer-reviewed publications reporting the use of this particular device in patient cohorts must be awaited to provide further guidance to the clinician, although one report exists of a similar device (from a different manufacturer and not marketed in the United States) that may be of assistance in this regard, which is discussed below.[49]

Efficacy

As noted previously, there are no published studies investigating the behavior of the Bilevel

Table 2
Parameters used by the BiPAP autoSV algorithm

Parameter	Range, if Operator Adjustable	Default Value
Low-pass filter time constant for computing average leak	n/a	Not specified
CSR Shape Index template	n/a	Triangle waveform
CSR Shape Index time span	n/a	2–5 min
CSR Severity Index time interval	n/a	Not specified
Pressure Support Index threshold	n/a	2 cm H_2O
Pressure Support Index time span	n/a	2–3 min or 2 CSR cycles
Time interval employed by proportional controller	n/a	"Few breaths"
Gain of proportional controller	n/a	9 cm H_2O per L/s
Equation to derive Peak Flow Target from CSR Shape Index, CSR Severity Index, and Pressure Support Index	n/a	Not specified
Internal limits of proportional controller	n/a	Not specified
Maximum PS	n/a	26 cm H_2O
Pressure waveform	n/a	Square wave with variable inspiratory rise time
Inspiratory rise time	0.1–0.6 s	Not specified
Inspiratory time	0.5–3 s, limited to prevent I:E >1:1 at selected respiratory rate	Not specified
EPAP (BiPAP auto SV only)	4–25 cm H_2O	Not specified
Minimum IPAP (BiPAP auto SV only)	4–30 cm H_2O	Not specified
Maximum IPAP (BiPAP auto SV only)	4–30 cm H_2O	Not specified
Transition from EPAP to IPAP	n/a	Accumulated inspiratory volume = 6 mL or expiratory air flow crosses "shape waveform"[a]
Transition from IPAP to EPAP	n/a	The lesser of when inspiratory air flow reaches a proportion of accumulated inspiratory volume or 3 s
Backup respiratory rate	Off; 4–30 breaths/min; Auto	Not specified

[a] See text for details.
Data from Refs.[44,82–88]

autoSV when subjected to bench testing against simulated breathing patterns, and thus far only a few published studies have appeared reporting efficacy in patients. In 2006, Kasai and colleagues[47] described their experience employing the device in the treatment of 4 patients with CHF and CSR/CSA. Two patients had been unsuccessfully treated with autotitrating CPAP, and 2 had not responded to bilevel PAP in spontaneous/timed mode. Treatment with ASV resulted in a decrease of mean ± SD AHI from 62.7 ± 10.1 at baseline to 5.9 ± 2.2, although it would appear from the figures that one patient still exhibited an AHI of just under 20 (individual data were not otherwise presented). The investigators do not give detailed information as to their titration protocol, only indicating that initial EPAP was set using values from the previous treatment with

Table 3
Additional parameters used by the BiPAP autoSV advanced algorithm

Parameter	Range, if Operator Adjustable	Default Value
BiFlex	"1"–"3" corresponding to additional increments of pressure relief; exact characteristics not specified	Not specified
Maximum Pressure	4–30 cm H_2O	Not specified
Minimum EPAP	4–25 cm H_2O[a]	Not specified
Maximum EPAP	4–25 cm H_2O[a]	Not specified
Pressure support minimum (PS or IPAP − EPAP)	0–26 cm H_2O	Not specified
Pressure support maximum (PS or IPAP − EPAP)	0–26 cm H_2O[b]	Not specified

[a] Settings above Maximum Pressure will not be accepted.
[b] Settings above Maximum Pressure-Maximum EPAP will not be accepted.
Data from Refs.[85–88]

autotitrating CPAP or bilevel PAP; when the latter was employed, minimum IPAP during ASV was set to the IPAP level that previously eliminated obstructive events. In all 4 cases, maximum IPAP was set to between 10 and 20 cm H_2O above the level used for the previous treatment with autotitrating CPAP or bilevel PAP. In the Japanese literature Kageshita and colleagues[93] reported the successful use of the Respironics "Heart PAP" ASV on one patient with CompSA (initially, OSA only but with the appearance of CSR/CSA as his heart disease worsened). Presumably this "Heart PAP" was similar or identical to the Bilevel autoSV marketed in the United States, but this is not certain. Arzt and colleagues[94] studied 14 male patients with severe systolic CHF and moderate to severe CSR/CSA during 3 consecutive nights in fixed order: a diagnostic night, a CPAP (10 patients) or bilevel PAP (4 patients) titration night, and then a Bilevel autoSV night. The optimal level of CPAP or EPAP from the second night was chosen as the value of EPAP during the ASV night, and maximum IPAP was set to 15 cm H_2O above EPAP. Mean ± SD AHI fell from 46 ± 4 at baseline, to 22 ± 4 with CPAP or bilevel PAP, and then declined further to 4 ± 1 on ASV; all 14 patients achieved an AHI of less than 15 while using ASV. The mean level of IPAP chosen by the ASV device was 8.0 ± 2.4 cm H_2O. Finally, Randerath and colleagues[95] applied this ASV device to a cohort of 10 men, naïve to PAP therapy, with moderate to severe CompSA (coronary artery disease, 3; CHF, 3; arterial hypertension, 2). Patients underwent baseline diagnostic laboratory NPSG, followed by a CPAP titration night and then an autoSV night. The level of CPAP determined to

suppress all obstructive phenomena (apneas, hypopneas, and snoring) was used as the EPAP and minimum IPAP settings for the following ASV night, and the value of maximum IPAP was set to EPAP + 10 cm H_2O. All patients proceeded to home treatment with ASV using settings derived from the ASV laboratory night for a period of 6 weeks. An important aspect of this study is the explicit description of how the results from the ASV night were used to set treatment parameters for the 6 weeks of in-home use. The minimum IPAP value was based on the machine-chosen IPAP values during the ASV night, as follows. (1) If machine-chosen IPAP remained at EPAP for at least one-third of the night, and within 2 cm H_2O for one-third of the night, then minimum IPAP was set to equal EPAP. (2) If IPAP exceeded EPAP by at least 2 cm H_2O for more than half the night, then minimum IPAP was set to EPAP + 2 cm H_2O. (3) If neither conditions 1 nor 2 were met, then minimum IPAP was set to EPAP + 1 cm H_2O. There apparently was some room for the physician to deviate from these guidelines in a given individual patient, the basis for which is not otherwise explained. Maximum IPAP was set to the IPAP that appeared to be most effective in suppressing CSA/CSR during the ASV night; this value was in the range of 15 to 20 cm H_2O and, in the main, not more than 5% of the ASV night was spent at higher IPAP levels than that chosen for maximum IPAP. If central apneas represented more than 30% of the total AHI, the study protocol called for using a fixed backup rate (only one patient met this criterion and a rate of 15 breaths/min was used); otherwise the automatic backup mode was employed. One patient also received an oxygen bleed due to a mean oxyhemoglobin saturation of 86% on room air. It is instructive to note that in this group of mildly overweight, middle-aged to elderly men, the mean ± SD for EPAP was 7.9 ± 2.3 cm H_2O, minimum IPAP was 9.1 ± 2.7 cm H_2O, and maximum IPAP was 16.3 ± 2.2 cm H_2O. After the 6 weeks of home use, another NPSG with ASV was performed and data from the baseline, ASV titration night, and 6 week follow up NPSG compared. Baseline mean ± SD total AHI was 48.9 ± 20.6, falling to 8.9 ± 6.2 during the first ASV night and 8.7 ± 7.4 during the 6-week ASV study. In one patient, AHI remained above 20 at the 6-week point but this was attributed to a persistent mask leak. Overall, there was a statistically significant increase in rapid eye movement as percent of total sleep time and a reduction in the percentages of stages 1 and 2. Even though it targets flow rather than recent average ventilation, the mechanism by which the AutoSV suppresses CSR/CSA is presumably similar to that attributed to the VPAP Adapt SV; that is, a component of ventilation is added that is anticyclic to the patient's own respiratory drive periodicity. This mechanism is demonstrated in **Fig. 1**, which depicts the behavior of the AutoSV in a patient with CSR: progressively increasing IPAP during the period of spontaneous breathing with waning flow, adding timed breaths at maximum IPAP during the apneic phase, and then progressively stepping down IPAP when spontaneous breathing resumes.

There is one published report of an ASV device similar to the BiPAP autoSV Advanced in that it automatically titrates both EPAP and IPAP.[49] This flow generator (SOMNOvent CR), not currently available in the United States, apparently combines an average ventilation algorithm similar to that of the ResMed VPAP Adapt plus a snoring and inspiratory flow profile method comparable to that of the BiPAP autoSV Advanced to determine IPAP and EPAP levels. This device differs from the others in that in addition to EPAP and IPAP, EEPAP is also titrated. In the study by Randerath and colleagues,[49] 12 patients with Comp-SA of moderate to severe degree (9 men; none with CHF but 7 with arterial hypertension and/or cardiac disease) underwent baseline laboratory NPSG, a night with ASV, used the device at

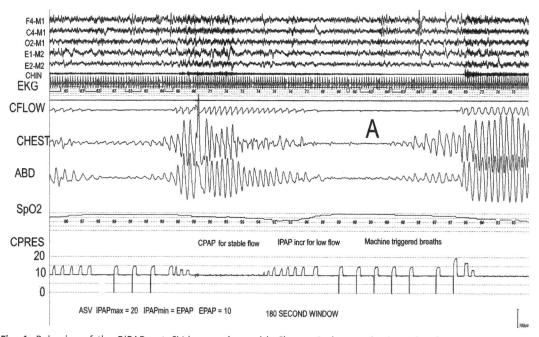

Fig. 1. Behavior of the BiPAP autoSV in a patient with Cheyne-Stokes respiration. The device is progressively increasing IPAP during the period of spontaneous breathing with waning flow, adding timed breaths at maximum IPAP during the apneic phase, and then progressively stepping down IPAP when spontaneous breathing resumes. Electroencephalogram and electrooculogram labels F4, C4, O2, E1, E2, M1, M2 indicate right frontal, right central, right occipital, left eye (outer canthus), right eye (outer canthus), left mastoid, right mastoid derivations, respectively. CHIN, submental electromyogram; EKG, electrocardiogram; CFLOW, instantaneous flow computed by bilevel PAP device; CHEST, ABD, chest and abdominal effort, respectively; SpO2, oxyhemoglobin saturation by pulse oximetry; CPRES, instantaneous pressure delivered by the bilevel PAP device. (*Courtesy of* Richard B. Berry MD.)

home for 19 $\pm$ 15 days, and then spent another laboratory NPSG night with their ASV. The settings chosen were EEPAP, 6 cm H_2O; maximum IPAP, 16 to 20 cm H_2O; and automatic backup rate. Mean $\pm$ SD for total AHI fell from 43.8 $\pm$ 24.0 at baseline to 4.0 $\pm$ 3.9 during the first ASV night, and then 2.1 $\pm$ 2.4 during the follow-up ASV night. It is not possible to speculate whether these data are transferable to practice using the BiPAP autoSV Advanced.

SUMMARY

Adaptive servo-ventilation applied noninvasively for the treatment of sleep apnea syndromes involves technology that is complex, cryptic, not necessarily intuitive, and possibly subject to change in subtle or material ways as a given product evolves. Published data on the whole suggests that these devices are capable of treating a wide variety of sleep-disordered breathing events, but may not necessarily suppress all events in any particular patient. For the most part, there is a paucity of literature particularly concerning randomized controlled trials. For the time being it would seem most wise to validate the use of any particular ASV device in any individual patient by systematic monitoring in the sleep laboratory before placing an order for treatment in the home.

REFERENCES

1. Chatburn RL. Computer control of mechanical ventilation. Respir Care 2004;49:507–15.
2. Menn SJ, Barnett GO, Schmechel D, et al. A computer program to assist in the care of acute respiratory failure. JAMA 1973;223:308–12.
3. Hernandez-Sande C, Moret-Bonillo V, Alonso-Betanzos A. ESTER: an expert system for management of respiratory weaning therapy. IEEE Trans Biomed Eng 1989;36:559–64.
4. East TD, Heermann LK, Bradshaw RL, et al. Efficacy of computerized decision support for mechanical ventilation: results of a prospective multi-center randomized trial. Proc AMIA Symp 1999;251–5.
5. Morris AH, Wallace CJ, Menlove RL, et al. Randomized clinical trial of pressure-controlled inverse ratio ventilation and extracorporeal CO_2 removal for adult respiratory distress syndrome. Am J Respir Crit Care Med 1994;149:295–305.
6. East TD, Böhm SH, Wallace CJ, et al. A successful computerized protocol for clinical management of pressure control inverse ratio ventilation in ARDS patients. Chest 1992;101:697–710.
7. Nemoto T, Hatzakis GE, Thorpe CW, et al. Automatic control of pressure support mechanical ventilation using fuzzy logic. Am J Respir Crit Care Med 1999;160:550–6.
8. Hewlett AM, Platt AS, Terry VG. Mandatory minute volume: a new concept in weaning from mechanical ventilation. Anaesthesia 1977;32:163–9.
9. Guthrie SO, Lynn C, Lafleur BJ, et al. A crossover analysis of mandatory minute ventilation compared to synchronized intermittent mandatory ventilation in neonates. J Perinatol 2005;25:643–6.
10. Branson RD, Johannigman JA. Innovations in mechanical ventilation. Respir Care 2009;54:933–47.
11. Yang KL, Tobin MJ. A prospective study of indexes predicting the outcome of trials of weaning from mechanical ventilation. N Engl J Med 1991;324: 1445–50.
12. Strickland JH, Hasson JH. A computer-controlled weaning system. A clinical trial. Chest 1993;103: 1220–6.
13. Laubscher TP, Heinrichs W, Weiler N, et al. An adaptive lung ventilation controller. IEEE Trans Biomed Eng 1994;41:51–9.
14. Dojat M, Pachet F, Guessoum Z, et al. NéoGanesh: a working system for the automated control of assisted ventilation in ICUs. Artif Intell Med 1997;11: 97–117.
15. Dojat M, Harf A, Touchard D, et al. Clinical evaluation of a computer-controlled pressure support mode. Am J Respir Crit Care Med 2000;161: 1161–6.
16. Anderson JR, East TD. A closed-loop controller for mechanical ventilation of patients with ARDS. Biomed Sci Instrum 2002;38:289–94.
17. Tehrani F, Rogers M, Lo T, et al. A dual closed-loop control system for mechanical ventilation. J Clin Monit 2004;18:111–29.
18. East TD, Wortelboer PJ, van Ark E, et al. Automated sulfur hexafluoride washout functional residual capacity measurement system for any mode of mechanical ventilation as well as spontaneous respiration. Crit Care Med 1990;18:84–91.
19. Brander L, Leong-Poi H, Beck J, et al. Titration and implementation of neurally adjusted ventilatory assist in critically ill patients. Chest 2009;135:695–703.
20. Branson RD. Dual control modes, closed loop ventilation, handguns, and tequila. Respir Care 2001;46: 232–3.
21. Berthon-Jones M. Feasibility of a self-setting CPAP machine. Sleep 1993;16(Suppl):S120–3.
22. Miles LE, Buschek GD, McClintock DP, et al. Development and application of automatic nasal CPAP calibration procedures for use in the unsupervised home environment. Sleep 1993; 16(Suppl):S118–9.
23. Behbehani K, Yen F-C, Burk JR, et al. Automatic control of airway pressure for treatment of obstructive sleep apnea. IEEE Trans Biomed Eng 1995;42: 1007–16.

24. Sackett D. Rules of evidence and clinical recommendations for the management of patients. Can J Cardiol 1993;9:487–9.
25. Morgenthaler TI, Aurora RN, Brown T, et al. Practice parameters for the use of autotitrating continuous positive airway pressure devices for titrating pressures and treating adult patients with obstructive sleep apnea syndrome. An update for 2007. Sleep 2008;31:141–7.
26. Eiken T, McCoy R. Performance of auto-adjust nasal CPAP devices in a simulation of varied patient breathing. The evolution of product performance. Sleep Rev 2006, May–June. Available at: http://www.sleepreviewmag.com/pdf/AA_Report.pdf. Accessed March 19, 2010.
27. Farré R, Montserrat JM, Rigau J, et al. Response of automatic continuous positive airway pressure devices to different sleep breathing patterns. A bench study. Am J Respir Crit Care Med 2002;166:469–73.
28. Abdenbi F, Chambille B, Escourrou P. Bench testing of auto-adjusting positive airway pressure devices. Eur Respir J 2004;24:649–58.
29. Rigau J, Montserrat JM, Wöhrle H, et al. Bench model to simulate upper airway obstruction for analyzing automatic continuous positive airway pressure devices. Chest 2006;130:350–61.
30. Lofaso F, Desmarais G, Leroux K, et al. Bench evaluation of flow limitation detection by automated continuous positive airway pressure devices. Chest 2006;130:343–9.
31. Rühle KH, Karweina D, Domanski U, et al. [Characteristics of auto-CPAP devices during the simulation of sleep-related breathing flow patterns]. Pneumologie 2009;63:390–8 [in German].
32. Husain AM. Evaluation and comparison of tranquility and autoset T autotitrating CPAP machines. J Clin Neurophysiol 2003;20:291–5.
33. Hertegonne KB, Proot PM, Pauwels RA, et al. Comfort and pressure profiles of two auto-adjustable positive airway pressure devices: a technical report. Respir Med 2003;97:903–8.
34. Pevernagie DA, Proot PM, Hertegonne KB, et al. Efficacy of flow- vs impedance-guided autoadjustable continuous positive airway pressure: a randomized cross-over trial. Chest 2004;126:25–30.
35. Shi HB, Cheng L, Nakayama M, et al. Effective comparison of two auto-CPAP devices for treatment of obstructive sleep apnea based on polysomnographic evaluation. Auris Nasus Larynx 2005;32:237–41.
36. Stammnitz A, Jerrentrup A, Penzel T, et al. Automatic CPAP titration with different self-setting devices in patients with obstructive sleep apnoea. Eur Respir J 2004;24:273–8.
37. Hertegonne KB, Rombaut B, Houtmeyers P, et al. Titration efficacy of two auto-adjustable continuous positive airway pressure devices using different flow limitation-based algorithms. Respiration 2008;75:48–54.
38. Sériès F, Plante J, Lacasse Y. Reliability of home CPAP titration with different automatic CPAP devices. Respir Res 2008;9:56.
39. Brown LK. Autotitrating CPAP. How shall we judge safety and efficacy of a "black box"? Chest 2006;130:312–4.
40. Brown LK. Filling in the gaps: the role of non-invasive adaptive servo-ventilation for heart failure-related central sleep apnea. Chest 2008;134:4–7.
41. Berthon-Jones M, Inventor; ResMed Ltd, assignee. Ventilatory assistance for treatment of cardiac failure and Cheyne-Stokes breathing. US Patent 6,532,959. March 18, 2003.
42. Teschler H, Dohring J, Wang YM, et al. Adaptive pressure support servo-ventilation: a novel treatment for Cheyne-Stokes respiration in heart failure. Am J Respir Crit Care Med 2001;164:614–9.
43. Morgenthaler TI, Gay PC, Gordon N, et al. Adaptive servo-ventilation versus non-invasive positive pressure ventilation for central, mixed, and complex sleep apnea syndromes. Sleep 2007;30:468–75.
44. Hill PD, inventor; Respironics Inc, assignee. Method and apparatus for providing variable positive airway pressure. US Patent 6,752,151. June 22, 2004.
45. U.S. Food and Drug Administration. 510(k) Summary (K063540). February 22, 2007. Available at: http://www.accessdata.fda.gov/cdrh_docs/pdf6/K063540.pdf. Accessed March 31, 2010.
46. U.S. Food and Drug Administration. 510(k) Summary—AutoSet CS2 (K051364). August 16, 2005. Available at: http://www.accessdata.fda.gov/cdrh_docs/pdf5/K051364.pdf. Accessed March 31, 2010.
47. Kasai T, Narui K, Dohi T, et al. First experience of using new adaptive servo-ventilation device for Cheyne-Stokes respiration with central sleep apnea among Japanese patients with congestive heart failure. Report of 4 clinical cases. Circ J 2006;70:1148–54.
48. Dedrick DL, Brown LK, Doggett JW, et al. Volume assured pressure support in adults with severe obstructive sleep apnea. Chest 2000;118:265S.
49. Randerath WJ, Galetke W, Kenter M, et al. Combined adaptive servo-ventilation and automatic positive airway pressure (anticyclic modulated ventilation) in co-existing obstructive and central sleep apnea syndrome and periodic breathing. Sleep Med 2009;10:898–903.
50. ResMed VP. Adapt SV clinical guide. Available at: http://www.resmed.com/us/assets/documents/product/vpap_adapt_sv/clinical_manual/228235_vpap-adapt-sv_clinical-manual_amer_eng.pdf. Accessed April 16, 2010.

51. ResMed VP. Adapt SV user guide. Available at: http://www.resmed.com/us/assets/documents/product/vpap_adapt_sv/user_guide/228234_vpap-adapt-sv_user-guide_amer_eng.pdf. Accessed April 2, 2010.

52. Brown S. Adaptive servo-ventilation using the ResMed VPAP Adapt SV. Sleep Diagn Ther 2007;2:20–2.

53. Pépin JL, Chouri-Pontarollo N, Tamisier R, et al. Cheyne-Stokes respiration with central sleep apnoea in chronic heart failure: proposals for a diagnostic and therapeutic strategy. Sleep Med Rev 2006;10:33–47.

54. ResMed. Adaptive servo-ventilation. Available at: http://www.resmed.com/us/clinicians/treatment/adapt_sv.html?nc=clinicians. Accessed April 6, 2010.

55. ResMed VP. Adapt SV and adaptive servo-ventilation. Technology fact sheet. Available at: http://www.resmed.com/us/documents/1010807r3-vpap-adapt-sv-tech-fact-sheet.pdf. Accessed April 6, 2010.

56. ResMed. Titration protocol for VPAP Adapt SV. Available at: http://www.resmed.com/us/documents/1011164r4-vpap-adapt-sv-protocol.pdf. Accessed April 8, 2010.

57. Kuzniar TJ, Golbin JM, Morgenthaler TI. Moving beyond empiric continuous positive airway pressure (CPAP) trials for central sleep apnea: a multimodality titration study. Sleep Breath 2007;11:259–66.

58. Sanders MH, Kern N. Obstructive sleep apnea treated by independently adjusted inspiratory and expiratory positive airway pressures via nasal mask. Physiologic and clinical implications. Chest 1990;98:317–24.

59. Philippe C, Stoïca-Herman M, Drouot X, et al. Compliance with and effectiveness of adaptive servoventilation versus continuous positive airway pressure in the treatment of Cheyne-Stokes respiration in heart failure over a six month period. Heart 2006;92:337–42.

60. Javaheri S, Malik A, Smith J, et al. Adaptive pressure support servoventilation; a novel treatment for sleep apnea associated with use of opioids. J Clin Sleep Med 2008;4:305–10.

61. Farney RJ, Walker JM, Boyle KM, et al. Adaptive servoventilation (ASV) in patients with sleep disordered breathing associated with chronic opioid medications for non-malignant pain. J Clin Sleep Med 2008;4:311–9.

62. Morganthaler TI, Kagramanov V, Hanak V, et al. Complex sleep apnea syndrome: is it a unique clinical syndrome? Sleep 2006;29:1203–9.

63. Gilmartin GS, Daly RW, Thomas RJ. Recognition and management of complex sleep-disordered breathing. Curr Opin Pulm Dis 2005;11:485–93.

64. Brown LK, Casey KR. Complex sleep apnea: the hedgehog and the fox. Curr Opin Pulm Med 2007;13:473–8.

65. Naughton M, Benard D, Tam A, et al. Role of hyperventilation in the pathogenesis of central sleep apneas in patients with congestive heart failure. Am Rev Respir Dis 1993;148:330–8.

66. Hanly PJ, Millar TW, Steljes DG, et al. The effect of oxygen on respiration and sleep in patients with congestive heart failure. Ann Intern Med 1989;111:777–82.

67. Naughton MT, Benard DC, Rutherford R, et al. Effect of continuous positive airway pressure on central sleep apnea and nocturnal pCO_2 in heart failure. Am J Respir Crit Care Med 1994;150:1598–604.

68. Khayat RN, Xie A, Patel AK, et al. Cardiorespiratory effects of added dead space in patients with heart failure and central sleep apnea. Chest 2003;123:1551–60.

69. Steens RD, Millar TW, Xiaoling S, et al. Effect of inhaled 3% CO_2 on Cheyne-Stokes respiration in congestive heart failure. Sleep 1994;17:61–8.

70. Takasaki Y, Orr D, Popkin J, et al. Effect of nasal continuous positive airway pressure on sleep apnea in congestive heart failure. Am Rev Respir Dis 1989;140:1578–84.

71. Schädlich S, Königs I, Kalbitz F, et al. Cardiac efficiency in patients with Cheyne-Stokes Respiration as a result of heart insufficiency during long-term nasal respiratory treatment with adaptive servo ventilation (AutoSet CS). Z Kardiol 2004;93:454–62.

72. Töpfer V, El-Sebai M, Wessendorf TE, et al. Adaptive servoventilation: effect on Cheyne-Stokes-respiration and on quality of life. Pneumologie 2004;58:28–32.

73. Banno K, Okamura K, Kryger MH. Adaptive servo-ventilation in patients with idiopathic Cheyne-Stokes breathing. J Clin Sleep Med 2006;2:181–6.

74. Zhang X, Yin K, Li X, et al. Efficacy of adaptive servoventilation in patients with congestive heart failure and Cheyne-Stokes respiration. Chin Med J 2006;119:622–7.

75. Szollosi I, O'Driscoll DM, Dayer MJ, et al. Adaptive servo-ventilation and deadspace: effects on central sleep apnoea. J Sleep Res 2006;15:199–205.

76. Bitter T, Westerheide N, Faber L, et al. Adaptive servoventilation in diastolic heart failure and Cheyne-Stokes respiration. Eur Respir J 2009. [Epub ahead of print]. DOI:10.1183/09031936.00045609.

77. Fietze I, Blau A, Glos M, et al. Bi-level positive pressure ventilation and adaptive servo ventilation in patients with heart failure and Cheyne-Stokes respiration. Sleep Med 2008;9:652–9.

78. Pepperell JC, Maskell NA, Jones DR, et al. A randomized controlled trial of adaptive ventilation

for Cheyne-Stokes breathing in heart failure. Am J Respir Crit Care Med 2003;168:1109–14.

79. Hastings PC, Vazir A, Meadows GE, et al. Adaptive servo-ventilation in heart failure patients with sleep apnea: a real world study. Int J Cardiol 2010;139: 17–24.

80. Morrell MJ, Meadows GE, Hastings P, et al. The effects of adaptive servo ventilation on cerebral vascular reactivity in patients with congestive heart failure and sleep-disordered breathing. Sleep 2007;30:648–52.

81. Yao SM, Zhang XL. Association between residual sleepiness and central sleep apnea events in patients with obstructive sleep apnea syndrome. Zhonghua Jie He He Hu Xi Za Zhi 2008;31: 664–9.

82. Respironics. BiPAP autoSV user manual. Available at: http://www.respironics.com/UserGuides/BiPAPautoSVUserManualPN1040200.pdf. Accessed April 13, 2010.

83. Respironics. BiPAP autoSV provider manual. Available at: http://www.internetage.ws/cpapdata/manuals/bipap_auto_sv/bipap_auto_sv_provider_manual.pdf. Accessed April 13, 2010.

84. Respironics. BiPAP autoSV Sleep therapy system setup guide. Available at: http://www.respironics.com/UserGuides/BiPAPautoSVSetUpGuidePN1043629.pdf. Accessed April 13, 2010.

85. Respironics. BiPAP autoSV advanced user manual. Available at: http://www.medical.philips.com/asset.aspx?alt=&p=http://www.medical.philips.com/pwc_hc/main/homehealth/sleep/bipapautosvadvanced/downloads/BiPAP_autoSV_Advanced_User_Manual.pdf. Accessed April 13, 2010.

86. Respironics. BiPAP autoSV advanced provider manual. Available at: http://www.internetage.ws/cpapdata/manuals/bipap_auto_sv_adv/provider_manual.pdf. Accessed April 13, 2010.

87. Zdrojkowski RJ, Estes M, inventors; Respironics Inc, assignee. Breathing gas delivery method and apparatus. US Patent 5,803,065. September 8, 1998.

88. Respironics. BiPAP autoSV advanced. Available at: http://bipapautosvadvanced.respironics.com. Accessed April 14, 2010.

89. Kakkar RK, Berry RB. Positive airway pressure treatment for obstructive sleep apnea. Chest 2007;132: 1057–72.

90. Hirshkowitz M, Sharafkhaneh A. Positive airway pressure therapy of OSA. Semin Respir Crit Care Med 2005;26:68–79.

91. Respironics. Auto algorithm. Available at: http://sleepapnea.respironics.com/technology/autoalgorithm.aspx. Accessed April 14, 2010.

92. Respironics. Taking the complexity out of complicated sleep-disordered breathing. Titration guide for BiPAP autoSV Sleep Therapy System. Available at: http://www.respironics.com/UserGuides/BiPAPautoSVTitrationGuidePN1042977.pdf. Accessed April 14, 2010.

93. Kageshita T, Maeda H, Kusakabe Y, et al. [HEART PAP (adapted-servo ventilation; ASV) is effective for the ventilation of chronic heart failure patient with Cheyne-Stokes respiration]. Nihon Kokyuki Gakkai Zasshi 2008;46:921–7 [in Japanese].

94. Arzt M, Wensel R, Montalvan S, et al. Effects of dynamic bilevel positive airway pressure support on central sleep apnea in men with heart failure. Chest 2008;134:61–6.

95. Randerath WJ, Galetke W, Stieglitz S, et al. Adaptive servo-ventilation in patients with coexisting obstructive sleep apnoea/hypopnea and Cheyne-Stokes respiration. Sleep Med 2008;9:823–30.

Positive Airway Pressure Therapy in Children

Sangeeta Chakravorty, MD[a],*, Jonathan D. Finder, MD[b]

KEYWORDS

- Child • Obstructive sleep apnea • Positive airway pressure
- Noninvasive positive pressure ventilation
- Neuromuscular disorders

Children with obstructive sleep apnea syndrome (OSAS) have recurrent episodes of partial or complete airway obstruction during sleep, resulting in hypoxemia, hypercapnia, and sleep disruption. The earliest and best description of pediatric obstructive apnea can be found in Sir William Osler's 1892 textbook, "The Principals and Practice of Medicine" in a chapter entitled "Chronic Tonsillitis"[1]:

"The direct effect of chronic tonsillar hypertrophy is the establishment of mouth-breathing. The indirect effects are deformation of the thorax, changes in the facial expression, and sometimes marked alteration in the mental condition… At night the child's sleep is greatly disturbed; the respirations are loud and snorting, and there are sometimes prolonged pauses, followed by deep, noisy inspirations. The child may wake up in a paroxysm of shortness of breath…"

Childhood OSAS is a common cause of morbidity in approximately 2% of children.[2] Because of the documented association of childhood OSAS with adverse neurocognitive, cardiovascular, metabolic, growth, and inflammatory sequelae, more children are being referred to sleep laboratories for polysomnography, based on the recommendations of the American Academy of Pediatrics (AAP) guidelines for management of OSAS.[3]

In the past, OSAS was primarily associated with adenotonsillar hypertrophy in children. However, because of the rising incidence of childhood obesity, this diagnosis increasingly affects the treatment and incidence of childhood OSAS. Obese children are more likely to have residual obstructive sleep apnea (OSA) after adenotonsillectomy. Tauman and colleagues[4] have shown that the polysomnogram may not always normalize after surgical resection. The use of noninvasive positive pressure ventilatory support using continuous positive airway pressure (CPAP) and nocturnal noninvasive positive pressure ventilation (NIPPV, also referred to as *BiPAP* or *bilevel PAP*) in children of all ages has increased in the past decade.

This article describes the use of pediatric positive airway pressure in the treatment of sleep-disordered breathing (SDB), highlighting pathophysiology and clinical practical considerations in the nonsurgical management of childhood OSAS and chronic respiratory failure.

PATHOPHYSIOLOGY OF SDB
OSAS

The essential feature of OSAS is increased upper airway resistance during sleep. In contrast to

There are no financial conflicts of interest to report.

[a] Pediatric Sleep Laboratory, Children's Hospital of Pittsburgh of UPMC, University of Pittsburgh School of Medicine, One Children's Hospital Drive, 4401 Penn Avenue, Pittsburgh, PA 15224, USA

[b] Pediatric Pulmonology, Children's Hospital of Pittsburgh of UPMC, University of Pittsburgh School of Medicine, One Children's Hospital Drive, 4401 Penn Avenue, Pittsburgh, PA 15224, USA

* Corresponding author.

E-mail address: sangeeta.chakravorty@chp.edu

Sleep Med Clin 5 (2010) 439–449
doi:10.1016/j.jsmc.2010.05.005

sleep.theclinics.com

adults, in whom OSAS occurs predominantly in men, prevalence of OSAS does not differ between the sexes during childhood.[5] Anatomic narrowing of the upper airway and neuromuscular tone of upper airway musculature determine the propensity for upper airway collapse during sleep. Narrowing of the nasopharynx caused by allergic rhinitis, turbinate hypertrophy, deviated nasal septum, and maxillary constriction can all increase resistance in the nasal compartment. Palatal factors, tongue-base collapse, macroglossia, and posterior displacement of the mandible in craniofacial syndromes may also contribute to narrowing of the oropharynx or hypopharynx and result in OSAS.

Adenotonsillar hypertrophy is the most common cause of OSA in children between 2 and 8 years of age.[6] Children with other comorbidities, such as obesity, Trisomy 21, and cerebral palsy, may concurrently have abnormal central arousal thresholds, disordered neural control or airway caliber, and decreased pharyngeal tone. Dynamic airway collapse may occur at multiple sites in children with OSA. Hence, this is a multifactorial disorder with overlapping influences that predispose patients to obstructed breathing. The combination of genetic influences, neuromuscular tone, and structural anatomic factors variably and additively affect the presentation and severity of OSA.[7]

Obesity is an increasingly important and common risk factor for OSA in children.[8] Upper airway narrowing results from deposition of adipose tissue around the neck and jaw with external compression. Respiratory mechanics are altered with decreased chest wall compliance and upward displacement of the diaphragm by the obese abdomen, especially in the supine position. Lung volumes are reduced during sleep, with increased risk of desaturation associated with obstructive events. Gas exchange abnormalities with hypercapnia and obesity-related hypoventilation can occur in children[9]; hence, monitoring for hypoventilation during sleep is mandated in pediatric polysomnography using end-tidal carbon dioxide (CO_2) or transcutaneous CO_2 monitoring devices according to the guidelines for testing published by the American Academy of Sleep Medicine (AASM) in 2007.[10]

Chronic obstructed breathing with chronic hypoxemia, hypercarbia, or both may eventually lead to pulmonary hypertension in severe OSA.[11] Cardiovascular morbidity, right heart strain, and cor pulmonale may then ensue. Children with OSAS show signs of increased sympathetic activity, autonomic dysfunction, endothelial dysfunction, and a trend toward higher arterial blood pressure.[12,13]

Impaired growth has been seen in some children with OSAS[14] and has been thought to be related to increased work of breathing during sleep. These children have been shown to have impaired secretion of nocturnal growth hormone. Secondary nocturnal enuresis can also be a consequence of OSA, which may be caused by brain natriuretic peptide or atrial natriuretic peptide secretion.[15] Neurocognitive consequences include a higher incidence of attention deficit-hyperactivity disorder[16] and impaired learning[17] and memory,[18] affecting daytime behaviors and school performance in vulnerable children. Chronic OSA can therefore have reversible and irreversible consequences for children. Many of the these morbidities have improved after treatment with adenotonsillectomy[19] and efficacious use of NIPPV in children.[20]

CHRONIC RESPIRATORY FAILURE

Children who are at risk for chronic respiratory failure as a result of neuromuscular weakness, scoliosis, cerebral palsy, or myopathic disorders may ventilate adequately when awake but may decompensate with hypoventilation during sleep (**Box 1, Table 1**). Normally, during sleep, a decrease in tidal volume occurs, especially during rapid-eye-movement (REM) sleep, with a reduction in the respiratory rate and central respiratory drive. The P_{CO_2} rises by 3 to 7 mm of Hg, and a corresponding drop in PaO_2 of 3 to 9 mm of Hg may occur, compared with the waking state. Hence, gas exchange abnormalities and relative hypercapnia become apparent in vulnerable individuals during sleep, leading to sleep disruption.[21,22]

CENTRAL SLEEP APNEA AND CENTRAL HYPOVENTILATION

Causes in children include prematurity (central sleep apnea), Arnold-Chiari malformation,[23] and congenital central hypoventilation syndrome. Children with congenital central hypoventilation syndrome (a genetic disorder caused by a mutation in the PHOX2B gene) may have decreased tidal volume or respiratory rate during sleep, but may not have frank central apnea. These disorders tend to present during infancy, although late diagnoses have been reported.[24]

DIAGNOSIS

A history of snoring is a sensitive, though not specific, symptom of OSAS. Primary snorers are those who snore but have no obstructive apnea, gas exchange abnormalities, or sleep

Box 1
Congenital and medical conditions associated with OSAS

Achondroplasia

Apert's syndrome

Beckwith-Wiedemann syndrome

Cerebral palsy

Choanal stenosis

Cleft palate patients after repair

Crouzon syndrome

Cystic hygroma

Down syndrome

Hallermann-Streiff syndrome

Hypothyroidism

Klippel-Feil syndrome

Mucopolysaccharidosis

Obesity

Osteopetrosis

Papillomatosis (oropharyngeal)

Pierre Robin sequence

Pfeiffer syndrome

Pharyngeal flap surgery

Prader-Willi syndrome

Sickle cell disease

Treacher Collins syndrome

Data from Sterni LM, Tunkel DE. Obstructive sleep apnea in children: an update. Pediatr Clin North Am 2003;50:427–43.

part of routine health maintenance. Children with a history of nightly snoring should be evaluated further with overnight polysomnography, which is the gold standard for diagnosing OSA in children. However, the criteria for the performance, scoring, and interpretation of pediatric versus adult polysomnograms have significant differences. A detailed explanation is beyond the scope of this article, but other reviews of this important topic are available.[26]

For pediatric polysomnography, based on the recommendations of the American Thoracic Society,[27] the following parameters must be continuously monitored:

1. Respiratory effort, assessed through abdominal and chest wall movement
2. Airflow at nose, mouth, or both
3. Arterial oxygen saturation
4. End-tidal CO_2 or transcutaneous CO_2 (to detect hypoventilation)
5. Electrocardiograph
6. Tibialis anterior electromyography to detect movement and arousal
7. Electroencephalography, electro-oculography, and chin muscle electromyography for sleep staging
8. Video recording of nocturnal events.

Data correlating polysomnography parameters with clinical outcomes in children are presently insufficient and no standard guidelines exist for classifying the severity of OSA in children. Polysomnography data from nonsnoring children defined OSA as more than one obstructive apnea event per hour of sleep. However, this classification does not take into consideration the duration of the obstructive event. Often obstructive apneas and hypopneas identified during a sleep study are combined to calculate the apnea–hypopnea index (AHI) defined as the number of discrete obstructive events per hour of sleep. Some sleep laboratories

fragmentation with multiple arousals on polysomnography (sleep study). Approximately 10% of children have primary snoring.[25] Screening children for OSA is recommended by the AAP as

Table 1
Severity of OSA based on polysomnography guidelines

	AHI	Oxygen Saturation Nadir
Normal	0–1 per h	>92%
Mild OSA	2–4 per h	
Moderate OSA	5–9 per h	
Severe OSA	>10 per h	<80%

Peak end-tidal CO_2 value greater than 60 mm Hg and percent of time spent with end-tidal CO_2 greater than 50 mm Hg should also be considered when assessing severity.

Abbreviations: AHI, apnea-hypopnea index.

Data from Halbower AC, Ishman SL, McGinley BM. Childhood obstructive sleep disordered breathing: a clinical update and discussion of technological innovations and challenges. Chest 2007;132(6):2030–41.

also report a respiratory disturbance index (RDI), which includes all the scored events (including central apneas) per hour. Ideally, only the AHI should be used to diagnose pediatric OSA.

The accepted consensus among many pediatric sleep specialists and laboratories is to use the guidelines in **Box 2** to assess severity of OSA based on polysomnography.

SURGICAL TREATMENT

Adenotonsillectomy is the preferred treatment for most children with OSAS. Sleep-related obstruction and quality of life measures are estimated to improve in more than 75% of children after adenotonsillectomy.[28] However, persistent respiratory abnormalities may be seen in a significant percentage of children varying between 25% and 70% on postoperative polysomnography.[4] Guilleminault and colleagues[29] estimate a cure rate after adenotonsillectomy of less than 50% in children. In their prospective survey, including questionnaires, clinical examination, polysomnography, and esophageal pressure monitoring, 94 of 199 children still had abnormal sleep recordings on repeat evaluation after adenotonsillectomy.

In another long-term follow-up of 615 preschool children, only half of the children who underwent surgery for SDB showed complete symptomatic improvement on follow-up.[30] In yet another study, a group of 79 healthy children with a mean age of 6 years was followed. Quality of life and AHI improved dramatically, but using the new pediatric guidelines for defining pediatric SDB, only 71% had normal polysomnography parameters after adenotonsillectomy.[31] Postoperative polysomnography may be indicated for children with craniofacial anomalies, obesity, and a preoperative AHI of greater than 10 per hour. Children with abnormal craniofacial anatomy or abnormal neuromotor tone may require additional treatment of persistent OSA, including pharyngeal surgery, uvulopalatopharyngoplasty, and tongue reduction procedures, and maxillomandibular advancement in syndromic children with obstructive macroglossia that results from craniofacial structural abnormalities.[32]

TREATMENT WITH POSITIVE AIRWAY PRESSURE

Nonsurgical treatment of SDB has a role in children undergoing positive airway pressure treatment. These modalities are used as second-line therapy in pediatrics, unlike in adults. The indications for CPAP/BiPAP therapy in children are as follows[33]:

Persistent symptomatic OSA after adenotonsillectomy

Contraindications to adenotonsillectomy

Family/patient preference for nonsurgical alternative

Complex sleep apnea with central and obstructive features

Preoperative management of patients with severe OSA while awaiting definitive treatment, postoperative management after surgery for severe OSA, or in patients with cardiovascular complications from OSA

Management of pulmonary hypertension and cor pulmonale.

Continuous positive airway pressure (CPAP) delivers a constant pressure to the airway; bilevel positive airway pressure (BiPAP) applies a pressure that decreases during exhalation (**Table 2**).

Mechanism of Action

The application of positive pressure mechanically stents the airway open, decreasing the negative forces that promote upper airway collapsibility and restores sleep continuity, improves functional residual capacity, stabilizes arterial oxygen saturation, and improves gas exchange, thus reversing many of the factors that disrupted the breathing during sleep. With the maintenance of a patent upper airway, the work of breathing is decreased, leading to rest of the respiratory muscles and improved tissue oxygenation from reversal of intermittent hypoxemia. Sleep fragmentation subsides with reduced arousal and sleep is more continuous and restful. The restorative function of sleep and subjective well-being are enhanced.

The level of positive pressure required to eliminate obstructive apneas and normalize ventilation and nighttime oxygen saturation in children is best accomplished by attended polysomnography with titration in a polysomnography laboratory manned by experienced technologists and expert interpreters.

CPAP in children has been studied for efficacy and safety and has been shown to relieve SDB.[34]

PRACTICAL GOALS OF POSITIVE PRESSURE TITRATION IN THE PEDIATRIC SLEEP LABORATORY

After SDB is diagnosed, when a therapeutic study is requested in the sleep laboratory, the physician must communicate the goals of the study clearly to the technologist. A therapeutic study involves measurement of the same parameters as in a diagnostic study. In addition, airflow is measured from

Box 2
Some causes of neuromuscular weakness and chronic respiratory failure

Myopathies
Muscular dystrophies
  Dystrophinopathies
  Duchenne's
  Becker's

Other muscular dystrophies
  Limb-girdle
  Emery-Dreifuss
  Facio-scapulo-humeral
  Congenital
  Myotonic dystrophy

Other myopathies
  Acid maltase deficiency
  Acid alpha glucocidase deficiency
  Mucopolysaccharidoses
  Mitochondrial myopathies

Inflammatory myopathies
  Polymyositis

Diseases of the myoneural junction
  Myasthenia gravis
  Congenital myasthenic syndromes
  Mixed connective tissue disease

Myopathies of systemic disease
  Cancer
  Cachexia/anorexia nervosa
  Medication-induced myopathy

Neurologic causes
Spinal muscular atrophy
Motor neuron diseases
Poliomyelitis
Neuropathies
  Hereditary sensory motor neuropathies
  Guillain-Barré syndrome

Multiple sclerosis
Disorders of supraspinal tone
  Friedreich's ataxia

Myelopathies
  Rheumatologic

Infectious
Vascular
Traumatic
Idiopathic

Static encephalopathies
  Arnold-Chiari malformation
  Syringomyelia
  Myelomeningocele
  Encephalitis

Data from Bach JB. Non-invasive mechanical ventilation. Philadelphia: Hanley and Belfus; 2002. p. 2.

the accurate internal flow sensor, which can show flow limitation. Clear parameters for oxygen saturation values and correction of hypercapnia, and the criteria for adding supplemental oxygen and conversion to BiPAP from CPAP, are helpful for judicious use of technologist time and satisfactory technical study performance.

The split-night study is discouraged in pediatric laboratories, because it can be rather frightening and uncomfortable for a child and parent to be awakened in the laboratory and to wear equipment, without adequate explanation and introduction earlier. Hence, most laboratories permit an interval of several days or weeks between the diagnostic and therapeutic sleep studies to allow time for the patient and family to understand the rationale for the proposed therapy and be prepared for positive airway pressure use when they arrive for the therapeutic study. The authors' practice has found home nasal CPAP mask desensitization to be very helpful in reducing anxiety, improving the child's cooperation, demystifying the experience of laboratory titration, and improving adherence to therapy in the long-term.

CPAP and BiPAP titrations may be performed as initial studies to ascertain the pressure required for treatment of patients with newly diagnosed SDB. The authors also periodically repeat the study when a previously stable and compliant CPAP user experiences symptom recurrence with snoring or excessive daytime somnolence (EDS) despite adequate documented compliance with therapy at home, or the CPAP user experiences a significant weight gain or loss. As the child grows, periodic reevaluations of therapy may become necessary, because the pressure required for maintaining airway patency may change with time, age, medications, and other medical comorbidities. All AASM certified laboratories and centers ideally should have written

Table 2
Complications of CPAP/BiPAP and ensuing treatment

Complications of CPAP/BiPAP	Treatment
Local discomfort or irritation from poor mask fit	Alternative mask trial
Eye irritation/conjunctivitis	Reduce leak, proper mask fit
Nasal congestion	Heated humidification
Skin irritation/ulceration	Barrier creams, tape, alternative mask
Aerophagy	Reduce pressures
Gastroesophageal reflux	Reduce pressures, medical therapy
Chest discomfort	Reduce pressures
Pneumothorax (not hitherto reported in children)	Reduce pressures
Midface hypoplasia with long-term use	Periodic cephalometry
Maxillary compression/dental misalignment	

Data from Schwengel DA, Sterni LM, et al. Perioperative management of children with obstructive sleep apnea. Anesth Analg 2009;109:60–75.

protocols for the positive airway pressure titration and oxygen supplementation procedures and all staff technologists should be trained to follow them.

A successful titration involves the documented resolution of apneas, hypopneas, snoring, arousals, and gas exchange abnormalities at the final pressure achieved in the laboratory. The technologist/interpreting physician should also document the interface used in the laboratory and note any leaks from the mask, and then after the titration assess the patient's response to the trial. The introduction of "smart cards" in positive airway pressure devices has improved the objective measurement of compliance data and provides a useful metric to monitor a patient's acceptance of and adherence to therapy.

Currently, data in the literature are insufficient to support the use of unattended autotitrating CPAP and BiPAP devices in the home setting, as is being done in adults.

TREATMENT OF BLOOD GAS ABNORMALITIES IN SDB

Hypoxemia is thought to play a central role in the neuronal injury, neuropsychological impairment,[35] and cardiovascular sequelae[36] of SDB. Infants have shown improved total sleep time, decreased periodic breathing, and decreased apnea with supplemental oxygen.[37] In children with a mean age of 4 years and significant OSA, supplemental oxygen significantly reduced the obstructive apnea index and paradoxic breathing but was considered a temporary treatment while awaiting

long-term therapy.[38] More research is needed to examine whether use of supplemental oxygen reduces cardiovascular risk and catecholamine release associated with hypertension in SDB.

Hypercapnia secondary to hypoventilation in obstructive hypoventilation and obesity–hypoventilation syndrome responds to treatment with BiPAP, with a higher span between inspiratory (IPAP) and expiratory (EPAP) positive airway pressures (>5 cm H_2O difference). Occasionally, a backup rate must be used to maintain minute ventilation if CPAP/BiPAP lead to development of central apneas during titration.[5] During titration, accurate measurement of end-tidal CO_2 values may be compromised by the difficulty in placing the end-tidal CO_2 cannula in conjunction with the chosen nasal interface, especially in young children. Correlation with a transcutaneous CO_2 monitor can be helpful in that circumstance.

POSITIVE PRESSURE TITRATION GUIDELINES

In April 2008, the positive airway pressure titration task force of the AASM published clinical guidelines for the manual titration of positive airway pressure in patients with OSA.[39] These recommendations are applicable to adult (defined by AASM as >12 years) and pediatric (<12 years) patients with a confirmed diagnosis of OSA (**Box 3**).

Although adult sleep physicians and laboratories have received these recommendations favorably, residual concerns remain because of the differing definitions for apnea, hypopnea, and severity of OSA in children. Furthermore, the

---

Box 3
Major recommendations of the positive airway pressure titration task force of the AASM

1. All potential PAP titration candidates should receive adequate PAP education, hands-on demonstration, careful mask fitting, and acclimatization before titration.

2. CPAP (IPAP or EPAP for BiPAP) should be increased until the following obstructive respiratory events are eliminated or the recommended maximum pressure is reached: apneas, hypopneas, respiratory effort–related arousals (RERA), snoring

3. The minimum recommended starting pressure for CPAP should be 4 cm H_2O for pediatric and adult patients, and the minimum starting IPAP and EPAP should be 8 and 4 cm H_2O, respectively, for BiPAP.

4. Maximum CPAP of 15 cm H_2O or IPAP of 20 cm H_2O (if patient on BiPAP) recommended for pediatric patients younger than 12 years. Maximum CPAP of 20 cm H_2O was recommended for patients older than 12 years.

5. Recommended IPAP–EPAP differential minimum during BiPAP titration was 4 cm H_2O and the recommended maximum was 10 cm H_2O

6. CPAP (IPAP or EPAP for patients on BiPAP, depending on the type of event) should be increased by at least 1 cm H_2O, with an interval no shorter than 5 minutes, with the goal of eliminating obstructive respiratory events.

7. CPAP (IPAP and EPAP for patients on BiPAP) should be increased from any level if at least one obstructive apnea is observed for patients younger than 12 years or two obstructive apneas are observed in patients older than 12 years.

8. CPAP (IPAP or patients on BiPAP) should be increased from any level if at least one obstructive hypopnea is observed for patients younger than 12 years or three obstructive hypopneas are observed in patients older than 12 years.

9. CPAP (IPAP for patients on BiPAP) should be increased from any level if at least three RERAs are observed for patients younger than 12 years, or five RERAs are observed in patients older than 12 years.

10. CPAP (IPAP for patients on BiPAP) may be increased from any level if at least 1 minute of unambiguous snoring is observed for patients younger than 12 years, or at least 3 minutes of unambiguous snoring are observed in patients older than 12 years.

11. The titration algorithm for split-night CPAP or BiPAP titration studies should be identical to that for full-night CPAP or BiPAP titration studies, respectively

12. If the patient is uncomfortable or intolerant of high pressures on CPAP, BiPAP may be tried. If obstructive events continue at CPAP 15 cm H_2O during the titration, the patient may be switched to BiPAP.

13. The pressure of CPAP or BiPAP selected for patient use after the titration study should reflect control of the patient's obstructive respiration by a low (preferably <5 per hour in patients >12 years) respiratory disturbance index (RDI) at the selected pressure, a minimum sea level oxygen saturation (SpO_2) greater than 90% at the pressure, and with a leak within acceptable parameters at the pressure.

14. An optimal titration reduces RDI to less than 5 for at least a 15-minute duration and should include supine REM sleep at the selected pressure that is not continually interrupted by spontaneous arousals or awakenings.

15. A good titration reduces RDI to less than 10 or by 50%. If the baseline RDI is less than 15, it should include supine REM sleep that is not continuously interrupted by spontaneous arousals or awakenings at the selected pressure.

16. An adequate titration does not reduce the RDI to less than 10, but rather reduces the RDI by 75% from baseline (especially in patients with severe OSA) or is one in which the titration grading criteria for optimal or good are met with the exception that supine REM sleep did not occur at the selected pressure.

17. An unacceptable titration is one that does not meet any of the above grades.

18. A repeat positive airway pressure titration study should be considered if the initial titration does not achieve a degree of optimal or good and, if it is a split-night polysomnography study, fails to meet AASM criteria (ie, titration duration should be >3 hours).

---

maximum pressures suggested in the guidelines are somewhat arbitrary, without sufficient evidence to support placing restrictions on the maximal pressure in children. More pediatric studies may be needed to better define the parameters of titration in children; however, these task force guidelines serve as a useful step in outlining

> **Box 4**
> **Factors influencing pediatric CPAP use**
>
> 1. Desensitization of children in the home setting before laboratory exposure to CPAP is helpful and advisable.
>
> 2. Some laboratories and programs use behavioral psychologists to help desensitize children and allow them to gradually overcome fears and discomfort.
>
> 3. Practitioners and parents should plan to use appropriate strategies to avoid escape behaviors and reinforce positive messages with interesting activities, education, and in-clinic demonstrations.
>
> 4. Many interfaces are available for pediatric CPAP; however, home use of nasal interfaces for SDB in young children (>7 years) and infants have not been approved by the U.S. Food Drug Administration (FDA).
>
> 5. Although ventilators are available for home use in infants, nasal interfaces for noninvasive use are not.
>
> 6. Because of their availability, nasal masks made for older children and adults are sometimes used as oronasal full-face masks in infants and younger children with neuromuscular disorders.
>
> 7. Little evidence shows that full-face masks are effective in treating OSA in children and adults. Full-face interfaces applied across the nasal and oral cavities cause equal pressure to be applied to the nasopharynx and oropharynx, which may not create the transmural pressure differential required to open the upper airway.
>
> 8. Very young children, children with neuromuscular weakness, those with gastroesophageal reflux, or those with developmental delays using a full-face mask are at risk with regard to aspiration of stomach contents. If they are unable to pull off the mask in an emergency, its use poses a risk. Hence, use of these interfaces should be discouraged except in rare circumstances when the benefits may outweigh the risk.
>
> 9. With the increased recognition of pediatric SDB and rising childhood obesity, evidence suggests that the use of NIPPV will increase in developed countries. The Pediatric Medical Device Safety and Improvement Act of 2007 (Title 111 for the FDA amendments Act of 2007) was passed to address this medical need.
>
> 10. Health care workers should put pressure on device manufacturers to improve the availability of suitable pediatric interfaces in the United States. Although CPAP is a safe and effective noninvasive alternative to tracheotomy, and is being used for infants and young children in other developed countries, the smallest pediatric devices are not commercially available in the United States because of a lack of profitability.
>
> *Data from* Halbower AC, Mc Ginley BM, et al. Treatment alternatives for sleep-disordered breathing in the pediatric population. Curr Opin Pulm Med 2008;14:551–8.

PAP protocols. The task force also elucidated that these recommendations should not be followed in a "cookbook" manner; instead, sleep technologists and clinicians should combine their experience and judgment with the application of these recommendations to attain the best possible titration outcome in any given patient.

SPECIAL CONSIDERATIONS FOR CPAP/BIPAP USE IN CHILDREN

As stated by Halbower and colleagues,[40] "CPAP use in children includes the training of the parents, whose complete support of the therapy is essential in order for the child to accept the use of the device." Several recommendations and factors can help achieve this goal, as listed in **Box 4**.

SPECIAL CONSIDERATIONS FOR THE NEUROMUSCULARLY WEAK CHILD

Noninvasive positive pressure ventilation has become increasingly accepted in patients with sleep hypoventilation secondary to neuromuscular weakness. The two major populations using bilevel pressure ventilation (BiPAP and VPAP) are those with Duchenne muscular dystrophy and spinal muscular atrophy. The boys and young men with Duchenne muscular dystrophy tend to develop hypoventilation in sleep once the restrictive defect reaches a threshold of approximately 30% of the predicted forced vital capacity.[41] Hypoventilation first occurs during REM sleep, with preservation of ventilation during non-REM sleep.[42]

Anticipation of the need for support of nocturnal ventilation is critical in this population, because the loss is inevitable but may be precipitated by acute illness. Therefore, routine polysomnography has been recommended annually for this patient population.[43] Use of bi-level ventilatory support in infants with spinal atrophy type I has recently become accepted therapy.[44] A lack of a spectrum of interfaces for infants has been the biggest challenge in initiating noninvasive support in those with spinal muscular atrophy type 1 (SMA-I). Aggressive management of infants with SMA-I has been shown to improve spontaneous daytime ventilation and avoid need for tracheostomy in this population.[45] Titration of bilevel ventilatory support should always be performed in the pediatric sleep laboratory, because brief hypoventilation and desaturation, which can interfere with REM sleep, are especially common in this population.

Other devices with modified BiPAP, such as average volume assured pressure support (AVAPS), which includes the ability to set a tidal volume and is thus similar to volume-controlled ventilation, are available commercially and may be beneficial for improving minute ventilation in patients with obesity hypoventilation.[46] No pediatric studies are available using this modality. Adaptive servoventilation may be considered if the patient is observed to have Cheyne-Stokes respiration, or if treatment-emergent central sleep apnea (ie, complex sleep apnea) during titration study is not eliminated by down-titration of pressure.[39]

NEWER THERAPIES IN DEVELOPMENT

A recent paper by McGinley and colleagues[47] showed the effectiveness of a high-flow, low-pressure, humidified nasal cannula for treating OSA in adults. When humidified air was delivered at 20 L/min through an open nasal cannula, the AHI in the adult research cohort with mild to moderate OSA dropped to fewer than 10 events per hour in most participants. The pressure increase in the oropharynx was only 2 cm H_2O, and therefore the mechanism for its effectiveness remains uncertain. Neural activation of dilatory muscles in the pharynx, increased lung volumes, or reduced dead space have been postulated as possible mechanisms. Studies examining its efficacy in children are in progress.

SUMMARY

Positive airway pressure therapy is playing an increasingly important role in the judicious management of a wide spectrum of childhood SDB. Positive airway pressure is effective and beneficial when prescribed and used correctly. Pediatric sleep specialists must advocate for their patients and demand better child-friendly devices and interfaces to improve adherence and compliance with therapy.

ACKNOWLEDGMENTS

The authors gratefully acknowledge the expert editorial assistance of Josephine Boyd.

REFERENCES

1. Osler W. Principles and practice of medicine. New York: D. Appleton and Company; 1892. p. 335–9.
2. Redline S, Tishler PV, Schluchter M, et al. Risk factors for sleep disordered breathing in children: associations with obesity, race and respiratory problems. Am J Respir Crit Care Med 1999;159:1527–32.
3. American Academy of Pediatrics. Clinical practice guideline: diagnosis and management of childhood obstructive sleep apnea syndrome. Pediatrics 2002; 109:704–12.
4. Tauman R, Gulliver TE, Krishna J, et al. Persistence of obstructive sleep apnea syndrome in children after adenotonsillectomy. J Pediatr 2006;149:803–8.
5. Liner LH, Marcus CL. Ventilatory management of sleep disordered breathing in children. Curr Opin Pediatr 2006;18:272–6.
6. Schecter MS; Section on Pediatric Pulmonology, Subcommittee on Obstructive Sleep Apnea Syndrome. Technical report: diagnosis and management of childhood obstructive sleep apnea syndrome. Pediatrics 2002;109:E69.
7. Arens R, Marcus CL. Pathophysiology of upper airway obstruction: a developmental perspective. Sleep 2004;27:997–1019.
8. Ng DK, Chow PY, Chan CH, et al. An update on childhood snoring. Acta Paediatr 2006;95(9):1029–35.
9. Kohler M, Lushington K, Couper R, et al. Obesity and risk of sleep-related obstruction in Caucasian children. J Clin Sleep Med 2008;4(2):129–36.
10. Redline S, Budhiraja R, Kapur V, et al. The scoring of respiratory events in sleep: reliability and validity. J Clin Sleep Med 2007;3:169–200.
11. Blum RH, McGowan FX Jr. Chronic upper airway obstruction and cardiac dysfunction: anatomy, pathophysiology and anesthetic implications. Paediatr Anaesth 2004;14:75–83.
12. Bixler EO, Vgontzas AN, Lin HM, et al. Blood pressure associated with sleep disordered breathing in a population sample of children. Hypertension 2008;52(5):841–6.
13. Enright PL, Goodwin JL, Sherrill DL, et al. Blood pressure elevation associated with sleep breathing disorder in a community sample of white and Hispanic children: the Tucson Children's assessment of sleep apnea study. Arch Pediatr Adolesc Med 2003;157(9):901–4.
14. Marcus CL, Carroll JL, Koerner CB, et al. Determinants of growth in children with the obstructive sleep apnea syndrome. J Pediatr 1994;125:556–62.
15. SansCapdevila O, Crabtree VM, Kheirandish-Gozal L, et al. Increased morning brain natriuretic peptide levels in children with nocturnal enuresis and sleep-disordered breathing: a community based study. Pediatrics 2008;121(5):e1208–14.

16. Chervin RD, Dillon JE, Bassetti C, et al. Symptoms of sleep disorders, inattention, hyperactivity in children. Sleep 1997;20(12):1185–92.

17. Kaeming KL, Pasvogel AE, Goodwin JL, et al. Learning in children and sleep disordered breathing: findings of the Tucson Children's assessment of sleep apnea (TuCASA) prospective cohort study. J Int Neuropsychol Soc 2003;9(7):1016–26.

18. Kheirandish L, Gozal D. Neurocognitive dysfunction in children with sleep disorders. Dev Sci 2006;9(4): 388–99.

19. Huang YS, Guilleminault C, Li HY, et al. Attention deficit/hyperactivity disorder with obstructive sleep apnea: a treatment outcome study. Sleep Med 2007;8(1):18–30.

20. Marcus CL, Ward SL, Mallory GB, et al. Use of nasal continuous positive airway pressure as treatment of childhood obstructive sleep apnea. J Pediatr 1995; 127:88–94.

21. Khan Y, Heckmatt JZ, Dubowitz V. Sleep studies and supportive ventilatory treatment in patients with congenital muscle disorders. Arch Dis Child 1996; 74(3):195–200.

22. Mellies U, Ragette R, Dohna Schwake C, et al. Long-term non-invasive ventilation in children and adolescents with neuromuscular disorders. Eur Respir J 2003;22(4):631–6.

23. Dauvilliers Y, Stal V, Abril B, et al. Chiari malformation and sleep breathing disorders. J Neurol Neurosurg Psychiatr 2007;78(12):1344–8.

24. Repetto GM, Corrales RJ, Abara SG, et al. Late onset congenital central hypoventilation syndrome due to a heterozygous 24-polyalanine expansion mutation in the PHOX2B gene. Acta Paediatr 2009; 98(1):192–5.

25. Corbo GM, Forastiere F, Agabiti N, et al. Snoring in 9-15 yr old children: risk factors and clinical relevance. Pediatrics 2001;108:1149–54.

26. Muzumdar H, Arens R. Diagnostic issues in pediatric obstructive sleep apnea. Proc Am Thorac Soc 2008;5(2):263–73.

27. American Thoracic Society. Standards and indications for cardiopulmonary sleep studies in children. Am J Respir Crit Care Med 1996,153:866–78.

28. Brietzke SE, Gallagher D. Effectiveness of tonsillectomy and adenoidectomy in the treatment of pediatric obstructive sleep apnea/hypopnea syndrome: a meta-analysis. Otolaryngol Head Neck Surg 2006;134:979–84.

29. Guilleminault C, Huang YS, Glamann C, et al. Adenotonsillectomy and obstructive sleep apnea in children: a prospective study. Otolaryngol Head Neck Surg 2007;136:169–75.

30. Lofstrand-Tidestrom B, Hulcrantz E. The development of snoring and sleep-related breathing distress from 4-6 yrs in a cohort of Swedish children. Int J Pediatr Otorhinolaryngol 2007;71:1025–33.

31. Mitchell RB. Adenotonsillectomy for obstructive sleep apnea in children: outcome evaluated by pre and postoperative polysomnography. Laryngoscope 2007;117:1025–33.

32. Kerschner JE, Lynch JB, Kleiner H, et al. Uvulopalatopharyngoplasty with tonsillectomy and adenoidectomy as a treatment for obstructive sleep apnea in neurologically impaired children. Int J Pediatr Otorhinolaryngol 2002;62:229–35.

33. Schwengel DA, Sterni LM, Tunkel DE, et al. Perioperative management of children with obstructive sleep apnea. Anesth Analg 2009;109:60–75.

34. Marcus CL, Rosen G, Ward SL, et al. Adherence to and effectiveness of positive airway pressure therapy in children with obstructive sleep apnea. Pediatrics 2006;117:e442–51.

35. Halbower AC, Degaonkar M, Barker PB, et al. Childhood obstructive sleep apnea associates with neuropsychological deficits and neuronal brain injury. PLoS Med 2006;3:e301.

36. Yamamoto H, Teramoto S, Yamaguchi Y, et al. Effect of nasal continuous positive airway pressure treatment on plasma adrenomodulin levels in patients with obstructive sleep apnea syndrome: roles of nocturnal hypoxia and oxidative stress. Hypertens Res 2007;30:1065–76.

37. Simakajornboon N, Beckerman RC, Mack C, et al. Effect of supplemental oxygen on sleep architecture and cardiorespiratory events in pre-term infants. Pediatrics 2002;110:884–8.

38. Aljadeff G, Gozal D, Bailey-Wahl SL, et al. Effects of overnight supplemental oxygen in obstructive sleep apnea in children. Am J Respir Crit Care Med 1996;153:51–5.

39. Kushida CA, Chediak A, Berry RB, et al. Clinical practice guidelines for manual titration of positive airway pressure in the treatment of obstructive sleep apnea. Consensus statement of the American Academy of Sleep Medicine PAP Task Force. J Clin Sleep Med 2008;4(2):157–71.

40. Halbower AC, McGinley BM, Smith PL. Treatment alternatives for sleep-disordered breathing in the pediatric population. Curr Opin Pulm Med 2008;14: 551–8.

41. Lyager S, Steffensen B, Juhl B. Indicators of need for mechanical ventilation in Duchenne muscular dystrophy and spinal muscular atrophy. Chest 1995;108:779–85.

42. Suresh S, Wales P, Dakin C, et al. Sleep-related breathing disorder in Duchenne muscular dystrophy: disease spectrum in the paediatric population. J Paediatr Child Health 2005;41: 500–3.

43. Finder JD, Birnkrant D, Carl J, et al. Respiratory care of the patient with Duchenne muscular dystrophy: an official ATS consensus statement. Am J Respir Crit Care Med 2004;170:456–65.

44. Wang CH, Finkel RS, Bertini ES, et al. Consensus statement for standard of care in spinal muscular atrophy. J Child Neurol 2007; 22:1027.

45. Bach JR, Niranjan V, Weaver B. Spinal muscular atrophy Type 1 A noninvasive respiratory management approach. Chest 2000;117:1100–5.

46. Storr JH, Seuth B, Fiechter R, et al. Average volume-assured pressure support in obesity hypoventilation: a randomized crossover trial. Chest 2006;130(3): 815–21.

47. McGinley BM, Patil SP, Kirkness JP, et al. A nasal cannula can be used to treat obstructive sleep apnea. Am J Respir Crit Care Med 2007;176:194–200.

Noninvasive Positive Airway Pressure in Hypercapnic Respiratory Failure in Noncardiac Medical Disorders

Charles A. Poon, MD[a], Kendra A. Becker, MD, MPH[a], Michael R. Littner, MD[a,b,*]

KEYWORDS

- Noninvasive positive pressure ventilation
- Chronic obstructive pulmonary disease • Cystic fibrosis
- Kyphoscoliosis • Neuromuscular disease

Noninvasive positive pressure ventilation (NIPPV) is commonly used to improve gas exchange in patients with various noncardiac medical conditions. This article discusses NIPPV in chronic obstructive pulmonary disease (COPD), cystic fibrosis (CF), kyphoscoliosis, and neuromuscular disorders, including amyotrophic lateral sclerosis (ALS), Duchenne muscular dystrophy (DMD), myasthenia gravis (MG), and postpolio syndrome (PPS). NIPPV is typically delivered by bilevel positive airway pressure (BPAP) or, in some cases, ventilatory support other than BPAP.

POSITIVE AIRWAY PRESSURE AS A TREATMENT MODALITY

Positive airway pressure (PAP) is delivered by medical devices that generate either a continuous PAP (CPAP) or a pressure gradient with different inspiratory and expiratory pressures, such as BPAP. BPAP is preferred in acute and chronic hypercapnic respiratory failure because it increases alveolar ventilation.

CPAP is effective in patients with obstructive sleep apnea (OSA) by increasing the extrathoracic airway pressure to a level above the atmospheric pressure, thereby preventing collapse of the upper airway. This process has been called a "pneumatic splint".[1]

CPAP may also increase the lung volume by increasing the functional residual capacity (FRC). This volume increase may improve oxygenation but may also increase hypercapnia by increasing respiratory dead space, which generally makes CPAP less effective for hypercapnic respiratory failure.[2]

BPAP may be effective for treating patients with hypercapnic respiratory failure. The inspiratory PAP to expiratory positive airway pressure (EPAP) differential provides a gradient to inflate and deflate the lungs. The EPAP is, in effect, a form of positive end-expiratory pressure that provides some of the benefits of CPAP (increase in FRC to improve oxygenation) combined with ventilatory support to reduce hypercapnia.[2]

NIPPV is delivered to patients through an interface that may include a nasal mask, nasal pillows,

[a] Pulmonary, Critical Care and Sleep Medicine, VA Greater Los Angeles Healthcare System (VA GLA), 16111 Plummer Street, Sepulveda, CA 91343, USA
[b] Department of Medicine, David Geffen School of Medicine at UCLA, Los Angeles, CA, USA
* Corresponding author. 10736 Des Moines Avenue, Porter Ranch, CA 91326.
E-mail address: mlittner@ucla.edu

Sleep Med Clin 5 (2010) 451–470
doi:10.1016/j.jsmc.2010.05.008
1556-407X/10/$ – see front matter. Published by Elsevier Inc.

a full-face mask, or an oral mouthpiece.[3] The complications of using a noninvasive interface, such as pressure sores, are beyond the scope of this article. Detailed methods of titration are also not covered in this article. However, the reader should be aware that inspiratory pressures greater than 20 cm may be required and ventilator support other than BPAP may be needed. Documentation of successful NIPPV is generally obtained through attended polysomnography (PSG), nocturnal monitoring of arterial oxygen hemoglobin saturation (saturation), transcutaneous partial pressure of carbon dioxide ($Paco_2$), or end-tidal CO_2.

PAP IN STABLE COPD

COPD is a treatable and preventable disease that results in airflow obstruction that is not fully (ie, partially) reversible.[4–6] The obstructive component of COPD is documented by spirometry with a post-bronchodilator forced expiratory volume in 1 second/forced vital capacity (FEV_1/FVC) ratio (in liters) of less than 0.70 (**Table 1**). The severity is determined in part by the FEV_1, with severe COPD being an FEV_1 of less than 50% predicted. COPD is primarily the result of cigarette smoking, a common cause of morbidity, and the fourth leading cause of mortality in the United States and the world.[4]

The clinical-pathologic conditions most associated with COPD are one or a combination of chronic bronchitis (chronic cough and sputum production) and emphysema. Symptoms may include dyspnea, COPD exacerbations, and fatigue.

Etiology and Pathophysiology

The pathologic results of exposure to cigarette smoke and the resulting neutrophil airway inflammation may include squamous metaplasia of the respiratory epithelium, respiratory ciliary loss and dysfunction, inflammation and fibrosis of airways, mucous gland hyperplasia and hypersecretion, increased airway smooth muscle, loss of alveolar attachments, and bronchoconstriction from vagally mediated release of acetylcholine.[4]

The differential diagnoses include asthma, bronchiectasis, bronchiolitis, upper airway obstruction (eg, from a tumor), postviral airway inflammation, eosinophilic bronchitis, and congestive heart failure.

Arterial blood gases are generally obtained only in borderline cases of hypoxemia (saturation $\leq 92\%$ by pulse oximetry) and to determine the presence of hypercapnia. Patients with very low FEV_1 levels (<30% predicted) are particularly at risk of having hypercapnia[4–6] and may be candidates for NIPPV.

Treatment of COPD

Pharmacologic treatment is primarily directed at relaxing the airway smooth muscle with bronchodilators. Attempts to reduce inflammation have not been obviously successful, but inhaled corticosteroids and phosphodiesterase inhibition (eg, theophylline) may have a limited anti-inflammatory effect. In addition, nonpharmacologic therapy includes pulmonary rehabilitation, smoking cessation, and long-term oxygen therapy (LTOT). The use

Table 1
Some measures of pulmonary function in obstructive and restrictive lung disease

Pulmonary Function	No Lung Disease	Obstruction	Restriction
FEV_1	80%–120% predicted	Normal or reduced	Normal or reduced
FVC	80%–120% predicted	Normal or reduced	Reduced
FEV_1/FVC	$\leq 0.7^a$	Reduced	Normal or increased
TLC	80%–120% predicted	Normal or increased	Reduced
DLCOsb	80%–120% predicted	Normal in chronic bronchitis, reduced in emphysema, may be increased in asthma	Normal or near normal in chest wall and neuromuscular disease, reduced in interstitial lung disease

Predicted ranges are approximate and should be modified according to specific patient populations. The abnormalities of pulmonary function are generalizations, individual patients may vary.
Abbreviations: DLCOsb, single breath diffusing capacity for carbon monoxide; TLC, total lung capacity.
[a] A rough rule of thumb, which may require adjustment based on the age of the patient.
Data from Global Initiative for Obstructive Lung Disease. Available at: www.goldcopd.org. Accessed April 2, 2010.

of LTOT, either continuous or nocturnal, should always be considered with the use of NIPPV for COPD. A comprehensive review of therapy for COPD is beyond the scope of this article. Refer for more detailed information to Refs.[4–6]

Comorbid Conditions

COPD is commonly associated with sleep complaints, such as insomnia and excessive sleepiness, and with comorbid conditions of OSA and gastroesophageal reflux disease, which may also produce sleep complaints. Patients with COPD and OSA (so-called overlap syndrome) have greater desaturation, although the severity of OSA is not otherwise substantially affected.[7] Treatment of the overlap syndrome is beyond the scope of this article, but health care providers should be aware that not all hypercapnic respiratory failure in COPD is solely the result of COPD.

Sleep Architecture and Arterial Oxygen Saturation

Patients with COPD have an apparent reduced sleep efficiency, increased time awake, increased arousals and awakenings, increased non–rapid eye movement (NREM) stage N1 sleep, and reduced stage N3 and REM sleep. However, depending on the study, these results do not appear to differ markedly from individuals of a similar age who do not have COPD.[8–11] REM sleep is characterized by reduced hypercapnic and hypoxic ventilatory responsiveness combined with hypotonia of the intercostal muscles,[12–14] which leads to hypoventilation as well as a reduction in resting lung volume (ie, a reduction in FRC) with an added component of ventilation/perfusion inequality. For these reasons, although there may be a general reduction in nocturnal saturation during sleep, the most vulnerable period is REM sleep, during which prolonged desaturation may occur.

Treatment of Stable COPD with NIPPV

Treatment of stable COPD patients begins with optimization of pharmacotherapy and assessment for hypoxemia (**Tables 2** and **3**). Hypoxemia is treated with LTOT, either continuous for daytime hypoxemia or nocturnal for isolated nocturnal hypoxemia. The effect of treatment of isolated nocturnal hypoxemia on patient outcomes is not well defined. One randomized controlled trial (RCT) of nocturnal oxygen in patients with isolated nocturnal hypoxemia had no reduction in mortality; however, the sample size was small.[15]

In patients with stable COPD and hypercapnia, nocturnal NIPPV may be indicated. Several clinical trials have addressed this question. The results are

mixed with limited benefits. A recent study of NIPPV suggested an improvement in mortality but a reduction in quality of life.[16] Evidence from a systematic review of RCTs up to 2002 supported improvements in health-related quality of life and dyspnea.[17] A meta-analysis of RCTs had essentially negative results on pulmonary function, blood gases, sleep efficiency, and 6-minute walking distance (see **Table 2**).[18]

Treatment in Acute Decompensation of COPD with NIPPV

Treatment of acute decompensation of COPD includes intensification of bronchodilator therapy and may include systemic corticosteroids and, if infection is suspected, antibiotics (see **Table 3**). NIPPV may be indicated if any of the following conditions are present[4]:

1. Moderate to severe dyspnea with the use of accessory muscles and paradoxic abdominal motion
2. Moderate to severe acidemia (pH <7.35) and/or hypercapnia ($Paco_2$ >45 mm Hg)
3. Respiratory rate greater than 25 breaths per minute

There are several contraindications to NIPPV[4]:

1. Respiratory arrest
2. Cardiovascular instability (hypotension, arrhythmias, myocardial infarction)
3. Diminished mental status
4. An inability or unwillingness of the patient to accept NIPPV
5. High aspiration risk
6. Viscous or copious secretions
7. Recent facial or gastroesophageal surgery
8. Craniofacial trauma
9. Fixed nasopharyngeal abnormalities
10. Burns
11. Extreme obesity.

There have been several studies to determine the efficacy of NIPPV in acutely decompensated COPD, generally because of an acute exacerbation of COPD. A meta-analysis was conducted of 8 RCTs, up to June 2002, of NIPPV in acute exacerbations of COPD with a $Paco_2$ of at least 45 mm Hg. NIPPV as an adjunct to usual care produced lower mortality, less intubation, less treatment failure, and greater improvements at 1 hour in pH, $Paco_2$, and respiratory rate. NIPPV resulted in fewer complications associated with treatment and shorter duration of stay in hospital.[19]

A meta-analysis was conducted of 13 RCTs of NIPPV in patients with acute exacerbations (as defined by the study investigators) of COPD up to

Table 2
NIPPV for stable COPD

Reference	FEV$_1$	Design	Age (yr)	n	Int	Cont	Outcome
McEvoy et al, 2009[16]	25%/23.1% predicted 0.63/0.55 L (Int/C)	RCT with mean 2.2-year follow-up. Most patients were hypercapnic	67.2/68.8 (Int/C)	72/72	NIPPV (Noct) + LTOT	LTOT	Possible survival improvement with NIPPV. Reduced quality of life with NIPPV
Kolodziej et al, 2007[17]	<1 L	Systematic review of 6 parallel RCTs and 9 Rcrossovers without concealment from <1 week to 6 months. Most patients were hypercapnic	63	351	NIPPV	No NIPPV	No benefit from parallel studies, benefit in Rcrossover studies in which patients are own controls in gas exchange, lung hyperinflation, HRQOL, dyspnea, MIPs, and MEPs (2 studies)
Wijkstra et al, 2003[18] Overlap of 3 studies with Kolodziej et al[17]	0.68–0.86 L	Meta-analysis of 3- to 12-month RCTs of hypercapnic COPD. Most patients were hypercapnic	NA	102	NIPPV (Noct)	No NIPPV	No significant benefit for arterial blood gases, 6MWD, PFTs, or sleep efficiency

Abbreviations: Cont, control; HRQOL, health-related quality of life; Int, intervention; Int/C, intervention/control; LTOT, long-term oxygen therapy; MEP, maximum expiratory respiratory pressure; MIP, maximum inspiratory respiratory pressure; n, number of patients; NA, not available; Noct, nocturnal; PFT, pulmonary function test; RCT, randomized controlled trial; Rcrossover, randomized crossover trial; 6MWD, 6-minute walk distance.

Table 3
NIPPV in COPD, CF, and kyphoscoliosis

Condition	NIPPV	Evidence
Stable hypercapnic COPD (also see **Table 2**)	Of limited use	Mixed with modest benefits when positive based on RCTs, meta-analyses, and systematic reviews
Acute respiratory failure in COPD	May prevent endotracheal intubation and reintubation	Well established for severe exacerbations based on 2 meta-analyses and 1 RCT. CPAP may be an alternative based on a retrospective study
Stable hypercapnic CF (an obstructive lung disease)	May be used for stable hypercapnic respiratory failure	Modest positive benefit based on several small studies and a meta-analysis of mostly short-term NIPPV
Acute respiratory failure in CF	May be used for acute hypercapnic respiratory failure	Minimal based on consensus and 1 Rcrossover when NIPPV is combined with chest physiotherapy
Kyphoscoliosis (a restrictive chest wall impairment)	May be used for hypercapnic respiratory failure	Several small studies (2 prospective, 1 retrospective) suggest improvement in symptoms, decreased hospitalizations, and possible improved survival with nocturnal NIPPV

Abbreviations: Rcrossover, randomized crossover trial; RCT, randomized controlled trial.

December 2002.[20] The overall results were similar to the meta-analysis of the 8 RCTs[19] (of note there was an overlap of RCTs with Ref.[19]). A post hoc analysis focused on studies of patients with a severe exacerbation (pH <7.30 or hospital mortality rate >10% in the control group). The results of these studies are similar to those of the overall group but with numerically greater benefit. There were 2 RCTs (in addition to the 13) with results of milder exacerbations. The results suggested that NIPPV had no benefit, but the number of subjects was substantially less (72 patients compared with 654 patients in the 13 studies that included patients with severe exacerbations).[19]

A retrospective study[21] focused on intensive care admissions for acute respiratory failure from an exacerbation of COPD. This study compared mask CPAP (not BPAP) in a cohort of 88 patients (initially 49 received CPAP, 22 were intubated, and 17 received medical therapy alone) from 1991 to 1995 with 2 other cohorts that did not have access to mask CPAP but were endotracheally intubated or treated medically without intubation. Mask CPAP was associated with a lower mortality compared with intubation, and a lower mortality and fewer subsequent intubations compared with medical therapy alone.

A recent RCT of NIPPV was conducted in 106 patients (70% of who had COPD) who remained hypercapnic after a successful spontaneous breathing trial and extubation. NIPPV led to a significant reduction in the reintubation rate and 90-day mortality.[22]

Summary

Nocturnal NIPPV is of limited usefulness for patients with severe stable hypercapnic COPD. NIPPV, usually with BPAP, is of benefit in reducing mortality and subsequent endotracheal intubation in appropriate patients with a severe exacerbation of COPD and acute respiratory failure. Noninvasive delivery of CPAP may be of benefit to reduce mortality and subsequent intubation. However, the evidence is retrospective and requires confirmation.

PAP in Stable CF

CF is an obstructive lung disease. CF is an autosomal recessive genetic disorder found frequently in white people of Northern European heritage. It is the most common lethal genetic disease, affecting 1 in 3000 white Americans.[23] The defect is a mutation in the gene that encodes the CF transmembrane conductance regulator (CFTR). CFTR is a cellular channel involved in the movement of mainly chloride ions across epithelial cellular membranes. CFTR can be found in the epithelial cell lining of the upper and lower airways, bowel and ducts of the pancreas, and reproductive tracts. The defective CFTR impairs the local movement of water by indirectly reducing the transport of sodium, which leads to lower aqueous volume and more viscous secretions in the lungs and other involved organs. The result is substantial morbidity and premature mortality from malfunction of the affected organs.[24] There has been excellent progress in the management of this disease, and average life expectancy has increased beyond infancy and childhood to a projected age greater than 50 years for patients with CF born in 2000.[25]

Pathophysiology

The greatest source of morbidity and mortality in CF is the effect on pulmonary function. The lungs appear normal at birth, and over time the airways become chronically obstructed by abnormal epithelial secretions, which promote repeated pulmonary infections from growth of bacteria such as *Pseudomonas aeruginosa*, including a mucoid type, *Haemophilus influenzae*, and *Staphylococcus aureus*. This repeated infection leads to bronchiectasis and remodeling of lung architecture, such as an increase in mucous gland volume.[26]   There   is   progressive   airway obstruction.[27] The combination of bronchiectasis and airway obstruction leads to chronic hypoxemia and hypercapnia, which contribute to respiratory failure and eventually death.[27]

Comorbid Sleep Conditions

Patients with CF commonly have reduced subjective sleep quality. For example, there is a significant reduction in sleep quality according to the Pittsburgh Sleep Quality Index (PSQI). There were also more awakenings reported for cough and bathroom usage in children with CF than for those in controls.[28,29] Further, difficulty with sleep initiation is a common complaint in patients with CF.[30,31]

Poor sleep quality is associated with abnormalities of sleep and pulmonary function. A reduction in sleep quality in children with CF may be associated with a reduced FEV_1.[30] Cough was present in patients with CF during sleep and independently predicted the degree of reduction in FEV_1.[30] Polysomnography has documented reduced sleep

efficiency in patients with CF compared with controls.[31,32] In 37 patients, aged 32 years, with CF and mostly severe lung disease, a reduced FEV_1 percentage predicted was associated with an increased (ie, poorer sleep quality) PSQI.[29] Severe reductions in FEV_1 associated with hypoxemia, including nocturnal hypoxemia, are a major factor in cor pulmonale in CF.[33,34] However, PSQI and symptoms, in general, do not reliably predict the degree of nocturnal hypoxemia, which supports the procurement of objective documentation on the need for nocturnal supplemental oxygen.

Sleep Architecture and Gas Exchange

In patients with CF, sleep is interrupted by respiratory events that are more frequent during REM sleep.[29,35–37] These events are typically hypopneas with negligible amounts of central, obstructive, or mixed apneic events.[36] There is a difference in the respiratory disturbance index (RDI) of apneas and hypopneas between REM and NREM sleep of between 11.5 and 12.6 events per hour.[36,37] A study of 32 patients with CF and moderate to severe lung disease found that a decrease in expiratory respiratory muscle strength correlated with an increase in RDI during REM.[36] The investigators suggested that because expiratory muscle strength is a significant measure of cough strength, a reduction may indicate impairment in clearing secretions.[36]

In a study of 21 patients, aged 27 years,[38] 8 had significant nocturnal desaturation and, as expected, these patients had the greatest impairment in pulmonary function (FEV_1, 31% vs 59% predicted) and lower awake saturations (90.9% vs 96.2%). In a study of 70 patients with CF aged 27 years with lung disease of a wide range of severity, 40% had saturations of less than 90% for more than 5% of the night.[39] Although an FEV_1 greater than 65% demonstrated a relative resistance to nocturnal desaturation (2 of 21 patients), only about half (25 of 49 patients) of those with FEV_1 of less than 65% had significant nocturnal desaturation.[39] These investigators concluded that nocturnal desaturation is more likely if the baseline awake saturation is less than 93%.[39] The previously cited study of 32 patients with moderate to severe CF also derived a formula for   expected   average   nocturnal   oxygen saturation.[36] The investigators observed that low bedtime partial pressure of arterial oxygen (Pao_2) plus elevated morning $Paco_2$ was the best combined predictor for nocturnal hypoxemia. FEV_1 and inspiratory muscle strength were also correlated with average overnight oxygenation.[36]

No statistical significance was found between FEV_1 and nocturnal saturation in a study of a healthier population with CF with average FEV_1 of 61%, suggesting that the sensitivity of this marker is reduced with less pulmonary impairment.[28] It is unclear whether milder cases of CF with more normal daytime saturation warrant investigation into sleep hypoxemia and what, if any, are the most sensitive screening markers in that population.

Episodic nocturnal desaturations in CF seem to be the result of a combination of factors. A low baseline oxygen saturation makes a patient susceptible to severe nocturnal hypoxemia with relatively brief reductions in ventilation. In the face of the obstructive pulmonary function in CF,[40] the hypotonia of accessory ventilatory muscles during REM sleep may lead to hypoventilation, a decrease in lung volume (FRC), and ventilation/perfusion mismatch similar to that in COPD. This condition may be exacerbated by respiratory muscle fatigue due to increased respiratory effort to overcome airway obstruction, including that from thick secretions and reduced respiratory muscle strength from malnutrition as a result of pancreatic insufficiency.[39]

$Paco_2$ has been found to increase during REM sleep in patients with CF.[29,31,32,35,36,41] Nocturnal hypercapnia was associated with significantly worse global, sleep efficiency–related, and sleep latency–related PSQI scores.[29] Reductions in FEV_1 and maximum expiratory respiratory pressure correlated with an increase in nocturnal transcutaneous PCO_2.[36] The significant association between these findings and nocturnal hypercapnia suggests that structural changes of the lung, specifically markers of airway obstruction, are predictors for nocturnal hypoventilation. This hypoventilation is exacerbated during REM and seems dependent on the degree of lung disease that is complicated by respiratory muscle weakness.

Nocturnal Oxygen Treatment for Stable CF

Nocturnal low-flow oxygen may maintain oxygen saturation throughout the night but does not improve[42] or may worsen[35] nocturnal hypercapnia. In addition, there are conflicting data on whether low-flow oxygen does[35] or does not[42] have beneficial effects on sleep architecture. In 7 patients, nasal CPAP significantly improved oxygen saturation and RDI frequency in NREM and REM sleep when compared with room air (4 patients) or nocturnal supplemental O_2 (3 patients) without CPAP.[43] However, there were no improvements in sleep architecture or hypercapnia.

NIPPV Treatment for Stable Hypercapnic CF

Treatment should include maximizing, as necessary, pharmacotherapy, including bronchodilators and human recombinant DNase as well as antibiotics plus supplemental oxygen as needed (see **Table 3**).

In a survey of 36 medical centers in France,[44] NIPPV was instituted for 7.6% of adult patients and 1.2% of pediatric patients with CF. NIPPV was used to treat severe hypercapnic respiratory exacerbations, and nocturnal NIPPV was used to treat patients with CF and stable daytime hypercapnia (mean $Paco_2$ of 48 mm Hg in adults). Compliance was 72% to 83%, with the most common complaints being difficulty sleeping with the device, feeling physically restricted, and perceived lack of benefit.

NIPPV (generally BPAP) is commonly used to treat selected patients with CF. However, there are few studies to confirm if NIPPV is efficacious in stable CF and virtually none to confirm in acute respiratory exacerbations of CF. Five studies analyzed nocturnal NIPPV in stable CF; these included 4 to 37 subjects[35,42,43,45,46] without long-term follow-up. Three of these studies originated from the same institution.[42,43,45] The use of BPAP ventilation, unlike low-flow oxygen, was found to significantly reduce nocturnal transcutaneous Pco_2[35,42] with a corresponding reduction in morning arterial acidosis.[42] Improvement in sleep architecture was not seen with NIPPV in one study,[41] but in another study there was an improvement in REM sleep minutes and percentage of total sleep time.[35] Subjective assessment of sleep quality was described as being improved in a 4-patient case series,[45] with patients describing that NIPPV provided rest for respiratory muscles and enabled better cough strength and daytime function. However, another study showed that most patients preferred low-flow oxygen alone, for reasons of comfort.[35] A 6-week crossover study of 37 patients suggested that nocturnal NIPPV improves chest symptoms, exertional dyspnea, nocturnal hypoventilation, and peak exercise capacity in adult patients with stable CF.[46] A Cochrane review[47] summarized 7 studies (6 single sessions and 1 6-week study) with 106 patients and concluded that NIPPV may improve sputum clearance, nocturnal saturation, and exercise performance. A prospective cohort study characterized the effects of long-term NIPPV in CF.[48] The study followed 12 patients for a mean of 5 months with severe pulmonary disease awaiting lung transplant. The study did not specifically mention time of day for NIPPV use but demonstrated significant progressive benefits in the

FEV$_1$, FVC, arterial blood gases, and stabilization of body mass index. Subjectively, these patients described a reduction in early morning headaches, improved sleep quality, and well being.

In a randomized crossover trial of 26 patients, chest physiotherapy was enhanced by NIPPV in acute respiratory exacerbations of CF to improve inspiratory muscle function, oxygen saturation, and dyspnea.[49]

Summary

Nocturnal NIPPV is commonly used to treat stable CF with severe hypercapnic respiratory failure and acute hypercapnic respiratory exacerbations of CF. The evidence for efficacy requires confirmation because of the limited number of studies and patients, and lack of sufficient long-term follow-up.

PAP in kyphoscoliosis

Kyphoscoliosis is a restrictive pulmonary disorder. Kyphosis is a deformity in the anteroposterior angle of the spine, whereas scoliosis is a lateral displacement of the spine. In severe cases, kyphoscoliosis can lead to impairment of respiratory muscles, upper airway obstruction, and eventually respiratory failure.

Kyphoscoliosis poses a problem in management with assisted ventilation. Intubation or tracheostomy can be difficult because of the curvature of the cervical spine and twisting of the trachea. Negative-pressure ventilators (such as iron lung and cuirass ventilators) can also induce upper airway collapse and cause further respiratory insufficiency. NIPPV overcomes some of these difficulties.

Etiology and Pathophysiology

Several conditions can cause kyphoscoliosis. Neuromuscular diseases, such as poliomyelitis, cerebral palsy, or muscular dystrophy, can lead to abnormal posture and deformity of the spinal column. Conditions that weaken the bony structure of the vertebral column may also cause kyphoscoliosis including Pott disease (tuberculosis of the spine), osteoporosis, and rickets. Other causes include connective tissue disorders or acquired abnormalities that directly deform the normal thoracic bony structures.

Approximately 80% of cases are idiopathic and begin in childhood. The diagnosis is often suspected based on clinical findings, although radiographs quantify the full impairment. The degree of spinal curvature best predicts future respiratory dysfunction, and deformity above T10 produces the greatest reduction in pulmonary function.[50]

Total lung capacity and vital capacity (VC) decrease without change in residual volume.[51] This decrease is from decreased compliance of the chest wall, which results in air trapping and recurring atelectasis. Eventually, the abnormal vertebral curvature impairs compliance of the lung and FRC decreases. These changes lead to the excessive use of the accessory muscle to help maintain minute ventilation.[52] The increased work of breathing progresses to respiratory muscle fatigue, hypoxemia, and hypercapnic respiratory failure.[53]

Treatment of Kyphoscoliosis

Mild disease often has a good prognosis and can be treated supportively. Severe disease, particularly patients with cor pulmonale, carries a worse prognosis.[54] Medical therapy for kyphoscoliosis includes optimization of respiratory function with pulmonary rehabilitation[55] and supplemental oxygen as needed for hypoxemia. Potential benefits of surgical intervention for adults are weighed against potential significant complications. Brace treatment and surgery have been helpful in improving FEV$_1$, FVC, inspiratory capacity, and 6-minute walking tests in adolescents.[56] Options for ventilator support of respiratory failure with kyphoscoliosis include tracheostomy and negative-pressure ventilators or NIPPV.

Comorbid Conditions

Kyphoscoliosis can be associated with significant upper airway obstruction caused by cervical and thoracic deformity. As a result, nocturnal oxygen desaturation occurs with frequent awakenings. These obstructive events and awakenings may occur first in REM sleep in milder cases before becoming prominent in NREM sleep in more severe cases. Excessive somnolence, snoring, and apneas may occur, similar to patients with OSA. The most severe cases of kyphoscoliosis and apnea are frequently associated with cor pulmonale, and polycythemia.[57]

Sleep Architecture, Arterial Oxygen Saturation, and NIPPV

Respiratory insufficiency and sleep apnea secondary to kyphoscoliosis can be improved with nocturnal NIPPV (see **Table 3**). The goal for NIPPV in these patients is primarily to reduce Paco$_2$. Additional end points may include improving symptoms of fatigue, dyspnea, impaired concentration, and daytime somnolence. When NIPPV is also required during daytime, an additional benefit of therapy is to avoid intubation and tracheostomy.

A limited number of studies have evaluated the long-term effects of nocturnal NIPPV for treatment of kyphoscoliotic respiratory insufficiency. A prospective case series[58] measured blood gas levels, respiratory muscle performance, and daytime symptoms in 16 patients with kyphoscoliosis treated with pressure-cycled or volume-cycled nocturnal NIPPV. These patients met the following criteria: $Paco_2$, less than or equal to 45 mm Hg; saturation (Sao_2), less than or equal to 88% for 5 consecutive minutes by nocturnal oximetry; maximal inspiratory pressure, less than 60 cm H_2O; or FVC, less than 50% of predicted. After a 3-year follow-up, there was a sustained decrease in hospitalizations and daytime symptoms and improved respiratory muscle performance and quality of life.[58] There was a nonsignificant trend to improved sleep efficiency and architecture after 6 months of therapy. There were significant improvements in the number of desaturations, baseline saturation, minimum saturation, and time spent below 90% saturation. Six patients received nocturnal oxygen therapy at 1 L/min, which further improved nocturnal oxygenation without increasing CO_2 levels.

A prospective case series of 7 excessively sleepy and hypercapnic patients demonstrated improvements in respiratory function with nocturnal CPAP (2 patients) or nocturnal NIPPV after 3 months.[59] There was significant improvement in respiratory muscle strength, daytime Pao_2, $Paco_2$, and nocturnal saturation, particularly during REM sleep. Sleep architecture and symptoms were improved with an increased duration of REM sleep and a reduction in daytime sleepiness.

PAP when used in conjunction with supplemental oxygen may also lead to improved long-term survival in patients with kyphoscoliosis. A retrospective analysis of 33 patients with hypercapnia evaluated the long-term effects of oxygen plus nocturnal NIPPV.[60] The results showed an improvement in survival at 1 year after starting treatment in patients using oxygen and NIPPV versus oxygen alone (100% vs 66%). There was improvement in respiratory muscle strength, an increase in Pao_2, a decrease in $Paco_2$, and an increase in VC. The investigators discuss that this retrospective analysis may have been affected by various factors, such as comorbid diseases, unaccounted treatments given, and severity of kyphoscoliosis. However, NIPPV seemed to be the only significant factor determining the improvement in survival.

Summary

The evidence for nocturnal NIPPV in kyphoscoliosis appears to show an improvement in daytime fatigue, daytime sleepiness, respiratory muscle function, sleep-related hypoxemia, quality of life and, possibly, sleep architecture. Survival may also be improved. Nocturnal NIPPV seems a safe and efficacious treatment for patients with respiratory failure secondary to kyphoscoliosis.

PAP in Neuromuscular Disorders

Neuromuscular disorders lead to restrictive pulmonary function from weakness of the respiratory muscles. A Cochrane review of 8 RCTs with 144 patients concluded that the therapeutic benefit of mechanical ventilation is weak but consistent, with alleviation of the symptoms of chronic hypercapnia in the short term. Prolongation of survival was mainly in patients with motor neuron diseases.[61] The following sections discuss the evidence regarding NIPPV in ALS, DMD, MG, and PPS.

ALS

ALS progressively leads to muscle weakness and death by degeneration of the upper and lower motor neurons. ALS is one of the most common neuromuscular diseases affecting 1 in 200,000 individuals per year. Typically, patients present with lower motor neuron signs, such as muscle weakness and fasciculations. Eventually there is muscle atrophy, complete weakness, and loss of control of voluntary muscles. Upper motor neuron signs are an increase in reflexes and spasticity. If the upper and lower motor neurons affect the cranial nerves there may be bulbar and pseudobulbar signs, including difficulty in speaking and swallowing. Patients may also show signs of pseudobulbar affect, such as inappropriate laughing and crying. ALS has a variable disease progression, but ends in an inability to ambulate and a respiratory insufficiency followed by death. The rate of symptom progression, bulbar onset, and older age portend a worse outcome. The median survival time from onset to death ranges from 20 to 48 months, but 10% to 20% of patients with ALS have a survival longer than 10 years.[62]

Respiratory system

Ultimately, in most patients, ALS results in respiratory muscle weakness, respiratory failure, and death. Respiratory muscle weakness and diaphragmatic paralysis impairs ventilation, which eventually leads to nocturnal hypoventilation and ultimately daytime respiratory failure. The hypoventilation may be worsened by bulbar dysfunction. Identifying patients early with nocturnal hypoventilation may delay the onset of daytime respiratory failure and prolong survival. Patients with ALS should undergo a full pulmonary workup, including pulmonary function tests and arterial blood gas determination as well as a sleep evaluation in selected patients. Of note, reduced quality of life seems to be related to respiratory muscle weakness rather than nocturnal events such as apneas, hypopneas, or disturbances in sleep architecture.[63]

Sleep

ALS often leads to insomnia, periodic limb movements/restless legs syndrome, and sleep-disordered breathing.[64] Sleep-disordered breathing is a well-documented consequence of ALS[65,66] even in the early stages of the disease. Seventeen patients with ALS with mild to severe bulbar involvement and 10 age-matched controls were studied with PSG.[65] Patients with ALS had a reduced total sleep time, more arousals, a greater NREM stage N1 sleep, and a higher apnea-hypopnea index (AHI; number of apneas and hypopneas per hour of sleep), particularly during REM sleep (22.1 in REM vs 2.9 during NREM). Eleven early-stage patients with ALS and bulbar involvement and 7 without the involvement were studied using ambulatory cardiorespiratory monitoring.[66] There were no significant differences between the 2 groups with respect to sleep-disordered breathing. However, 3 patients with bulbar involvement had an AHI greater than 5 (9.5, 18.7, and 38.8). Patients with ALS, particularly those with bulbar involvement, complaining of excessive daytime sleepiness, disrupted sleep, snoring, and witnessed apnea, or with CO_2 retention should generally undergo an evaluation for a sleep disorder, including polysomnography. Treatment of fatigue and daytime sleepiness in patients with ALS, in addition to treatment of sleep-disordered breathing, may include modafinil. A 2-week open-label study of modafinil in 15 patients found a reduced fatigue scale and reduced Epworth Sleepiness Scale.[67]

Disruptions of sleep architecture may be related to the presence of diaphragmatic dysfunction.[68] Thirteen patients with ALS and impaired diaphragmatic function were compared with 8 patients with ALS and preserved diaphragmatic function. Patients with ALS and preserved function had normal REM sleep duration. In contrast, REM sleep was reduced in those with impaired function, including 5 patients with less than 3 minutes of REM sleep. In those with impaired function, there was more awakening after sleep onset, a trend toward longer sleep latency, less total sleep time, and a greater AHI. Although both groups averaged an AHI of less than 5, 1 of the patients with impaired function had an AHI of 19. Of note, survival was substantially less in those with impaired function. Another PSG study of 11 patients with ALS and preserved diaphragmatic

function did not confirm these results.[69] REM sleep was reduced overall and was normal in only 3 of the 11 patients. There was mild desaturation in most with an AHI greater than 5 in 3, including 1 with an AHI of 118.

Treatment with NIPPV

Studies have demonstrated improvement in survival in patients started on NIPPV, and current practice parameters from the American Academy of Neurology recommend the use of NIPPV when FVC is less than 50% of predicted, sniff nasal pressure (SNP) is less than 40 cm H_2O, or maximal inspiratory respiratory pressure is less than −60 cm H_2O (**Table 4**).[115] NIPPV decreases the work of breathing, supports weakened respiratory muscle function, and improves gas exchange. A retrospective chart review was conducted of 122 patients with ALS with FEV_1 less than 50% of predicted or a recent decrease of 15% in FEV_1 within a 3-month period.[70] The results suggested that BPAP (time of day not specified but implied that it was predominantly nocturnal) can significantly prolong survival and slow the decline of FVC in patients with ALS, particularly in those who tolerated BPAP for greater than 4 hours per day. Survival was increased from a mean of 4.6 to 14.2 months, including in patients with poor bulbar function. An RCT was conducted in 41 patients with one or both of symptomatic daytime hypercapnia or a maximum inspiratory respiratory muscle pressure less than 60% predicted and orthopnea. The results demonstrated that patients using nocturnal NIPPV experienced a median overall survival benefit of 205 days as well as a general improvement in the quality of life. There was improvement in sleep symptoms but no survival benefit in a subgroup with poor bulbar function.[71] However, these patients used BPAP for 3.8 h/d versus 9.3 h/d in the patients with good bulbar function, suggesting that reduced compliance with NIPPV may have led to the poorer outcome. A non-RCT in 9 patients with ALS with reduced VC, daytime hypercapnia ($Paco_2$ >49 mm Hg), nocturnal hypopnea with arousals, and daytime hypersomnolence were treated with 6 weeks of NIPPV, and showed improvement on cognitive testing compared with baseline. A control group of 10 patients with ALS without respiratory or sleep complaints and not requiring NIPPV did not improve during the 6 weeks.[72]

Optimal timing of commencing NIPPV is still unresolved. Current evidence has led to a recommendation that NIPPV is of benefit in symptomatic

Table 4
NIPPV in neuromuscular disorders

Condition	NIPPV	Evidence
ALS	Recommended by American Academy Neurology Guidelines for hypercapnia and FVC <50% predicted and possibly for early ALS	Level of evidence for established respiratory compromise is B (A being highest) and C for early intervention.[115] Improves survival, reduces rate of decline of pulmonary function, and improves quality of life
DMD	Routinely used for nocturnal and continuous hypercapnic respiratory failure. Not recommended for patients without daytime and/or nocturnal hypercapnia because there may be an increase in mortality	Recommended by at least 2 guidelines.[86,87] Supported by an RCT and several prospective and retrospective cohort studies and case series
MG	May be used for selected patients with myasthenic crisis with modest hypercapnia	Three retrospective studies support the use to prevent endotracheal intubation and support the patient until the crisis is resolved
PPS	Routinely used for nocturnal and continuous hypercapnia	Two retrospective case series and 1 polysomnographic study support the use to convert patients from body ventilators, prevent endotracheal intubation and tracheostomy, and improve pulmonary function and sleep architecture. In some patients with predominant OSA, nocturnal CPAP rather than NIPPV may be appropriate therapy

patients with hypercapnia or an FVC less than 50% of the predicted value. However, there is reason to consider that NIPPV initiated early in the ALS disease course may be of benefit. The American Academy of Neurology practice parameters suggest that early initiation may improve NIPPV compliance.[115] In addition, NIPPV is likely to reduce respiratory muscle work at all levels of ALS severity associated with respiratory muscle weakness and to possibly reduce the rate of decline of pulmonary function. A study examined the cost effectiveness of earlier NIPPV treatment based on patient perceptions of the impact on quality of life. The results indicate that NIPPV would be a cost-effective treatment, if begun before currently recommended levels of severity, and if it improves health-related quality of life in patients with ALS by at least 13.5%.[73] In fact, a study randomized patients with ALS to either an FVC of greater than 70% predicted (early intervention based, in part, on at least 1 minute of nocturnal desaturation <90%) or an FVC of less than 50% predicted (standard of care). There was an improvement in the vitality subscale of a quality-of-life Short Form 36 (SF-36) in 5 of 6 patients randomized to early intervention.[74]

Other treatment options
Unfortunately, ALS is universally fatal with minimal therapeutic options. As discussed, NIPPV is the major ventilatory intervention that improves survival. Mechanical ventilation (via a tracheostomy tube) is used in later-stage patients with ALS. Percutaneous endoscopic gastrotomy is usually needed to provide nutrition. Riluzole is the only Food and Drug Administration–approved drug for the treatment of ALS. Riluzole has been shown to slow disease progression to a modest degree.[75]

Summary
ALS may lead to insomnia and sleep-disordered breathing characterized by apneas and hypopneas. Patients with bulbar involvement are more likely to have daytime sleepiness and disrupted sleep. REM sleep is a vulnerable period for sleep-disordered breathing, particularly in patients with bulbar involvement. REM sleep may be selectively reduced in patients with diaphragmatic dysfunction; however, the supporting data are inconclusive. Treatment with NIPPV for up to 24 h/d is recommended in patients with an FVC of less than 50% predicted or evidence of substantial

respiratory muscle dysfunction, such as a maximal inspiratory respiratory pressure less than −60 cm H_2O. NIPPV can prolong survival, particularly in those patients without bulbar involvement, and may slow the rate of decline of pulmonary function. Cognitive function may also be improved by NIPPV. Early intervention with NIPPV in patients with more preserved function may have benefits in compliance and quality of life.

DMD

DMD is an X-linked recessive disorder caused by a mutation of the locus gene at Xp21. The DMD gene was named *dystrophin*. Dystrophin protein is essential to the structural stability of the myofiber, and without dystrophin, muscles are susceptible to mechanical injury and undergo repeated cycles of necrosis and regeneration until the ability to regenerate is lost. The functional loss of dystrophin protein initiates a series of events, including loss of other components of the dystrophin-associated glycoprotein complex, sarcolemmal breakdown with attendant calcium ion influx, phospholipase activation, oxidative cellular injury, and ultimately, myonecrosis.[76]

DMD is characterized by rapid progression of muscle degeneration, eventually leading to loss of ambulation and death. It affects 1 in 3500 males, making it the most prevalent of the muscular dystrophies. Symptoms of proximal muscle weakness can appear as early as infancy, with more obvious symptoms by 6 years of age, and with the inability to walk by 10 or 12 years. Death is the result of cardiac or respiratory failure.[77]

Respiratory system

Respiratory muscle weakness, often accompanied by thoracic scoliosis and decline in VC, usually starts by age 10 years. Respiratory failure and death generally occur by the second decade of life. Respiratory failure is nearly inevitable when the VC decreases to less than 20% predicted, with 74% of patients with DMD dying of respiratory insufficiency.[78] Measurement of VC, erect and supine, a chest radiograph, arterial blood gas tensions, and nocturnal oximetry have been recommended for each patient with potential respiratory compromise.[79] Additional measurements may include maximal inspiratory and expiratory respiratory pressures and maximal SNP. Polysomnography should be reserved for suspected sleep-disordered breathing.

Sleep

Respiratory failure is often preceded by sleep-disordered breathing. Nocturnal hypoventilation occurs during sleep because of inspiratory muscle

weakness and a decrease in ventilatory drive, which ultimately progresses to daytime hypoventilation. In DMD, daytime hypercapnia results in death, usually within 1 year without ventilatory assistance.[80] There are few PSG studies of patients with DMD. A study of 6 patients with a VC of 27% predicted, without daytime hypercapnia or significant hypoxemia, and between the ages of 12 and 20 years demonstrated an average total sleep time of 376 minutes, sleep efficiency of 82%, 16% of NREM stage N1, 47% N2, and 24% N3, 12% REM, and an AHI of 11 per hour of sleep (65/h during REM). A higher AHI was associated with more daytime symptoms, such as insomnia.[81] In addition, the patients spent 25% of the night with a saturation of greater than 5% below baseline. A second PSG study was conducted of 21 patients with DMD, average age 15 years, VC 35% predicted, and Sao_2 96%, and 12 normal controls of average age 14 years.[82] Total sleep time was 439 minutes, REM time 84 minutes, sleep efficiency 93%, and awake after sleep onset 20 minutes. There were several desaturations greater than 5% below baseline in 12 of the 21 patients with DMD and greater than 10% below baseline in 10 of these 12 patients. These results occurred most often in REM sleep, averaging 6 per hour versus 1 per hour in NREM sleep. Sleep hypoxemia was not obviously related to daytime or sleep symptoms. One of the patients (age 23) had continuous hypoxemia during sleep and died 2 months after being studied. Follow-up of 9 patients with DMD showed an increase in desaturation events with a shift from obstructive to central events in 2 patients. Sleep architecture in control subjects was similar to that in patients with DMD. There were central apneas in these subjects, averaging 2.9 per hour of sleep. However, there was only 1 subject with obstructive apnea, and this subject had the only 2 desaturations greater than 5% below baseline.

Treatment with NIPPV

In 35 patients, quality-of-life scores by the SF-36 Medical Outcomes Study Survey questionnaire were, as expected, substantially reduced for physical function in patients who were spontaneously breathing or on NIPPV (FVC, 48% predicted vs 12% predicted) (see **Table 4**). However, in this cross-sectional study, role-emotional, social function, and mental health scores were nearly normal and did not differ between spontaneously breathing patients (n = 21) and those with NIPPV (n = 14).[83] This observation suggests that the use of NIPPV promotes a quality of life similar to that of those who do not require NIPPV.

Treatment with NIPPV can delay onset of respiratory failure with daytime hypercapnia. In a review of 20 years of publications, there was evidence to support early (nocturnal hypercapnia alone) and late (daytime and nocturnal hypercapnia) initiation of NIPPV but not to support the use of prophylactic (normocapnia day and night) NIPPV. One study of prophylactic NIPPV was associated with an increase in mortality.[84]

Early initiation with nocturnal hypercapnia alone was supported by a 2-year RCT[85] in which 9 patients on nocturnal NIPPV for nocturnal hypercapnia had an improvement in quality of life and did not subsequently present with acute hypercapnic decompensation. Seven of 10 patients within 12 months and 2 more within 24 months who were randomized to the control group developed daytime hypercapnia ($Paco_2>49$ mm Hg) or met other preset criteria and were placed on NIPPV. This study indicates that ventilatory support for patients with nocturnal hypercapnia is inevitable, generally within 2 years. Early initiation of NIPPV is likely to reduce the possibility of acute hypercapnic decompensation requiring ventilatory support and improve the quality of life in these patients.

Late initiation of NIPPV for patients with daytime hypercapnia ($Paco_2>45$ mm Hg) (these patients frequently have an FVC of <20% predicted) is recommended by several guidelines.[86,87] A prospective cohort study using a nasal and mouthpiece interface used 24 hours a day had 51% of patients surviving for 7 years after initiation of NIPPV with a mean age at death of 31 years.[88] A case series of 23 patients with DMD has suggested that nocturnal NIPPV improves survival in patients with daytime hypercapnia. One-year and 5-year survival rates were 85% and 73%, respectively, as compared with historical survival rates of 1 year or less.[80] A non-RCT of NIPPV had a 2-year survival for 5 of 5 patients with DMD when compared with the survival of 1 of 5 DMD patients who declined NIPPV. Of note, FVC and maximum voluntary ventilation were better maintained in the ventilated patients.[89]

A retrospective longitudinal study[90] up to 1995 studied 15 patients with DMD who were ventilated by NIPPV (mean 22 months), 10 of whom eventually required tracheostomies.

In a retrospective case series of 91 patients with DMD with NIPPV combined with oximetry checks, use of a mechanical assisted cough device and access to a portable volume ventilator was associated with greater survival than use of NIPPV alone.[77]

Medical treatment
There is no known cure for DMD. Since inflammation has been implicated in the pathogenesis of DMD, steroids have been one of the mainstays of therapy. A Cochrane review of RCTs provided evidence that glucocorticoid therapy in DMD improves muscle strength and function from 6 months to 2 years.[91] Ultimately, supportive care with a multidisciplinary team, including occupational and physical therapy, plays an important role in the care of patients with DMD.

Summary
DMD may lead to sleep-disordered breathing, which often precedes ventilatory failure. The presence of sleep-disordered breathing may increase symptoms of daytime sleepiness and insomnia. Nocturnal desaturation is common even in patients without daytime hypoxemia or hypercapnia, and REM sleep is the most vulnerable sleep stage. Daytime hypercapnia is an ominous sign foretelling death, typically within 1 year without ventilatory support. Once nocturnal hypercapnia develops, daytime hypercapnia requiring at least nocturnal ventilation is inevitable, generally within 2 years to prolong survival. Early use of nocturnal NIPPV for nocturnal hypercapnia can improve the quality of life and potentially reduce the possibility of subsequent acute hypercapnic decompensation. Nocturnal and eventually continuous NIPPV for daytime hypercapnia improve survival. Such patients have a quality of life similar to patients with DMD who do not require NIPPV. Adjunctive measures, such as an assisted cough device, monitoring with nocturnal oximetry, and access to a portable ventilator to supplement NIPPV, may improve survival. Prophylactic NIPPV for daytime and nocturnal normocapnic patients is not recommended and may lead to an increase in mortality.

MG

MG is the most common neuromuscular disorder. MG results from a loss of acetylcholine receptors at the neuromuscular junction from autoimmune antibodies. Patients develop profound weakness from loss of acetylcholine receptors in bulbar, ocular, limb, and respiratory muscles. The incidence of this disorder is 10 to 20 new cases per million people per year, with an overall prevalence of 100 to 200 per million people.[92] MG occurs at all ages and has a bimodal distribution. An early peak occurs in the second or third decades in mostly females. A second peak occurs in the sixth to eighth decade primarily in males. The diagnosis of MG can be made by both clinical and serologic testing.

Pathophysiology
Acetylcholine is stored in nerve terminals and, when released, produces muscle contraction.

Acetylcholinesterase hydrolyzes acetylcholine, which halts the contraction. The loss of acetylcholine receptors in MG and the normal acetylcholine rundown (reduction in the amount of acetylcholine release per neurologic impulse) leads to reduced muscle contraction and muscle fatigue.[93]

As mentioned, the loss of muscle acetylcholine receptors in MG is caused by antibodies against acetylcholine receptors.[93] Approximately 80% to 90% of patients with MG have an autoimmune serum antibody directed at the acetylcholine receptor. This antibody affects the ocular, bulbar, limb, and respiratory muscles. Although the serum concentration of this antibody does not correlate with disease severity, a decrease in the antibody level often correlates with clinical remission.[94] Those patients who test negative for antiacetylcholine receptor antibodies often test positive for muscle-specific receptor tyrosine kinase.[95,96] This antibody also produces a reduction in the number of acetylcholine receptors.

Approximately 75% of patients with MG also have an abnormal thymus. Sixty-five percent of these patients have findings on histologic examination of thymic hyperplasia. Muscle-like cells within the abnormal thymus tissue may therefore bear acetylcholine receptors that initiate the autoimmune response in MG. In addition, 10% of patients have thymic tumors, mostly thymomas.[94] Thymectomy often improves symptoms of generalized MG and may also be effective in the absence of a thymoma.[97]

Comorbid sleep conditions

Patients with MG are prone to hypopneas during sleep because of preexisting reduced respiratory muscle tone during sleep and REM sleep–related loss of nondiaphragmatic muscle tone. Although studies show a predominance of nonobstructive events, these patients may also be prone to upper airway obstruction due to weakness of bulbar and pharyngeal muscles.

Sleep complaints of patients with MG resemble symptoms in other forms of sleep disordered breathing. These symptoms can include morning headaches, excessive daytime somnolence, and a sensation of breathlessness at night. Respiratory muscle weakness may be sufficient to cause hypercapnia. The occurrence of these symptoms typically correlates with advanced age, increased weight, diminished total lung capacity, and abnormal daytime blood gas.[98] Overall, symptoms may be subtle and require a degree of suspicion for sleep-disordered breathing.[99] The adequacy of respiratory muscle strength in the daytime should not preclude the possibility of diminished muscle strength at night.

Treatment including NIPPV

Current medical therapeutic strategies for MG improve outcomes and achieve remission in most patients (see **Table 4**). There are 4 main goals of treatment: symptomatic treatment with anticholinesterase agents, rapid immunomodulating therapy, chronic immunomodulating therapy, and surgical treatment with thymectomy. These therapies are beyond the scope of this article.

As previously reviewed, NIPPV has been successfully used in patients with acute and chronic respiratory failure to avoid the need for invasive ventilation or to reduce long-term mortality.[100] However, because of the remitting nature of MG, there are essentially no studies of long-term NIPPV in MG.

Myasthenic crisis is defined as an acute exacerbation of myasthenic weakness, causing respiratory failure and requiring mechanical ventilation.[101] The condition is estimated to occur in at least 15% to 20% of patients with MG. Treatments often consist of immunotherapy, endotracheal intubation, and mechanical ventilation. At this time there are no generally accepted clinical criteria for initiation of NIPPV in myasthenic crisis or for when to safely discontinue NIPPV. However, a limited number of studies suggest NIPPV may be a useful alternative to endotracheal intubation in some patients.

A retrospective review documented that NIPPV prevented intubation in 7 of 11 episodes of myasthenic crisis. The presence of hypercapnia greater than 50 mm Hg predicted NIPPV failure with subsequent endotracheal intubation.[102] A retrospective study examined 41 patients who received ventilatory support, 14 of whom received NIPPV initially. Successful NIPPV was defined as patients free from intubation during hospitalization. Of the 14 patients, 6 required subsequent intubation and 8 remained free of intubation. Of 33 patients (including the 6 initially receiving NIPPV) who were intubated and subsequently extubated, 13 required reintubation. Based on a post hoc analysis, the investigators concluded that NIPPV may be used in patients with a low Acute Physiology and Chronic Health Evaluation II score (<6) and a lesser degree of metabolic compensation for respiratory acidosis (a serum bicarbonate level <30).[103] A study reviewed 60 episodes in 52 patients on ventilatory support for myasthenic crisis.[104] NIPPV was used in 24 episodes, and endotracheal intubation with ventilation was used in 36 episodes. Intubation was avoided in 14 of the 24 cases treated with NIPPV. The only predictor of subsequent intubation was a $Paco_2$ level greater than 45 mm Hg. Length of ventilatory support was 5.6 days in those treated initially with NIPPV and 13.6 days in those initially intubated.

Summary

In general, patients with MG with severe gas exchange abnormalities, compromised airway, or with urgent requirement for intubation should not use NIPPV in the acute setting. However, NIPPV, when selectively administered, can reduce the number of endotracheal intubations and time of ventilatory support while patients receive medical treatment for a myasthenic respiratory crisis.

PAP in PPS

PPS is estimated to occur in 25% to 50% of postpolio survivors approximately 15 to 30 years after recovery from the initial illness. PPS is the new-onset weakness of muscles that were originally affected as well as muscles that may have been originally unaffected, accompanied by fatigue. Joint degeneration, muscle atrophy, and skeletal deformities such as scoliosis can occur. Respiratory difficulties commonly arise from chronic microatelectasis, reduced pulmonary compliance (stiff lungs), chronic alveolar hypoventilation as indicated by hypercapnia, decreased cough, and reduced clearing of secretions. Weakness of bulbar swallowing muscles may lead to aspiration pneumonia. Severity of PPS is usually related to the severity in the initial illness. One possible cause of PPS is decompensation of a chronic denervation and reinnervation process. The remaining healthy motor neurons can no longer maintain new sprouts so that denervation exceeds reinnervation.[105] Other potential causes are reactivation of a latent virus or an autoimmune reaction. In addition, comorbid conditions such as COPD may contribute.[106] Diagnosis is based on clinical evaluation meeting the following criteria[107]:

1. A prior episode of poliomyelitis with residual motor neuron loss
2. A period (usually at least 15 years) of neurologic and functional stability after recovery from the acute illness
3. The gradual or rarely abrupt onset of new weakness or abnormal muscle fatigue, muscle atrophy, or generalized fatigue
4. Exclusion of other conditions that could cause similar manifestations.

Laboratory tests such as arterial blood gases, pulmonary function, and sniff nasal inspiratory pressure measurements are usually performed to determine severity.[106]

Comorbid Sleep Conditions and Sleep Architecture

Sleep apnea is common in PPS patients, particularly those with residual bulbar dysfunction. OSA occurs because of decreased respiratory muscle strength, pharyngeal weakness, and increased musculoskeletal deformities from scoliosis. PPS can lead to chronic alveolar hypoventilation and respiratory failure. Central sleep apnea can also occur in PPS because of a residual dysfunction of the surviving bulbar reticular neurons.

Sleep architecture may be affected in PPS by possible damage to the pontine tegmentum of the brainstem, an area known to influence REM sleep. Although the exact pathology is unknown, there is an increased latency to REM sleep in patients with PPS with bulbar dysfunction but no significant difference in patients with PPS without bulbar dysfunction as compared with controls.[108] One study documented disturbed sleep second to abnormal movements in sleep, such as nocturnal myoclonus, periodic limb movements, and ballistic movements, particularly during stage N2 of NREM sleep.[109]

Another study evaluated the most common clinical manifestations in patients with PPS with sleep-disordered breathing. Hypersomnolence was present in 32 of the 35 patients with sleep-disordered breathing and PPS. Snoring was noted in 100% of patients with OSA, 0% of those with PPS hypoventilation, and 67% of those with combined OSA and hypoventilation.[110] Part of the evaluation of PPS should include a detailed evaluation for possible OSA.

Treatment with NIPPV

A trial of NIPPV may reduce the risk of endotracheal intubation or tracheostomy (see **Table 4**). Respiratory insufficiency becomes evident with progressive nocturnal hypoventilation followed by daytime hypercapnia. Traditionally, patients with chronic alveolar hypoventilation were treated with tracheostomies or body ventilators, such as an iron lung, rocking bed, or cuirass. Studies suggest that NIPPV may be an alternative approach. A retrospective review[90] found that 1 of 20 patients with PPS on NIPPV required tracheostomy compared with 14 of 25 who were on body ventilation. A retrospective case series documented an improvement in arterial blood gases and pulmonary function during long-term treatment with nocturnal NIPPV in patients with neuromuscular disease, including 18 with PPS.[111]

Five patients with PPS requiring ventilatory assistance on rocking beds had PSG.[112] These patients had consistently poor sleep quality with decreased total sleep time, decreased sleep efficiency with increased arousals, and decreased slow wave sleep, NREM stage N2 sleep, and REM sleep. Sleep-disordered breathing occurred and was greatest in REM sleep. These patients did not tolerate CPAP as an alternative to rocking bed. However, they had improvement in sleep architecture and arterial blood gases when placed on NIPPV and all were able to switch successfully from rocking beds to NIPPV. There were also 5 patients who had poor sleep architecture but did not require ventilatory assistance. These patients had predominantly sleep-disordered breathing consistent with OSA, and 4 were successfully treated with CPAP rather than NIPPV.

Non-NIPPV Treatment

Unfortunately, there are few options regarding treatment in PPS. Patients are offered physical and occupational therapy to maintain muscle strength. Anticholinesterases have had some success in improving muscle strength in some patients. Treatment with intravenous immunoglobulin (IVIG) is under investigation. A small RCT pilot study showed no effect with IVIG treatment on muscle strength and fatigue. However, IVIG-treated patients with PPS reported significantly less pain after 3 months of treatment.[113] An RCT was conducted to determine whether modafinil could improve fatigue and quality of life in patients with PPS, but demonstrated no difference in a comparison with controls.[114]

SUMMARY

NIPPV, which may include both daytime and nocturnal use, is effective for patients with PPS with hypercapnic respiratory failure. NIPPV may prevent tracheostomy and may improve sleep architecture and arterial blood gases. Sleep-disordered breathing is common in patients with PPS, particularly during REM sleep, and, if no other ventilatory assistance is required, may be treated with nocturnal CPAP rather than NIPPV.

REFERENCES

1. Sullivan CE, Issa FG, Berthon-Jones M, et al. Reversal of obstructive sleep apnoea by continuous positive airway pressure applied through the nares. Lancet 1981;1(8225):862–5.
2. Pérez de Llano LA, Golpe R, Ortiz Piquer M, et al. Short-term and long-term effects of nasal intermittent positive pressure ventilation in patients with obesity-hypoventilation syndrome. Chest 2005; 128:587–94.
3. Mehta S, Hill NS. Noninvasive ventilation. Am J Respir Crit Care Med 2001;163:540–77.
4. Global Initiative for Obstructive Lung Disease. Available at: www.goldcopd.org. Accessed February 4, 2010.
5. American Thoracic Society/European Respiratory Society COPD guidelines. Available at: http://www.copd-ats-ers.org/copddoc.pdf. Accessed February 10, 2010.
6. Department of Veterans Affairs/Department of Defense COPD guidelines Ver. 2.0. Available at: http://www.healthquality.va.gov/Chronic_Obstructive_Pulmonary_Disease_COPD.asp. Accessed February 4, 2010.
7. Sanders MH, Newman AB, Haggerty CL, et al. Sleep and sleep-disordered breathing in adults with predominantly mild obstructive airway disease. Am J Respir Crit Care Med 2003;167:7–14.
8. Bonnet MH, Arand DL. EEG arousal norms by age. J Clin Sleep Med 2007;3:271–4.
9. Phillips B, Berry D, Schmitt F, et al. Sleep quality and pulmonary function in the healthy elderly. Chest 1989;95:60–4.
10. Sahlin C, Franklin KA, Stenlund H, et al. Sleep in women: normal values for sleep stages and position and the effect of age, obesity, sleep apnea, smoking, alcohol and hypertension. Sleep Med 2009;10:1025–30.
11. Ohayon MM, Carskadon MA, Guilleminault C, et al. Meta-analysis of quantitative sleep parameters from childhood to old age in healthy individuals: developing normative sleep values across the human lifespan. Sleep 2004;1(27):1255–73.
12. Ballard RD, Clover CW, Suh BY. Influence of sleep on respiratory function in emphysema. Am J Respir Crit Care Med 1995;151:945–51.
13. Marrone O, Salvaggio A, Insalaco G. Respiratory disorders during sleep in chronic obstructive pulmonary disease. Int J Chron Obstruct Pulmon Dis 2006;1:363–72.
14. Littner MR, McGinty DJ, Arand DL. Determinants of oxygen desaturation in the course of ventilation during sleep in chronic obstructive pulmonary disease. Am Rev Respir Dis 1980;122:849–57.
15. Fletcher EC, Luckett RA, Goodnight-White S, et al. A double-blind trial of nocturnal supplemental oxygen for sleep desaturation in patients with chronic obstructive pulmonary disease and a daytime PaO_2 above 60 mm Hg. Am Rev Respir Dis 1992;145:1070–6.
16. McEvoy RD, Pierce RJ, Hillman D, et al. Nocturnal non-invasive nasal ventilation in stable hypercapnic COPD: a randomised controlled trial. Thorax 2009;64:561–6.
17. Kolodziej MA, Jensen L, Rowe B, et al. Systematic review of noninvasive positive pressure ventilation in severe stable COPD. Eur Respir J 2007;30: 293–306.
18. Wijkstra PJ, Lacasse Y, Guyatt GH, et al. A meta-analysis of nocturnal noninvasive positive pressure ventilation in patients with stable COPD. Chest 2003;124:337–43.

19. Lightowler JV, Wedzicha JA, Elliott MW, et al. Non-invasive positive pressure ventilation to treat respiratory failure resulting from exacerbations of chronic obstructive pulmonary disease: Cochrane systematic review and meta-analysis. BMJ 2003;326:185–9.

20. Keenan SP, Sinuff T, Cook DJ, et al. Which patients with acute exacerbation of chronic obstructive pulmonary disease benefit from noninvasive positive-pressure ventilation? A systematic review of the literature. Ann Intern Med 2003;138:861–70.

21. Dial S, Menzies D. Is there a role for mask continuous positive airway pressure in acute respiratory failure due to COPD? Lessons from a retrospective audit of 3 different cohorts. Int J Chron Obstruct Pulmon Dis 2006;1:65–72.

22. Ferrer M, Sellarés J, Valencia M, et al. Non-invasive ventilation after extubation in hypercapnic patients with chronic respiratory disorders: randomised controlled trial. Lancet 2009;374(9695):1082–8.

23. Walters S, Mehta A. Epidemiology of cystic fibrosis. In: Hodson M, Geddes DM, Bush A, editors. Cystic fibrosis. 3rd edition. London: Edward Arnold Ltd; 2007. p. 21–45.

24. Davies JC, Alton EW, Bush A. Cystic fibrosis. BMJ 2007;335:1255–9.

25. Dodge JA, Lewis PA, Stanton M, et al. Cystic fibrosis mortality and survival in the UK: 1947–2003. Eur Respir J 2007;29:522–6.

26. O'Sullivan BP, Freedman SD. Cystic fibrosis. Lancet 2009;373(9678):1891–904.

27. Davis PB. Pathophysiology of the lung disease in cystic fibrosis. In: Davis PB, editor. Cystic fibrosis. New York: Marcel Dekker; 1993. p. 193.

28. Jankelowitz L, Reid KJ, Wolfe L, et al. Cystic fibrosis patients have poor sleep quality despite normal sleep latency and efficiency. Chest 2005;127:1593–9.

29. Milross MA, Piper AJ, Norman M, et al. Subjective sleep quality in cystic fibrosis. Sleep Med 2002;3:205–12.

30. Amin R, Bean J, Burklow K, et al. The relationship between sleep disturbance and pulmonary function in stable pediatric cystic fibrosis patients. Chest 2005;128:1357–63.

31. Naqvi SK, Sotelo C, Murry L, et al. Sleep architecture in children and adolescents with cystic fibrosis and the association with severity of lung disease. Sleep Breath 2008;12:77–83.

32. Bradley S, Solin P, Wilson J, et al. Hypoxemia and hypercapnia during exercise and sleep in patients with cystic fibrosis. Chest 1999;116:647–54.

33. Francis PW, Muller NL, Gurwitz D, et al. Hemoglobin desaturation: its occurrence during sleep in patients with cystic fibrosis. Am J Dis Child 1980;134:734–40.

34. Fraser KL, Tullis DE, Sasson Z, et al. Pulmonary hypertension and cardiac function in adult cystic fibrosis: role of hypoxemia. Chest 1999;115:1321–8.

35. Gozal D. Nocturnal ventilatory support in patients with cystic fibrosis: comparison with supplemental oxygen. Eur Respir J 1997;10:1999–2003.

36. Milross MA, Piper AJ, Norman M, et al. Predicting sleep-disordered breathing in patients with cystic fibrosis. Chest 2001;120:1239–45.

37. Milross MA, Piper AJ, Norman M, et al. Night-to-night variability in sleep in cystic fibrosis. Sleep Med 2002;3:213–9.

38. Coffey MJ, FitzGerald MX, McNicholas WT. Comparison of oxygen desaturation during sleep and exercise in patients with cystic fibrosis. Chest 1991;100:659–62.

39. Frangolias DD, Wilcox PG. Predictability of oxygen desaturation during sleep in patients with cystic fibrosis: clinical, spirometric, and exercise parameters. Chest 2001;119:434–41.

40. Bell SC, Saunders MJ, Elborn JS, et al. Resting energy expenditure and oxygen cost of breathing in patients with cystic fibrosis. Thorax 1996;51:126–31.

41. Tepper RS, Skatrud JB, Dempsey JA. Ventilation and oxygenation changes during sleep in cystic fibrosis. Chest 1983;84:388–93.

42. Milross MA, Piper AJ, Norman M, et al. Low-flow oxygen and bilevel ventilatory support: effects on ventilation during sleep in cystic fibrosis. Am J Respir Crit Care Med 2001;163:129–34.

43. Regnis JA, Piper AJ, Henke KG, et al. Benefits of nocturnal nasal CPAP in patients with cystic fibrosis. Chest 1994;106:1717–24.

44. Fauroux B, Burgel P, Boelle P, et al. Practice of noninvasive ventilation for cystic fibrosis: a nationwide survey in France. Respir Care 2008;53:1482–9.

45. Piper AJ, Parker S, Torzillo PJ, et al. Nocturnal nasal IPPV stabilizes patients with cystic fibrosis and hypercapnic respiratory failure. Chest 1992;102:846–50.

46. Young AC, Wilson JW, Kotsimbos TC, et al. Randomised placebo controlled trial of non-invasive ventilation for hypercapnia in cystic fibrosis. Thorax 2008;63:72–7.

47. Moran F, Bradley JM, Piper AJ. Non-invasive ventilation for cystic fibrosis. Cochrane Database Syst Rev 2009;1:CD002769.

48. Hill AT, Edenborough FP, Cayton RM, et al. Long-term nasal intermittent positive pressure ventilation in patients with cystic fibrosis and hypercapnic respiratory failure (1991–1996). Respir Med 1998;92:523–6.

49. Holland AE, Denehy L, Ntoumenopoulos G, et al. Non-invasive ventilation assists chest physiotherapy in adults with acute exacerbations of cystic fibrosis. Thorax 2003;58:880–4.

50. McMaster MJ, Glasby MA, Singh H, et al. Lung function in congenital kyphosis and kyphoscoliosis. J Spinal Disord Tech 2007;20:203–8.

51. Weber B, Smith JP, Briscoe WA, et al. Pulmonary function in asymptomatic adolescents with idiopathic scoliosis. Am Rev Respir Dis 1975;111:389–97.

52. Lisboa C, Moreno R, Fava M, et al. Inspiratory muscle function in patients with severe kyphoscoliosis. Am Rev Respir Dis 1985;132:48–52.

53. Di Bari M, Chiarlone M, Matteuzzi D, et al. Thoracic kyphosis and ventilatory dysfunction in unselected older persons: an epidemiological study in Dicomano, Italy. J Am Geriatr Soc 2004;52:909–15.

54. Bergofsky EH, Turino GM, Fishman AP. Cardiorespiratory failure in kyphoscoliosis. Medicine (Baltimore) 1959;38:263–317.

55. dos Santos Alves VL, Stirbulov R, Avanzi O. Impact of a physical rehabilitation program on the respiratory function of adolescents with idiopathic scoliosis. Chest 2006;130:500–5.

56. Pehrsson K, Danielsson A, Nachemson A. Pulmonary function in adolescent idiopathic scoliosis: a 25 year follow up after surgery or start of brace treatment. Thorax 2001;56:388–93.

57. Mezon BL, West P, Israels J, et al. Sleep breathing abnormalities in kyphoscoliosis. Am Rev Respir Dis 1980;122:617–21.

58. Gonzalez C, Ferris G, Diaz J, et al. Kyphoscoliotic ventilatory insufficiency: effects of long-term intermittent positive-pressure ventilation. Chest 2003;124:857–62.

59. Ellis ER, Grunstein RR, Chan S, et al. Noninvasive ventilatory support during sleep improves respiratory failure in kyphoscoliosis. Chest 1988;94:811–5.

60. Buyse B, Meersseman W, Demedts M. Treatment of chronic respiratory failure in kyphoscoliosis: oxygen or ventilation? Eur Respir J 2003;22:525–8.

61. Annane D, Orlikowski D, Chevret S, et al. Nocturnal mechanical ventilation for chronic hypoventilation in patients with neuromuscular and chest wall disorders. Cochrane Database Syst Rev 2007;(4):CD001941.

62. Chio A, Logroscino G, Hardiman O, et al. Prognostic factors in ALS: a critical review. Amyotroph Lateral Scler 2009;10:310–23.

63. Bourke SC, Bullock RE, Williams TL, et al. Noninvasive ventilation in ALS: indications and effect on quality of life. Neurology 2003;61:171–7.

64. George CF, Guilleminault C. Sleep and neuromuscular diseases. Chapter 69. In: Kryger MH, Roth T III, Dement WC, editors. Principals and practice of sleep medicine. 4th edition. Philadelphia: Elsevier; 2005. p. 830–52.

65. Ferguson KA, Strong MJ, Ahmad D, et al. Sleep-disordered breathing in amyotrophic lateral sclerosis. Chest 1996;110:664–9.

66. Kimura K, Tachibana N, Kimura J, et al. Sleep-disordered breathing at an early stage of amyotrophic lateral sclerosis. J Neurol Sci 1999;164:37–43.

67. Carter GT, Weiss MD, Lou JS, et al. Modafinil to treat fatigue in amyotrophic lateral sclerosis: an open label pilot study. Am J Hosp Palliat Care 2005;22:55–9.

68. Arnulf I, Similowski T, Salachas F, et al. Sleep disorders and diaphragmatic function in patients with amyotrophic lateral sclerosis. Am J Respir Crit Care Med 2000;161:849–56.

69. Atalaia A, De Carvalho M, Evangelista T, et al. Sleep characteristics of amyotrophic lateral sclerosis in patients with preserved diaphragmatic function. Amyotroph Lateral Scler 2007;8:101–5.

70. Kleopa KA, Sherman M, Neal B. BIPAP improves survival and rate of pulmonary function decline in patients with ALS. J Neurol Sci 1999;164:82–8.

71. Bourke SC, Tomlinson M, Williams TL, et al. Effects of non-invasive ventilation on survival and quality of life in patients with amyotrophic lateral sclerosis: a randomised controlled trial. Lancet Neurol 2006;5:140–7.

72. Newsom-Davis IC, Lyall RA, Leigh PN, et al. The effect of non-invasive positive pressure ventilation (NIPPV) on cognitive function in amyotrophic lateral sclerosis (ALS): a prospective study. J Neurol Neurosurg Psychiatr 2001;71:482–7.

73. Gruis KL, Chernew ME, Brown DL. The cost-effectiveness of early noninvasive ventilation for ALS patients. BMC Health Serv Res 2005;5:58.

74. Jackson CE, Rosenfeld J, Moore DH, et al. A preliminary evaluation of a prospective study of pulmonary function studies and symptoms of hypoventilation in ALS/MND patients. J Neurol Sci 2001;191:75–8.

75. Miller RG, Mitchell JD, Lyon M, et al. Riluzole for amyotrophic lateral sclerosis (ALS)/motor neuron disease (MND). Cochrane Database Syst Rev 2007;1:CD001447.

76. Mellion M, Tseng B. Dystrophinopathies. Available at: http://emedicine.medscape.com/article/1173204-overview. Accessed February 4, 2010.

77. Gomez-Merino E, Bach JR. Duchenne muscular dystrophy: prolongation of life by noninvasive ventilation and mechanically assisted coughing. Am J Phys Med Rehabil 2002;81:411–5.

78. Baydur A, Gilgoff I, Prentice W, et al. Decline in respiratory function and experience with long-term assisted ventilation in advanced Duchenne's muscular dystrophy. Chest 1990;97:884–9.

79. Howard RS, Davidson C. Long term ventilation in neurogenic respiratory failure. J Neurol Neurosurg Psychiatr 2003;74(Suppl 3):iii24–30.

80. Simonds AK, Muntoni F, Heather S, et al. Impact of nasal ventilation on survival in hypercapnic Duchenne muscular dystrophy. Thorax 1998;53:949–52.

81. Barbé F, Quera-Salva MA, McCann C, et al. Sleep-related respiratory disturbances in patients with Duchenne muscular dystrophy. Eur Respir J 1994;7:1403–8.

82. Khan Y, Heckmatt JZ. Obstructive apnoeas in Duchenne muscular dystrophy. Thorax 1994;49: 157–61.

83. Kohler M, Clarenbach CF, Böni L, et al. Quality of life, physical disability, and respiratory impairment in Duchenne muscular dystrophy. Am J Respir Crit Care Med 2005;172:1032–6.

84. Toussaint M, Chatwin M, Soudon P. Mechanical ventilation in Duchenne patients with chronic respiratory insufficiency: clinical implications of 20 years published experience. Chron Respir Dis 2007;4: 167–77.

85. Ward S, Chatwin M, Heather S, et al. Randomised controlled trial of non-invasive ventilation (NIV) for nocturnal hypoventilation in neuromuscular and chest wall disease patients with daytime normocapnia. Thorax 2005;60:1019–24.

86. Anonymous. Clinical indications for noninvasive positive pressure ventilation in chronic respiratory failure due to restrictive lung disease, COPD, and nocturnal hypoventilation—a consensus conference report. Chest 1999;116:521–34.

87. Robert D, Willig TN, Leger P, et al. Long-term nasal ventilation in neuromuscular disorders: report of a consensus conference. Eur Respir J 1993;6: 599–606.

88. Toussaint M, Steens M, Wasteels G, et al. Diurnal ventilation via mouthpiece: survival in end-stage Duchenne patients. Eur Respir J 2006;28:549–55.

89. Vianello A, Bevilacqua M, Salvador V, et al. Long-term nasal intermittent positive pressure ventilation in advanced Duchenne's muscular dystrophy. Chest 1994;105:445–8.

90. Baydur A, Layne E, Aral H, et al. Long term noninvasive ventilation in the community for patients with musculoskeletal disorders: 46 year experience and review. Thorax 2000;55:4–11.

91. Manzur AY, Kuntzer T, Pike M, et al. Glucocorticoid corticosteroids for Duchenne muscular dystrophy. Cochrane Database Syst Rev 2008;(1):CD003725.

92. Phillips LH. The epidemiology of myasthenia gravis. Semin Neurol 2004;24:17–20.

93. Drachman DB. Myasthenia gravis. N Engl J Med 1994;330:1797–810.

94. Vincent A. Unravelling the pathogenesis of myasthenia gravis. Nat Rev Immunol 2002;2: 797–804.

95. Vincent A, McConville J, Farrugia ME, et al. Antibodies in myasthenia gravis and related disorders. Ann N Y Acad Sci 2003;998:324–35.

96. Hoch W, McConville J, Helms S, et al. Auto-antibodies to the receptor tyrosine kinase MuSK in patients with myasthenia gravis without acetylcholine receptor antibodies. Nat Med 2001;7:365–8.

97. Gronseth GS, Barohn RJ. Practice parameter: thymectomy for autoimmune myasthenia gravis (an evidence-based review): report of the Quality Standards Subcommittee of the American Academy of Neurology. Neurology 2000; 55:7–15.

98. Quera-Salva MA, Guilleminault C, Chevret S, et al. Breathing disorders during sleep in myasthenia gravis. Ann Neurol 1992;31:86–92.

99. Keesey JC. Does myasthenia gravis affect the brain? J Neurol Sci 1999;170:77–89.

100. Shneerson JM, Simonds AK. Noninvasive ventilation for chest wall and neuromuscular disorders. Eur Respir J 2002;20:480–7.

101. Bedlack RS, Sanders DB. On the concept of myasthenic crisis. J Clin Neuromuscul Dis 2002;4:40–2.

102. Rabinstein A, Wijdicks EF. BiPAP in acute respiratory failure due to myasthenic crisis may prevent intubation. Neurology 2002;59:1647–9.

103. Wu JY, Kuo PH, Fan PC, et al. The role of noninvasive ventilation and factors predicting extubation outcome in myasthenic crisis. Neurocrit Care 2009;10(1):35–42.

104. Seneviratne J, Mandrekar J, Wijdicks EF, et al. Noninvasive ventilation in myasthenic crisis. Arch Neurol 2008;65:54–8.

105. Gonzalez H, Ottervald J, Nilsson KC, et al. Identification of novel candidate protein biomarkers for the post-polio syndrome—implications for diagnosis, neurodegeneration and neuroinflammation. J Proteomics 2009;71:670–81.

106. Soliman MG, Higgins SE, El-Kabir DR, et al. Noninvasive assessment of respiratory muscle strength in patients with previous poliomyelitis. Respir Med 2005;99:1217–22.

107. Jubelt B, Agre JC. Characteristics and management of postpolio syndrome. JAMA 2000;26(284): 412–4.

108. Siegel H, McCutchen C, Dalakas MC, et al. Physiologic events initiating REM sleep in patients with the postpolio syndrome. Neurology 1999;52:516–22.

109. Bruno RL. Abnormal movements in sleep as a postpolio sequelae. Am J Phys Med Rehabil 1998;77: 339–43.

110. Hsu AA, Staats BA. Postpolio sequelae and sleep-related disordered breathing. Mayo Clin Proc 1998; 73:216–24.

111. Duiverman ML, Bladder G, Meinesz AF, et al. Home mechanical ventilatory support in patients with restrictive ventilatory disorders: a 48-year experience. Respir Med 2006;100: 56–65.

112. Steljes DG, Kryger MH, Kirk BW, et al. Sleep in postpolio syndrome. Chest 1990;98:133–40.

113. Farbu E, Rekand T, Vik-Mo E, et al. Post-polio syndrome patients treated with intravenous immunoglobulin: a double-blinded randomized controlled pilot study. Eur J Neurol 2007;14:60–5.

114. Vasconcelos OM, Prokhorenko OA, Salajegheh MK, et al. Modafinil for treatment of fatigue in post-polio syndrome: a randomized controlled trial. Neurology 2007;15(68):1680–6.

115. Miller RG, Jackson CE, Kasarskis EJ, et al. Practice parameter update: the care of the patient with amyotrophic lateral sclerosis: drug, nutritional, and respiratory therapies (an evidence-based review): report of the Quality Standards Subcommittee of the American Academy of Neurology. Neurology 2009;73: 1218–26.

Noninvasive Positive Pressure Ventilation in the Treatment of Hypoventilation in Children

Iris A. Perez, MD[a,b], Thomas G. Keens, MD[a,b],
Sally L. Davidson Ward, MD[b,c],*

KEYWORDS

- Hypoventilation • Chronic respiratory failure
- Noninvasive ventilation • NPPV
- Bilevel positive airway pressure • Neuromuscular disease
- Ventilatory muscle weakness

Adequate ventilation requires sufficiently robust central respiratory control and ventilatory muscle function to overcome the workload imposed by the pulmonary mechanics and properties of the upper airway. Hypoventilation due to chronic respiratory failure (CRF) in childhood therefore can result from dysfunction of each of these components of the respiratory system. Noninvasive positive pressure ventilation (NPPV) can provide ventilatory support for children with hypoventilation or CRF caused by a variety of underlying clinical entities. Children with CRF stemming from central respiratory control abnormalities, ventilatory muscle weakness or, in some circumstances, restrictive or obstructive lung disease can be managed successfully with NPPV. Although NPPV offers the advantage of not requiring a tracheostomy with the attendant complications, it is not appropriate for all children with CRF because use is generally not well tolerated during wakefulness and the devices have limited portability. Successful use requires cooperation on the part of the child, thus making introduction of the therapy and selection of the interface critical for

adherence. Management of CRF requires a multidisciplinary approach to educate and support the patient and family, and to ensure patient safety and quality of life. When NPPV is used for CRF caused by a progressive disease, periodic retitration of pressures is required as well as a consideration of the ongoing appropriateness of noninvasive ventilation. Although NPPV has wide applicability in the pediatric intensive care unit setting for acute respiratory failure, this topic is beyond the scope of this discussion.

PHYSIOLOGY OF CHRONIC RESPIRATORY FAILURE IN CHILDREN

The ability to sustain spontaneous ventilation requires adequate function of neurologic control of breathing, ventilatory muscles, and lung mechanics. Significant dysfunction of any of these 3 components of the respiratory system may impair a child's ability to breathe spontaneously. Respiratory failure occurs when central respiratory drive and/or ventilatory muscle power are inadequate to overcome the respiratory load (**Fig. 1**).

[a] Childrens Hospital Los Angeles, 4650 Sunset Boulevard, Los Angeles, CA 90027, USA
[b] Keck School of Medicine, University of Southern California, Los Angeles, CA, USA
[c] Division of Pediatric Pulmonology, Childrens Hospital Los Angeles, Mailstop #83, 4650 Sunset Boulevard, Los Angeles, CA 90027, USA
* Corresponding author. Division of Pediatric Pulmonology, Childrens Hospital Los Angeles, Mailstop #83, 4650 Sunset Boulevard, Los Angeles, CA 90027.
E-mail address: sward@chla.usc.edu

Sleep Med Clin 5 (2010) 471–484
doi:10.1016/j.jsmc.2010.05.013
1556-407X/10/$ – see front matter © 2010 Elsevier Inc. All rights reserved.

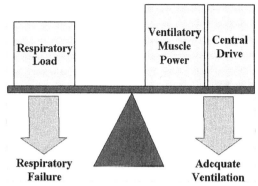

Fig. 1. The respiratory balance. In normal individuals, ventilatory muscle power and central drive are more than adequate to overcome the respiratory load, tipping the balance to the right, which results in adequate ventilation. However, when ventilatory muscle power and/or central drive are sufficiently decreased and/or the respiratory load is sufficiently increased, or some combination thereof, ventilatory muscle power and central drive may not be sufficient to overcome the respiratory load. The balance will tip to the left, and respiratory failure will result.

CRF occurs if the cause of this imbalance is not reversible, and chronic ventilatory support will therefore be required.[1–6]

CRF implies that a chronic, perhaps irreversible, underlying respiratory disorder is causing respiratory insufficiency that results in inadequate ventilation or hypoxia.[1] The diagnosis of CRF is usually made once repeated attempts to wean from assisted ventilation have failed for at least 1 month in a patient without superimposed acute respiratory disease, or in a patient who has a diagnosis with no prospect of being weaned from the ventilator. This article focuses on CRF, which means that the patient has been determined to be ventilator dependent, and that he or she cannot be weaned from assisted ventilation at the near future.

CENTRAL HYPOVENTILATION SYNDROMES

The cause of CRF in children with central hypoventilation syndromes is inadequate central respiratory drive, either congenital or acquired.[7–13] The congenital form may be genetic (congenital central hypoventilation syndrome) or result from an identifiable brainstem lesion.[7,11–16] Acquired forms of central hypoventilation syndrome may be caused by brainstem trauma, tumor, hemorrhage, stroke, or infection.[8,16]

The primary components of respiratory control are oxygen and CO_2 sensors, integration of input from receptors, and a motor response (**Fig. 2**). The central chemoreceptor, located in the medulla, is sensitive to changes in $P_{a}CO_2$. CO_2

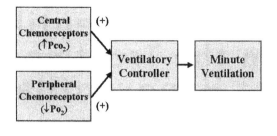

Sensors   Integration   Motor Response

Fig. 2. Neurologic control of breathing. Neurologic control of breathing can be divided into sensors, integration, and motor response. The most important sensors are central and peripheral chemoreceptors, which sense CO_2 and oxygen, respectively. This information is integrated in the brainstem and other areas of the brain. The motor response is minute ventilation or breathing.

in arterial blood diffuses across the blood-brain barrier, increasing H^+ concentration in cerebral spinal fluid (CSF). Central chemoreceptor cells respond to changes in CSF H^+. This mechanism comprises a dynamic system sensitive to small P_{CO_2} changes. Minute ventilation increases linearly with increasing $P_{a}CO_2$. Therefore, central chemoreceptors are responsible for breathing minute to minute. Blood H^+ and HCO_3^- ions do not readily diffuse across the blood-brain barrier. However, with time, if P_{CO_2} remains chronically elevated, resulting in a chronic elevation of CSF H^+, renal conservation of HCO_3^- will determine a new CSF H^+ baseline. In this way, central chemoreceptors may habituate to high P_{CO_2} values, as evidenced by a normal arterial pH in the presence of an elevated $P_{a}CO_2$. Peripheral chemoreceptors, located in the carotid bodies at the bifurcation carotid arteries, are sensitive to changes in $P_{a}O_2$, large changes in pH, and large changes in $P_{a}CO_2$. Peripheral chemoreceptor function is tied closest to the hypoxic ventilatory response. Minute ventilation increases exponentially as $P_{a}O_2$ decreases and linearly as $S_{a}O_2$ decreases. Central and peripheral chemoreceptors act synergistically so that in a patient with both hypercapnia and hypoxia, ventilation will be stimulated more than by hypercapnia or hypoxia alone. Note that central and peripheral chemoreceptors are in anatomically distinct sites. Therefore, damage to the brainstem does not affect afferent peripheral chemoreceptor function.

Based on the function of the chemoreceptors, one can predict the clinical picture associated with central hypoventilation syndromes due to isolated chemoreceptor dysfunction. Patients with central chemoreceptor dysfunction cannot precisely control ventilation minute to minute. Therefore, P_aco_2 should increase until sufficient hypoxia triggers peripheral chemoreceptor stimulation. In general, these patients would have abnormal blood gases at all times, but they will be worse in sleep than in wakefulness, because there are multiple nonrespiratory stimuli for ventilation that are active during wakefulness. Cortical influences, specifically arousal, fear anxiety, fever, and pain, can all stimulate breathing.

All receptors input to the ventilatory controller in the brain. While it is believed that the location of the ventilatory controller is primarily in the brainstem, it is now apparent that other brain structures participate in ventilatory control as well, notably the cerebellum.[17–20] Input from oxygen and CO_2 sensors is processed and integrated in the ventilatory controller. Patients with abnormalities of the ventilatory controller would be predicted to have absent ventilatory responses to both hypoxia and hypercapnia. Patients with congenital central hypoventilation syndrome (CCHS) primarily have a defect in the integration of chemoreceptor input to the ventilatory controller, although they have reasonably preserved mechanoreceptor function.[15,21,22]

While subtle clinical differences may exist between different types of central hypoventilation syndromes, in those severe enough to cause CRF there are more similarities than differences. In general, these patients have no subjective or objective response to hypoxia or hypercapnia whether they are awake or asleep (**Fig. 3**).[15,16,23] Therefore, ventilation is inadequate at all times. However, because ventilation is uniformly compromised during sleep compared with wakefulness, all children with central hypoventilation syndromes have more severe hypoxia and hypercapnia during sleep.

VENTILATORY MUSCLE WEAKNESS AND NEUROMUSCULAR DISEASE

The diaphragm is the major muscle of breathing.[24] The intercostal and accessory muscles optimize diaphragm function in normal individuals. Ventilatory muscle weakness has several physiologic consequences. Inspiratory muscle weakness prevents children from inspiring deeply, resulting in atelectasis. Expiratory muscle weakness prevents effective coughing, resulting in decreased removal of pulmonary secretions and foreign material from the lungs. In combination, these increase the incidence and severity of pneumonia, which is the leading cause of morbidity and mortality in children with neuromuscular disease (NMD).

Ventilatory muscles are skeletal muscles; thus, they can fatigue.[24,25] For a muscle to perform work, it must be able to produce energy. If the diaphragm generates more than 40% of its maximal transdiaphragmatic pressure on each breath, it will fatigue.[24] Normal individuals require less than 5% of maximal transdiaphragmatic pressure on each breath, indicating considerable reserve. For a normal individual to show diaphragmatic fatigue, there would have to be a substantial increase in the respiratory load. With ventilatory muscle weakness, even a normal respiratory load may require greater than 40% of maximal transdiaphragmatic pressure, and diaphragm fatigue and respiratory failure will result. Pharmacologic agents cannot restore ventilatory muscle strength.

It should be noted that several conditions can predispose the diaphragm to fatigue, and attention

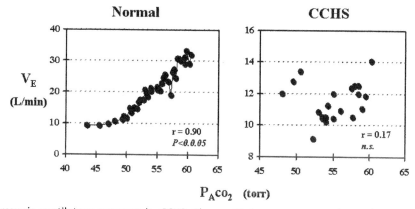

Fig. 3. Hypercapnic ventilatory response in CCHS. The ventilatory response to increasing CO_2 is shown for a normal individual and for a patient with CCHS. Minute ventilation (V_E) is plotted on the ordinate, and alveolar (end-tidal) Pco_2 (P_Aco_2) is plotted on the abscissa. Whereas normal individuals have a tight linear increase in V_E with P_Aco_2, the CCHS patient has no relationship between V_E and P_Aco_2.

should be paid to try and minimize them to the extent possible. Hypoxia decreases the ability of muscle to produce energy, as anaerobic energy production is much less efficient than aerobic energy production. Hypercapnia and acidosis interfere with excitation-coupling of muscle. Hyperinflation puts the diaphragm at a mechanical disadvantage, due to shortened muscle fibers, thus decreasing strength. Malnutrition decreases strength by decreasing muscle mass, and it decreases endurance by decreasing muscle oxidative enzymes to produce energy.[26,27] Increased respiratory loads decrease the ability of ventilatory muscles to achieve adequate ventilation. For those patients who have been ventilator dependent for some time, disuse can decrease both strength and endurance.[26,28] Minimizing these conditions may improve ventilatory muscle function to the point that less ventilatory support is required.

Two basic types of ventilatory muscle weakness are seen in NMD: progressive and nonprogressive. In progressive NMD, such as spinal muscular atrophy or muscular dystrophy, muscle weakness worsens with time, resulting in an inevitable and predictable development of CRF.[4,29–33] In nonprogressive NMDs, such as congenital myopathies, the muscle weakness per se does not progress. However, there may be a relative progression of impairment, because muscle strength cannot increase to overcome the increasing functional demands as the body grows. Many children with static neuromuscular disorders become nonambulatory and ventilator dependent at or near puberty, because of the marked increase in body mass associated with the pubertal growth spurt.

Children with chronically elevated P_{CO_2} greater than 55 to 60 mm Hg, due to ventilatory muscle weakness, will develop progressive pulmonary hypertension. Although oxygen administration improves the P_aO_2 and relieves hypoxia, this treatment alone is inadequate, as hypoventilation persists with resulting pulmonary hypertension. Thus, these children require home mechanical ventilation.[29–31,33]

IMPACT OF OBESITY ON THE RESPIRATORY SYSTEM

Although obesity is not strictly an NMD, it can result in CRF as a consequence of altered pulmonary mechanics, hypoventilation during sleep, and obstructive sleep apnea. Obesity decreases the compliance of the chest wall and lung by as much as two-thirds compared with individuals of normal weight, and compliance is further decreased in the recumbent position. Lung volumes are reduced and there is relative underventilation at the bases of the lungs, leading to ventilation perfusion mismatch and hypoxemia. Obesity also causes airways obstruction and mechanical disadvantage of the diaphragm, thus increasing the work of breathing and predisposing to fatigue.[34–37] Severe obstructive sleep apnea often accompanies obesity, thus further compromising the respiratory system. Long-standing gas exchange abnormalities during sleep can lead to daytime hypoventilation. With the pediatric obesity epidemic, the obesity hypoventilation syndrome is no longer limited to adults, and has become well described in children. These patients are excellent candidates for NPPV, and adequate ventilation during sleep will usually correct the waking hypoventilation and daytime sleepiness.

CHRONIC PULMONARY DISEASE

Chronic pulmonary disease due to intrinsic lung disease may increase the work of breathing to a level higher than can be sustained by spontaneous ventilation. Often the underlying lung disease is intrinsically unstable, requiring frequent adjustments in ventilator settings. Some children with chronic pulmonary disease will stabilize to the point where home mechanical ventilation is possible, but are generally not candidates for NPPV and are best managed by positive pressure ventilation via tracheostomy.[1,2,38–42] However, NPPV has been used in children with advanced obstructive lung disease, such as cystic fibrosis, as a bridge to lung transplantation.[40] Restrictive lung disease stemming from thoracic dysplasia or scoliosis resulting in CRF can be managed by NPPV in some pediatric patients. CRF in young children may be supported by initially by NPPV, but with growth, as metabolic needs increase, they may need invasive ventilation. In older children with thoracic restriction who have reached skeletal maturity, NPPV can be a long-term option to support ventilation.[43]

PATIENT SELECTION AND CLINICAL PRESENTATION

The choice of NPPV for treatment of children with CRF is based on the child's underlying medical diagnoses, condition, and the goal of therapy, based on discussion with the family. In general, a candidate for NPPV should have a stable airway and good airway protection, that is, effective cough, normal swallowing function, and ability to handle the secretions adequately. The patient should require assisted ventilation only during sleep and must not require frequent pediatric intensive care unit admissions and intubation for respiratory infections or exacerbations.[43] The bilevel positive airway pressure device is not as powerful as home mechanical ventilators via tracheostomy, thus unstable patients are not candidates for noninvasive ventilation unless used as a form of palliation. The next sections describe examples of patients who may benefit from NPPV.

CENTRAL HYPOVENTILATION SYNDROMES

Central hypoventilation can be congenital or acquired.[8,44–47] Whereas central respiratory drive is impaired in central hypoventilation syndromes, the lungs and ventilatory muscles may be nearly normal, permitting reasonably stable ventilator settings to achieve adequate gas exchange. This group of patients can be offered a variety of modalities for ventilatory support, including NPPV.[2,7,8,12]

Congenital Central Hypoventilation Syndrome

CCHS is a rare disorder of failure of automatic central control of breathing[48,49] caused by the mutation of the PHOX2B gene.[13,50,51] Most CCHS patients manifest symptoms in the newborn period as failure to breathe in the delivery room or failure to be extubated from assisted ventilation. Others present in the first few months of life with episodes of severe apnea, apparent life-threatening event, or respiratory arrest. Occasionally they may present with feeding difficulty or breath-holding spells.[7,11–13,15,52] CCHS patients require life-long assisted ventilation during sleep and approximately 30% of patients require ventilatory support 24 hours a day. Positive pressure ventilation (PPV) via tracheostomy is the most common method of providing assisted ventilation.[7,8] Some patients are candidates for NPPV.[14,53,54] Although NPPV is used in very young patients in other centers, at the Childrens Hospital Los Angeles the authors ventilate patients via tracheostomy and mechanical home ventilation until they are about 5 years of age. Then, if the family desires, patients can be transitioned to diaphragm pacing or NPPV with backup rate and the tracheostomy removed.

Myelomeningocoele/Arnold-Chiari Malformation II

Almost all patients with myelomeningocoele (MMC) have Arnold-Chiari malformation (Chiari II malformation; ACM) characterized by downward displacement of the cerebellar tonsils and medulla.[55,56] This malformation of the brainstem affects respiratory control. In infancy, major manifestations include abnormal vocal cord mobility with resultant obstructive sleep apneas,[57–59] clinically significant hypoventilation, central apneas, and breath-holding spells.[60–62] Patients with myelomeningocele and ACM had blunted ventilatory responses to hypercapnia and hypoxia and had abnormal arousal responses to hypoxia and hypercapnia.[16,62–64] With very abnormal central respiratory control, patients may require ventilatory support. Those who require ventilatory support only during sleep can be managed with NPPV.[65]

Prader-Willi Syndrome

Prader Willi syndrome (PWS) is a disorder caused by deletion of the long arm of paternally derived chromosome 15, resulting in abnormalities of the hypothalamic function such as hyperphagia, obesity, hypogonadism, and behavioral and sleep disorders. During sleep, patients with PWS have obstructive sleep apnea syndrome (OSAS), hypoventilation, hypoxia, and abnormalities of sleep architecture.[8,66] It is unclear as to what might be the relative contributions of obesity versus the intrinsic disorder of ventilatory control, but patients with OSAS with or without hypoventilation can be supported with NPPV even from a young age.[67–69]

Acquired Central Hypoventilation Syndrome/ROHHAD

Rapid-onset obesity with hypothalamic dysfunction, hypoventilation, and autonomic dysregulation syndrome (ROHHAD) is a disorder that causes severe hypoventilation. The most characteristic manifestations include presentation of rapid-onset obesity in the first 10 years of life, followed by hypothalamic dysfunction and onset of symptoms of autonomic dysregulation, with later onset of alveolar hypoventilation. Patients do not have mutations of the PHOX2B gene or other CCHS candidate genes. Ize-Ludlow and colleagues[70] noted that 60% of patients had cardiorespiratory arrest and had evidence of abnormal respiratory control, with obstructive sleep apnea, cyanosis, or oxygen desaturation occurring before the arrest. In this group of patients, 47% were on 24-hour assisted ventilation requiring tracheostomy and the remainder were on night-time ventilation via NPPV.

Obesity Hypoventilation Syndrome

Children with morbid obesity increasingly present with severe OSAS and significant hypoventilation. Some children and adolescents experience excessive daytime sleepiness that interferes with daily life. Systemic and pulmonary hypertension may be present due to prolonged hypoventilation and hypercapnia. In addition, unlike the majority of children with OSAS, respiratory control can be altered with resetting of chemoreceptor function, resulting in daytime hypoventilation.[8] In these children, NPPV can be used to improve to improve sleep quality, normalize gas exchange, and reverse excessive daytime sleepiness.

Neuromuscular Disorders

Children with ventilatory muscle weakness make good candidates for home mechanical ventilation. Because the cause of their respiratory failure is primary muscle weakness, these patients usually do not have significant lung disease, which would require the need for frequent changes in ventilator settings. These children usually are much more stable on home mechanical ventilation, and have less frequent pneumonias and hospital admissions than they did before the institution of home mechanical ventilation.[3,29–32]

Duchenne muscular dystrophy (DMD) is a disease characterized by progressive loss of muscle strength, eventually resulting in loss of ambulation, loss of ventilatory muscle strength, and death from respiratory insufficiency. Respiratory failure occurs at an average age of 13 years and is the cause of death in 90% of individuals before the age of 20 years. The majority of patients develop cardiomyopathy.[71] Significant sleep related hypoxemia with profound oxygen desaturation may occur with normal diurnal ventilation in advanced DMD.[72] Predictors of sleep hypoventilation include forced expiratory volume in 1 second of less than 40% and a Pco_2 and of 45 mm Hg or greater.[73] More recently, Toussaint and colleagues[74] showed that vital capacity of less than 680 mL predicts daytime hypercapnea. NPPV has been used to treat patients with DMD with CRF. NPPV has been shown to improve dyspnea, respiratory disturbance, arousals from sleep, and sleep quality, and to normalize gas exchange.[75–78]

Spinal muscular atrophy (SMA) is an autosomal recessive disease of the anterior horn cells. Affected children present with hypotonia and weakness of the distal muscles of the upper and lower extremities, and progressive involvement of the chest wall muscles. The severity of the weakness generally correlates with the age of onset. The most severe type presents in infancy. Milder types present with later onset, and the course is more insidious. Type 1 SMA (Werdnig-Hoffman disease) patients have impaired head control, with a weak cry and cough. Weakness

and hypotonia in the limbs and trunk are eventually accompanied by intercostal muscle weakness. Respiratory failure is progressive and patients die before 2 or 3 years of age unless they receive assisted ventilation. Many families opt for comfort care and accept natural death for their infants with SMA Type 1. NPPV as part of comfort care is an individual family decision. SMA Type 2 patients have delayed motor milestones. Sitting is achieved, but standing and ambulation without aids are never obtained. Bulbar weakness with swallowing dysfunction may lead to poor weight gain. Patients have difficulty coughing and clearing secretions. Scoliosis eventually develops. Type 3 (Kugelberg-Welander disease) or juvenile SMA has later and variable age of onset. All patients achieve independent walking ability. Swallowing dysfunction, cough, and nocturnal hypoventilation are less common.[79]

For SMA patients, NPPV can be provided as routine therapy or as a palliative tool. NPPV can be used to achieve adequate inspiratory chest wall expansion and air entry, and normalization of gas exchange.[76,80–82] In a randomized controlled trial using mixed groups of patients with NMD with nocturnal hypoventilation and daytime normocapnia, noninvasive ventilation significantly improved nocturnal blood gas tensions.[76] NPPV may aid in chest wall development in SMA.[82]

Congenital myopathies are a heterogeneous group of disorders that usually present at birth or in early infancy with hypotonia and muscle weakness. In addition, there may be an associated respiratory control abnormality.[83,84] Several reports show a good response to night-time NPPV in patients with congenital myopathy.[83–87] Nemaline rod myopathy (NM) is a clinically and genetically heterogeneous condition characterized by abundance of rod-like structures in skeletal muscle. The clinical spectrum ranges from severe cases with prenatal or neonatal onset and early death to late-onset cases with only slow progression. In infancy, the most common presentation is hypotonia and general weakness, predominantly affecting facial and axial muscles, and disproportionate feeding and respiratory difficulties. Mortality is high in those presenting before 28 days of age.[88,89] In the series of Ryan and colleagues,[88] ventilatory failure at delivery and arthrogryosis multiplex congenita were associated with very high mortality. Myotubular myopathies are characterized histologically by the presence of small, rounded muscle fibers with centrally located nuclei. The X-linked recessive myotubular myopathy presents in the neonatal period with profound hypotonia and inability to establish spontaneous respiration. Female carriers of the disorder have a high incidence of miscarriages and stillbirths. Death usually occurs from respiratory failure in infancy or early childhood. In the study by McEntagart and colleagues,[90] 75% of survivors were on assisted ventilation, with most patients on full-time PPV via tracheostomy. The autosomal dominant and recessive forms of myotubular myopathy have mostly a later age of onset and milder clinical course.[91]

Cystic Fibrosis

Cystic fibrosis (CF) is an autosomal recessive disorder caused by a mutation in the gene (CF gene) that encodes for the cystic fibrosis transmembrane conductance regulator protein (CFTR).[92] The defective transport of sodium and chloride across the respiratory epithelial cell membrane predisposes to recurrent infection and inflammation of the airways. With persistent infection, progressive lung disease develops.[93,94] Patients die of respiratory failure despite advances in respiratory care. To date, the average life span is 36.9 years.[95] NPPV has been used in CF as a bridge to lung transplantation.[40] To date, studies have shown that NPPV can result in improvements in symptoms, gas exchange, pulmonary function, and increased exercise performance.[96–100]

INITIATION OF NPPV

In the ideal circumstance, NPPV is instituted electively when hypoventilation has become evident, but before acute respiratory develops.[101] However, this is not always possible, and patients who are candidates for NPPV may not present until acute respiratory failure occurs. In the retrospective study by Sritippayawan and colleagues[32] evaluating the presentation of CRF in pediatric patients with NMD receiving chronic mechanical ventilation, only 21% of NMD patients had assisted ventilation instituted electively. Thus the first use of NPPV may be in an intensive care unit setting with no time for advance discussion, education, and planning of therapy with the patient and family.[102] This scenario emphasizes that the first aspect of appropriate initiation of NPPV is early identification of patients, education of patients and families about the availability for assisted ventilation with disease progression, and creating an understanding within the medical community that most families do not view ventilatory support of their child as a choice or option, but as a necessary treatment.[43,103] Elective initiation of NPPV can be accomplished in the sleep laboratory or during an admission to the hospital.[43]

SLEEP LABORATORY TITRATION

In the authors' experience, patients are candidates for titration in the sleep laboratory setting if they have less severe hypoventilation (arterial or capillary P_{CO_2} <60 mm Hg), are not acutely ill, do not have major atelectasis, and are developmentally able to cooperate with the therapy. Most details of NPPV titration are similar to adult patients, as outlined in the article by Berry elsewhere in this issue. The most important areas that distinguish adult from pediatric patients are the level of cooperation and understanding, both of which vary with the age and developmental level of the child. The patient and family should be educated in advance about the titration study and the NPPV equipment and interface, with verbal and written material.[104] The medical care team must convey a high level of confidence and trust in the parents' abilities to master the techniques, and more importantly in their ability to work with their child in using the therapy each night. A parental approach that is consistent, committed, and calm should be emphasized. Patients should be fitted with and given an appropriate interface to wear at home at bedtime for practice and desensitization prior to the study. Parents are encouraged to build this into the child's usual bedtime routine. An age-appropriate reward system for wearing the interface is often helpful. In this way when the patient arrives for the titration study, the focus can be on identifying the correct settings to achieve adequate gas exchange, normal respiratory pattern, and optimal sleep quality.

Other aspects of pediatric NPPV titration that deserve to be highlighted include pressure selection, the importance of end-tidal CO_2 monitoring, and the use of the timed mode. Younger children generally do not tolerate maximal inspiratory pressures of greater than 20 cm of water pressure; higher pressures result in discomfort and sleep disruption, especially during the initial titration and months of use. However, the authors have seen children with progressive neuromuscular disorders who are well adapted to NPPV tolerate higher pressures as their disease progresses. Children are also poorly tolerant of painful procedures, thus noninvasive monitoring is preferred when possible. The use of end-tidal CO_2 monitoring during the titration study will often provide an accurate measure of ventilation and avoid the use of arterial or capillary blood gas collection. A small end-tidal CO_2 catheter can be placed at one of the nares under the mask interface. Readings are deemed accurate when a plateau is present in the waveform. If the plateau is lost, the catheter can be repositioned at the first wakefulness opportunity. Because the catheter is quite small, the interface seal is not disrupted. However, subjects who use nasal prongs or pillows as their preferred interface cannot be monitored in this way and gas exchange must be inferred from Spo_2 measurements, transcutaneous CO_2 measurements, or intermittent blood gas sampling.

Special mention is warranted for the use of the timed mode in pediatric patients. The timed mode can be particularly useful in subjects who are unable to reliably trigger machine-generated breaths and thus are better ventilated with a set rate and inspiratory time for all breaths. Pediatric patients who may benefit from the timed mode for NPPV include those with congenital and acquired central respiratory control abnormalities and those patients who are profoundly weak, for example, SMA Type 1 and advanced DMD patients. Age-appropriate respiratory rate and inspiratory times are selected and then titrated along with pressures to achieve adequate gas exchange and sleep quality.

Some children are very young or have developmental disabilities, and thus cannot communicate with the polysomnographic technician or respiratory therapist to express discomfort with the interface or the pressures. Technicians and therapists who are skilled in working with children of all ages and abilities are required for a successful NPPV titration. Understanding that a patient's discomfort can have different origins, and working carefully with the child and parent to minimize fear and maximize comfort, require patience and skills that develop over years of experience. Reducing pressures, selecting a different interface, and changing the patient's position should all be tried. However, there are occasions, despite advance preparation, when the child's inability to cooperate prevents completion of an adequate titration. If hypoventilation is not severe, a further period of time acclimating in the home setting can be tried. The NPPV interface and device can be used for a short time each night in the home on the best-tolerated pressure levels identified during the study, with a gradual increase in the time used each night. When use has increased to more than 4 to 6 hours per night, the laboratory titration can be repeated to identify optimal pressures. If the clinical situation dictates a more rapid initiation of therapy, hospitalization is indicated.

HOSPITAL TITRATION

NPPV titration in the inpatient setting is indicated for patients who have failed titration as an outpatient or those who are too unstable to wait for an elective laboratory-based titration. Children in the latter category include those who have daytime hypoventilation, have comorbidities such as pulmonary hypertension, nutritional failure, or severe excessive daytime sleepiness, or with pulmonary abnormalities such as major atelectasis or pneumonia. Some patients may be so unstable as to require initial care in the intensive care unit.[102] Adequacy of ventilation is determined by blood gases, pulse oximetry, measurements of exhaled minute ventilation and tidal volume provided by the graphic display of the NPPV device, and by physical examination of the patient while wearing the device. It may take several days or longer to optimize gas exchange while settings are adjusted and the pulmonary mechanics and acid-base balance are correct. Initially, patients may require support during both sleep and wakefulness. Careful attention to skin integrity under the interface is extremely important, especially with extended or continuous use. Skin erosions are painful, limit acceptance of the device, and can lead to disfiguring scars. Careful fitting of the mask, periodic loosening of the headgear, alternating between a mask interface and nasal prongs, and cushioning of the bridge of the nose can help prevent skin breakdown. Hydrocolloid dressings (eg, Duoderm, Comfeel) are useful to protect the nasal bridge. Child Life specialists can assist children who are struggling with the device by play therapy and calming techniques.

Some patients who present with CRF may also be in nutritional failure. Malnutrition decreases ventilatory muscle strength and endurance, and should be addressed during the hospital admission for NPPV titration. Patients with ventilatory muscle weakness often have oral motor dysfunction, which decreases their ability to take in adequate calories. These patients may also be at risk for aspiration from above due to abnormal swallowing coordination. An assessment by the dysphagia team and registered dietitian are part of the multidisciplinary approach to care.

Patients can be discharged home when they: (1) are successfully using the NPPV device, (2) are able to breath spontaneously during wakefulness for the majority of wakefulness, and (3) have a safe route for feeding that provides adequate calories for growth. Some patients may continue to need supplemental oxygen during wakefulness, due to coexisting pulmonary disease, but hypoventilation during wakefulness should not be treated by supplemental oxygen. Discharge planning involves ordering home equipment and transitioning the patient to the home NPPV. The patient's own home unit should be used for 1 to 2 nights with ongoing monitoring prior to discharge on the settings identified. The family must be educated in how to use the NPPV and related therapy by the home care vendor, and demonstrate proficiency. After discharge, a formal titration study in the sleep laboratory can be performed to confirm that settings remain appropriate.

OUTPATIENT MANAGEMENT

After discharge from the sleep laboratory or from the hospital, patients on NPPV are followed closely to ensure adherence and to address issues that may have arisen after the initiation of therapy. Routine evaluation is required to meet the needs of the growing child. In general, patents are seen within a few weeks after initiation of NPPV, then every 3 to 4 months for follow-up. At follow- up, potential problems are explored including issues with equipment and interface, and possible complications associated with the therapy that may interfere with usage. Adherence can be determined objectively via machine download information. Complications with NPPV use, such as nasal dryness, epistaxis, eye irritation and conjunctivitis due to air leak from the mask, skin ulceration, gastric distention, emesis in those using a full face mask, and mouth breathing in those using nasal mask or prongs, are addressed. Nasal steroids or humidification can help relieve nasal obstruction and improve compliance. In addition to the positive airway pressure machine, other home equipment such as oxygen, pulse oximeter, and humidifier are ordered as needed on the follow-up visit. Facial complications can be avoided by regular follow-up to assess mask fit or by changing the interface from time to time. Facial growth assessments by craniofacial experts have been suggested because of the possible risk of midface hypoplasia.[53] Pneumothorax has been reported in patients with DMD on NPPV, and the authors have encountered this complication, with the anecdotal observation that poor nutrition may be an additional risk factor.[105]

Even the most stable patients may be exposed to alveolar hypoventilation and hypoxemia during sleep or while breathing spontaneously while awake. Thus, screening for pulmonary hypertension with echocardiography every 1 to 2 years, and more frequently if indicated, is recommended. When signs of pulmonary hypertension are discovered, it should be assumed that the ventilation is not adequate and settings need to be adjusted. This adjustment may require repeat overnight polysomnography for retitration, or admission to the hospital for gas exchange monitoring and settings adjustment.

Success of long-term NPPV involves a multidisciplinary team approach that would include a pulmonologist or sleep specialist with expertise in PPV, a nurse coordinator, a dietitian, a social worker, and an expert home vendor. The home care vendor must respond promptly to equipment concerns and be willing to assist the health care team in ongoing education for the patient and family. Regular communication between the health care team and the home care vendor is critical. Patients should have access to a psychologist or psychiatrist when appropriate to provide either psychological support or behavioral therapy to improve compliance. Some patients may require the services of a physical therapist, dysphagia team including speech and language therapist, or occupational therapist.

RESPIRATORY CARE

Patients with neuromuscular weakness have ineffective cough and impaired airways clearance and secretion mobilization. At each visit, adequacy of cough, work of breathing, presence of paradoxic breathing, and chest deformity need to be reviewed. When cough is inadequate and chest percussion is insufficient to maintain comfort and prevent atelectasis, additional equipment can be ordered such as mechanical insufflation-exsufflation or cough assist device. Many patients benefit from aerosolized bronchodilators to facilitate airways clearance. Pulse oximetry for home use can be ordered to screen for hypoxemia associated with atelectasis or respiratory tract infection, and help caregivers know when to intensify therapy.

NUTRITION

Some patients with CRF are at risk for malnutrition or obesity. Regular involvement of a dietitian can facilitate maintenance of ideal body weight. When adequate nutrition cannot be achieved safely by oral feedings, gastrostomy tube placement may be indicated, as malnutrition will further weaken ventilatory muscles.

Regular monitoring for disease progression is critical during follow-up visits, and includes daytime blood gas monitoring to assess development of diurnal hypoventilation. Presence of daytime hypoventilation would indicate the need for full ventilatory assistance. For appropriate patients, monitoring would also include pulmonary function testing. Patients on NPPV should have periodic polysomnography with end-tidal CO_2 and oxygen saturation monitoring to assess adequacy of the ventilatory support they receive at home. When full polysomnography is not readily available, alternative monitoring with overnight pulse oximetry or capillary blood gas on arousal in the morning can be done.[29,106,107]

MANAGEMENT OF INTERCURRENT ILLNESS

During acute an illness, patients with CRF are at increased risk for pulmonary complications. These patients may require antibiotics, oxygen, increased use of airways clearance aids, aerosol treatments, or increased NPPV use. If the noninvasive approach fails, patients require hospitalization and even intubation.[106,108] Patients with severe muscle wasting from any disorder are at risk for hypoglycemia and electrolyte imbalance in the setting of fasting[109,110]; thus during an acute illness prolonged fasting should be avoided, and nutritional intake and hydration should be optimized.

Common illnesses pose a unique threat to children with CRF. Children with CCHSs will not increase respiratory effort, tidal volume, or respiratory rate, as they do not experience subjective dyspnea. Thus, even a relatively trivial upper airway infection may compromise a ventilator-assisted child.[8]

A significant clinical problem when treating children with central hypoventilation syndromes is the difficulty in recognizing hypoxia and hypercapnia clinically. Caregivers must be alert to subtle signs of dysfunction, therefore objective gas exchange monitoring (pulse oximetry and end-tidal P_{CO_2} monitoring) is necessary.

SUMMARY

CRF in children can result from inadequacy of central respiratory control, ventilatory muscle function, obesity, thoracic restriction, or intrinsic lung disease. NPPV is a useful treatment modality for children with CRF who can be stabilized with ventilatory support during sleep. Careful introduction of the interface and equipment are key to successful long-term use of therapy, and initial treatment may be best accomplished during a hospital stay, although some patients can have NPPV initiated in the sleep laboratory. Outpatient follow-up requires a multidisciplinary approach to support the family and patient, and to ensure safety and quality of life. Periodic reassessment of NPPV settings is needed as patients grow and disease status changes. Intercurrent respiratory illnesses require careful attention to airway clearance, and may require intubation and ventilation in the intensive care unit. If patients lose the ability to protect their airway or require multiple admissions for intubation and ventilation, transition to PPV via tracheostomy should be entertained. As technology advances with improved interface comfort, patient-ventilator synchrony, and monitoring of the effectiveness of ventilation, it is anticipated that more patients will be supported by NPPV.

REFERENCES

1. Make BJ, Hill NS, Goldberg AI, et al. Mechanical ventilation beyond the intensive care unit: report of a Consensus Conference of the American College of Chest Physicians. Chest 1998;113: 289S–344S.
2. Keens TG, Kun SS, Ward SLD. Chronic respiratory failure. Chapter 47. In: Nichols DG, editor. Rogers' textbook of pediatric intensive care. 4th edition. Philadelphia: Lippincott, Williams, and Wilkins; 2008. p. 753–66.
3. Fauroux B, Boffa C, Desguerre I, et al. Long-term noninvasive mechanical ventilation for children at home: a national survey. Pediatr Pulmonol 2003;5: 119–25.
4. Simonds AK, Ward S, Heather S, et al. Outcome of paediatric domiciliary mask ventilation in neuromuscular and skeletal disease. Eur Respir J 2000;16:476–81.
5. Paditz E. Nocturnal nasal mask ventilation in childhood. Pneumologie 1994;48:744–9.
6. Teague WG. Non-invasive positive pressure ventilation: current status in paediatric patients. Paediatr Respir Rev 2005;6:52–60.
7. Chen ML, Keens TG. Congenital central hypoventilation syndrome: not just another rare disorder. Paediatr Respir Rev 2004;5:182–9.
8. Keens TG, Davidson Ward SL. Syndromes affecting respiratory control during sleep. In: Loughlin GM, Marcus CL, Carroll JL, editors. Sleep and breathing in children: a developmental approach. Lung biology in health and disease series. New York: Marcel Dekker, Inc.; 2000. p. 525–53.
9. Kerbl R, Litscher H, Grubbbauer HM, et al. Congenital central hypoventilation syndrome (Ondine's curse syndrome) in two siblings: delayed diagnosis and successful noninvasive treatment. Eur J Pediatr 1996;155:977–80.
10. Marcus CL. Ventilator management of abnormal breathing during sleep: continuous positive airway pressure and nocturnal noninvasive intermittent positive pressure ventilation. In: Loughlin GM, Marcus CL, Carroll JL, editors. Sleep and breathing in children: a developmental approach. Lung biology in health and disease series. New York: Marcel Dekker, Inc.; 2000. p. 797–811.

11. Marcus CL, Jansen MT, Poulsen MK, et al. Medical and psychosocial outcome of children with congenital central hypoventilation syndrome. J Pediatr 1991;119:888–95.

12. Weese-Mayer DE, Shannon DC, Keens TG, et al. Idiopathic congenital central hypoventilation syndrome: diagnosis and management. Am J Respir Crit Care Med 1999;160:368–73.

13. Weese-Mayer DE, Rand CM, Berry-Kravis EM, et al. Congenital central hypoventilation syndrome from past to future: model for translational and transitional autonomic medicine. Pediatr Pulmonol 2009;44:521–35.

14. Villa MP, Dotta A, Castello D, et al. Bi-level positive airway pressure (BiPAP) ventilation in an infant with central hypoventilation syndrome. Pediatr Pulmonol 1997;24:66–9.

15. Paton JY, Swaminathan S, Sargent CW, et al. Hypoxic and hypercapnic ventilatory responses in awake children with congenital central hypoventilation syndrome. Am Rev Respir Dis 1989;140:368–72.

16. Swaminathan S, Paton JY, Ward SL, et al. Abnormal control of ventilation in adolescents with myelodysplasia. J Pediatr 1989;115:898–903.

17. Macey PM, Woo MA, Macey KE, et al. Hypoxia reveals posterior thalamic, cerebellar, midbrain and limbic deficits in congenital central hypoventilation syndrome. J Appl Physiol 2005;98:958–69.

18. Harper RM, Macey PM, Woo MA, et al. Hypercapnic exposure in congenital hypoventilation syndrome reveals CNS respiratory control mechanisms. J Neurophysiol 2005;93:1647–58.

19. Kumar R, Macey PM, Woo MA, et al. Neuroanatomic deficits in congenital central hypoventilation syndrome. J Comp Neurol 2005;487:361–71.

20. Woo MA, Macey PM, Macey KE, et al. FMRI responses to hyperoxia in congenital central hypoventilation syndrome. Pediatr Res 2005;57:510–8.

21. Paton JY, Swaminathan S, Sargent CW, et al. Ventilatory response to exercise in children with congenital central hypoventilation syndrome. Am Rev Respir Dis 1993;147:1185–91.

22. Shea SA, Andres LP, Paydarfar B, et al. Effect of mental activity on breathing in congenital central hypoventilation syndrome. Respir Physiol 1993;94:251–63.

23. Shea SA, Andres LP, Shannon DC, et al. Respiratory sensations in subjects who lack a ventilatory response to CO_2. Respir Physiol 1993;93:203–91.

24. Roussos CS, Macklem PT. Diaphragmatic fatigue in man. J Appl Physiol 1977;43:189–97.

25. Nickerson BG, Keens TG. Measuring ventilatory muscle endurance in humans as sustainable inspiratory pressure. J Appl Physiol 1982;52:768–72.

26. Keens TG, Bryan AC, Levison H, et al. Developmental pattern of muscle fiber types in human ventilatory muscles. J Appl Physiol 1978;44:909–13.

27. Scott CB, Nickerson BG, Sargent CW, et al. Developmental pattern of maximal transdiaphragmatic pressure in infants during crying. Pediatr Res 1983;17:707–9.

28. Keens TG, Krastins IR, Wannamaker EM, et al. Ventilatory muscle endurance training in normal subjects and patients with cystic fibrosis. Am Rev Respir Dis 1977;116:853–60.

29. Finder JD, Birnkrant D, Carl J, et al. Respiratory care of the patient with Duchenne muscular dystrophy: ATS consensus statement. Am J Respir Crit Care Med 2004;170:456–65.

30. Gilgoff RL, Gilgoff IS. Long-term follow-up of home mechanical ventilation in young children with spinal cord injury and neuromuscular conditions. J Pediatr 2003;142:476–80.

31. Lyager S, Steffensen B, Juhl B. Indicators of need for mechanical ventilation in Duchenne muscular dystrophy and spinal muscular atrophy. Chest 1995;108:779–85.

32. Sritippayawan S, Kun SS, Keens TG, et al. Initiation of home mechanical ventilation in children with neuromuscular diseases. J Pediatr 2003;142:481–5.

33. Gilgoff IS, Kahlstrom E, MacLaughlin E, et al. Long-term ventilatory support in spinal muscular atrophy. J Pediatr 1989;115:904–9.

34. Deane S, Thomson A. Obesity and the pulmonologist. Arch Dis Child 2006;91:188–91.

35. Beuther DA, Weiss ST, Sutherland ER. Obesity and asthma. Am J Respir Crit Care Med 2006;174:112–9.

36. Parameswaran K, Todd DC, Soth M. Altered respiratory physiology in obesity. Can Respir J 2006;13:203–10.

37. Shore SA. Obesity and asthma: lessons from animal models. J Appl Physiol 2007;102:516–28.

38. Appierto L, Cori M, Bianchi R, et al. Home care for chronic respiratory failure in children: 15 years experience. Paediatr Anaesth 2002;12:345–50.

39. Faroux B, Sardet A, Foret D. Home treatment for chronic respiratory failure in children: a prospective study. Eur Respir J 1995;8:2062–6.

40. Hodson ME, Madden BP, Steven MH, et al. Noninvasive mechanical ventilation for cystic fibrosis patients – a potential bridge to transplantation. Eur Respir J 1991;4:524–7.

41. Jardine E, O'Toole M, Paton JY, et al. Current status of long term ventilation of children in the United Kingdom: questionnaire survey. BMJ 1999;318:295–9.

42. Kamm M, Burger R, Rimensberger P, et al. Survey of children supported by long-term mechanical ventilation in Switzerland. Swiss Med Wkly 2001;131:261–6.

43. Mehta S, Hill NS. Noninvasive ventilation. Am J Respir Crit Care Med 2001;163:540–77.

44. Chen ML, Witmans MB, Tablizo MA, et al. Disordered respiratory control in children with partial cerebellar resections. Pediatr Pulmonol 2005;40:88–91.

45. Hui SH, Wing YK, Poon W, et al. Alveolar hypoventilation syndrome in brainstem glioma with improvement after surgical resection. Chest 2000;118:266–8.

46. Lee DK, Wahl GW, Swinburne AJ, et al. Recurrent acoustic neuroma presenting as central hypoventilation. Chest 1994;105:949–50.

47. Rosen GM, Bendel AE, Neglia JP, et al. Sleep in children with neoplasms of the central nervous system: case review of 14 children. Pediatrics 2003;112(1 Pt 1):e46–54.

48. Deonna T, Arczynska W, Torrado A. Congenital failure of automatic ventilation (Ondine's curse): a case report. J Pediatr 1974;84:710–4.

49. Mellins RB, Balfour HH Jr, Turino GM, et al. Failure of automatic control of ventilation (Ondine's curse). Report of an infant born with this syndrome and review of the literature. Medicine 1970;49:487–504.

50. Amiel J, Laudier B, Attie-Bitach T, et al. Polyalanine expansion and frameshift mutations of the paired-like homeobox gene PHOX2B in congenital central hypoventilation syndrome. Nat Genet 2003;33:459–61.

51. Weese-Mayer DE, Berry-Kravis EM, Zhou L, et al. Idiopathic congenital central hypoventilation syndrome: analysis of genes pertinent to early autonomic nervous system embryologic development and identification of mutations in PHOX2B. Am J Med Genet A 2003;123:267–78.

52. Weese-Mayer DE, Silvestri JM, Menzies LJ, et al. Congenital central hypoventilation syndrome: diagnosis, management, and long-term outcome in thirty-two children. J Pediatr 1992;120:381–7.

53. Tibballs J, Henning RD. Noninvasive ventilatory strategies in the management of a newborn infant and three children with congenital central hypoventilation syndrome. Pediatr Pulmonol 2003;36:544–8.

54. Migliori C, Cavazza A, Motta M, et al. Early use of nasal-BiPAP in two infants with congenital central hypoventilation syndrome. Acta Paediatr 2003;92:823–6.

55. Schut L, Bruce DA. The Arnold Chiari malformation. Orthop Clin North Am 1978;9:913–21.

56. Gilbert JN, Jones KL, Rorke LB, et al. Central nervous system anomalies associated with meningomyelocele, hydrocephalus, and the Arnold-Chiari malformation: reappraisal of theories regarding the pathogenesis of posterior neural tube closure defects. Neurosurgery 1986;18:559–64.

57. Hays RM, Jordan RA, McLaughlin JF, et al. Central ventilatory dysfunction in myelodysplasia: an independent determinant of survival. Dev Med Child Neurol 1989;31:366–70.

58. Krieger AJ, Detwiler JS, Trooskin SZ. Respiratory function in infants with Arnold-Chiari malformation. Laryngoscope 1976;86:718–23.

59. Holinger PC, Holinger LD, Reichert TJ, et al. Respiratory obstruction and apnea in infants with bilateral abductor vocal cord paralysis, meningomyelocoele, hydrocephalus, and Arnold Chiari malformation. J Pediatr 1978;92:368–73.

60. Oren J, Kelly DH, Todres ID, et al. Respiratory complications in patients with myelodysplasia and Arnold-Chiari malformation. Am J Dis Child 1986;140:221–4.

61. Waters KA, Forbes P, Morielli A, et al. Sleep-disordered breathing in children with myelomeningocoele. J Pediatr 1998;132:672–81.

62. Davidson Ward SL, Jacobs RA, Gates EP, et al. Abnormal ventilatory patterns during sleep in infants with myelomeningocoele. J Pediatr 1986;109:631–4.

63. Gozal D, Arens R, Omlin KJ, et al. Peripheral chemoreceptor function in children with myelomeningocoele and Arnold-Chiari malformation type 2. Chest 1995;108:425–31.

64. Ward SL, Nickerson BG, Van der Hal A, et al. Absent hypoxic and hypercapneic arousal responses in children with myelomeningocoele and apnea. Pediatrics 1986;78:44–50.

65. Kirk VG, Morielli A, Gozal D, et al. Treatment of sleep-disordered breathing in children with myelomeningocoele. Pediatr Pulmonol 2000;30:445–52.

66. Hertz G, Cataletto M, Feinsilver SH, et al. Sleep and breathing patterns is patients with Prader Willi (PWS): effects of age and gender. Sleep 1993;16:366–71.

67. Arens R, Gozal D, Omlin KJ, et al. Hypoxic and hypercapnic ventilatory responses in Prader-Willi syndrome. J Appl Physiol 1994;77:222–30.

68. Gozal D, Arens R, Omlin KJ, et al. Absent peripheral chemosensitivity in the Prader-Willi syndrome. J Appl Physiol 1994;77:2231–6.

69. Nixon GM, Brouillette RT. Sleep and breathing in Prader-Willi syndrome. Pediatr Pulmonol 2002;34:209–17.

70. Ize-Ludlow D, Gray JA, Sperling MA, et al. Rapid-onset obesity with hypothalamic dysfunction, hypoventilation and autonomic dysregulation presenting in childhood. Pediatrics 2007;120:e179–88.

71. Brooke MH, Fenichel GM, Griggs RC, et al. Duchenne muscular dystrophy: pattern of clinical progression and effects of supportive therapy. Neurology 1989;39:475–81.

72. Smith PE, Calverley PM, Edwards RH. Hypoxemia during sleep in Duchenne muscular dystrophy. Am Rev Respir Dis 1988;137:884–8.

73. Hukins CA, Hillman DR. Daytime predictors of sleep hypoventilation in Duchenne muscular dystrophy. Am J Respir Crit Care Med 2000;161: 166–70.

74. Toussaint M, Steens M, Soudon P. Lung function accurately predicts hypercapnia in patients with Duchenne muscular dystrophy. Chest 2007;131: 368–75.

75. Toussaint M, Chatwin M, Soudon P. Mechanical ventilation in Duchenne patients with chronic respiratory insufficiency: clinical implication of 20 years published experience. Chron Respir Dis 2007;4: 167–77.

76. Ward S, Chatwin M, Heather S, et al. Randomized controlled trial of non-invasive ventilation (NIV) for nocturnal hypoventilation in neuromuscular disease and chest wall disease patients with daytime normocapnia. Thorax 2005;60: 1019–24.

77. Mellies U, Ragette R, Dohna Schwake C, et al. Long-term noninvasive ventilation in children and adolescents with neuromuscular disorders. Eur Respir J 2003;22:631–6.

78. Toussaint M, Soudon P, Kinnear W. Effect of non-invasive ventilation on respiratory muscle loading and endurance in patients with Duchenne muscular dystrophy. Thorax 2008;63:430–4.

79. Han JJ, McDonald CM. Diagnosis and clinical management of spinal muscular atrophy. Phys Med Rehabil Clin N Am 2008;19:661–80, xii.

80. Bach JR, Wang TG. Noninvasive long-term ventilatory support for individuals with spinal muscular atrophy and functional bulbar musculature. Arch Phys Med Rehabil 1995;76:213–7.

81. Petrone A, Pavone M, Testa MB, et al. Noninvasive ventilation in children with spinal muscular atrophy types 1 and 2. Am J Phys Med Rehabil 2007;86: 216–21.

82. Bach JR, Bianchi C. Prevention of pectus excavatum for children with spinal muscular atrophy type 1. Am J Phys Med Rehabil 2003;82:815–9.

83. Schweitzer C, Danet V, Polu E, et al. Nemaline myopathy and early respiratory failure. Eur J Pediatr 2003;162:216–7.

84. Riley DJ, Santiago TV, Daniele RP, et al. Blunted respiratory drive in congenital myopathy. Am J Med 1977;63:459–66.

85. Sasaki M, Takeda M, Kobayashi K, et al. Respiratory failure in nemaline myopathy. Pediatr Neurol 1997;16:344–6.

86. Khan Y, Heckmatt JZ, Dubowitz V. Sleep studies and supportive ventilatory treatment in patients with congenital muscle disorders. Arch Dis Child 1996;34:195–200.

87. Jungbluth H, Sewry CA, Brown SC, et al. Mild phenotype pf nemaline myopathy with sleep hypoventilation due to a mutation in the skeletal muscle

α-actin (ACTA1) gene. Neuromuscul Disord 2001; 11:35–40.

88. Ryan MM, Schnell C, Strickland CD, et al. Nemaline myopathy: a clinical study of 143 cases. Ann Neurol 2001;50:312–20.

89. Wallgren-Pettersson C. Congenital nemaline myopathy. A clinical follow-up of 12 patients. J Neurol Sci 1989;89:1–14.

90. McEntagart M, Parsons G, Buj-Bello A, et al. Genotype-phenotype correlation in X-linked myotubular myopathy. Neuruomuscul Disord 2002;12:939–46.

91. Akiyama C, Nonaka I. A follow-up study of congenital non-progressive myopathies. Brain Dev 1996; 18:404–8.

92. Riordan JR, Rommens JM, Kerem B, et al. Identification of the cystic fibrosis gene: cloning an characterization of complementary DNA. Science 1989;245:1066–73.

93. Gibson RL, Burns JL, Ramsey BW. Pathophysiology and management of pulmonary infections in cystic fibrosis. Am J Respir Crit Care Med 2003; 168:918–51.

94. Davis PB. Cystic fibrosis since 1938. Am J Respir Crit Care Med 2006;173:475–82.

95. CFF, 2006. Cystic Fibrosis Foundation, Patient registry 2005, Annual report. Cystic Fibrosis Foundation annual data report. Bethesda (MD): Cystic Fibrosis Foundation; 2005. p. 2–3.

96. Gozal D. Nocturnal ventilatory support in patients with cystic fibrosis: comparison with supplemental oxygen. Eur Respir J 1997;10:1999–2003.

97. Serra A, Polese G, Braggion C, et al. Non-invasive proportional assist and pressure support ventilation in patients with cystic fibrosis and chronic respiratory failure. Thorax 2002;57:50–4.

98. Fauroux B, Le Roux E, Ravilly S, et al. Long-term noninvasive ventilation in cystic fibrosis. Respiration 2008;76:168–74.

99. Young AC, Wilson JW, Kotsimbos TC, et al. Randomized placebo controlled trial of non-invasive ventilation for hypercapnia in cystic fibrosis. Thorax 2008;63:72–7.

100. Moran F, Bradley JM, Piper AJ. Non-invasive ventilation for cystic fibrosis. Cochrane Database Syst Rev 2009;1:CD002769.

101. Norregaard O. Noninvasive ventilation in children. Eur Respir J 2002;20:1332–42.

102. Piastra M, Antonelli M, Caresta E, et al. Noninvasive ventilation in childhood acute neuromuscular respiratory failure: a pilot study. Respiration 2006; 73:791–8.

103. Carnevale FA, Alexander E, Davis M, et al. Daily living with distress and enrichment: the moral experience of families with ventilator assisted children at home. Pediatrics 2006;117:e48–60.

104. Marcus CL, Rosen G, Ward SL, et al. Adherence to and effectiveness of positive airway pressure

therapy in children with obstructive sleep apnea. Pediatrics 2006;117:e442–51.

105. Vianello A, Arcaro G, Gallan F, et al. Pneumothorax associated with long-term non-invasive positive pressure ventilation in Duchenne muscular dystrophy. Neuromuscul Disord 2004;14:353–5.

106. Wang CH, Finkel RS, Bertini ES, et al. Consensus statement for standard of care in spinal muscular atrophy. J Child Neurol 2007; 22:1027–49.

107. Bushby K, Finkel R, Birnkrant DJ, et al. Diagnosis and management of Duchenne muscular dystrophy, part 2: implementation of multidisciplinary care. Lancet Neurol 2010;9:177–89.

108. Schroth MK. Special considerations in the respiratory management of spinal muscular atrophy. Pediatrics 2009;123(Suppl 4):S245–9.

109. Bruce AK, Jacobsen E, Dossing H, et al. Hypoglycaemia in spinal muscular atrophy. Lancet 1995; 346:609–10.

110. Orngreen MC, Zacho M, Hebert A, et al. Patients with severe muscle wasting are prone to develop hypoglycemia during fasting. Neurology 2003;61: 997–1000.

Noninvasive Positive Pressure Ventilation Titration and Treatment Initiation for Chronic Hypoventilation Syndromes

Richard B. Berry, MD

KEYWORDS

- Noninvasive positive pressure ventilation • Titration
- Treatment • Chronic hypoventilation syndromes

Noninvasive positive airway pressure (NPPV) via mask during sleep is increasingly used to treat adults and children with chronic diurnal alveolar hypoventilation (CAH) syndromes.[1–45] In addition, patients who have significant hypoventilation only during sleep may also benefit from nocturnal NPPV. The benefits of NPPV include improved sleep quality, improved diurnal and nocturnal arterial PCO_2 and PO_2, reduced nocturnal dyspnea, and improved quality of life. NPPV treatment has been used in CAH syndromes (**Box 1**) secondary to restrictive thoracic cage disorders (RTCD), neuromuscular diseases (NMD), central respiratory control disturbances (CRCD), and the obesity hypoventilation syndrome (OHS). NPPV during sleep has also been used with mixed success in patients with chronic obstructive pulmonary disease (COPD) and to manage patients with acute respiratory failure. The

initiation and use of NPPV in these two settings is not discussed in this article.

Application of NPPV via a mask interface avoids the morbidity involved with tracheostomy. Many of the initial studies of NPPV used volume ventilators with a mask interface. The volume ventilators were set at high tidal volumes (10–15 mL/kg) to compensate for leak. Today, the most common approach is to use a BPAP device that delivers separately adjustable inspiratory positive airway pressure (IPAP) and expiratory positive airway pressure (EPAP).[46] The IPAP and EPAP are adjusted to maintain upper airway patency and the IPAP-EPAP difference provides pressure support (PS) to augment tidal volume. The delivered tidal volume may vary depending on respiratory system impedance and the patient's ventilatory effort. However, BPAP devices are leak tolerant and are thus preferred for use with

Acknowledgments: The other members of the American Academy of Sleep Medicine NPPV Titration Task Force include Alejandro Chediak, MD, Lee K. Brown, MD, Jonathan Finder, MD, David Gozal, MD, Conrad Iber, MD, Clete A. Kushida, MD, PhD, RPSGT, Timothy Morgenthaler, MD, James A. Rowley, MD, and Sally L. Davidson-Ward, MD. Many of the suggestions for titration and NPPV treatment initiation presented in this chapter were formulated as a group effort of the task force. However, it should be emphasized that the suggestions for NPPV titration presented in this chapter are preliminary thoughts and a work in progress. The final recommendations may differ and include additional material. The reader should review the finalized NPPV titration guidelines when approved and published.

Division of Pulmonary, Critical Care, and Sleep Medicine, University of Florida, Box 100225 HSC, Gainesville, FL 32610-0225, USA
E-mail address: sleep_doc@msn.com

Sleep Med Clin 5 (2010) 485–505
doi:10.1016/j.jsmc.2010.05.002
1556-407X/10/$ – see front matter. Published by Elsevier Inc.

limits) as well as the respiratory rate. BPAP in the spontaneous-timed (ST) mode provides a backup rate to ensure a minimum respiratory rate (**Fig. 1**). If the patient fails to initiate an IPAP/EPAP cycle within a time window based on the backup rate, the device will deliver a machine-triggered IPAP cycle for the set inspiratory time (IPAPtime). For example, if the backup rate is 15 bpm, the time window following the previous breath is 4 seconds. If a spontaneous breath does not occur within this time window, the device provides a machine-triggered breath. For BPAP in the timed mode, the device delivers IPAP/EPAP cycles at a set respiratory rate with a set IPAPtime. Volume-targeted BPAP (VT-BPAP) is a new mode of NPPV that automatically adjusts the IPAP-EPAP difference to deliver a target tidal volume.[44,45]

Many clinicians routinely use the ST mode in patients with NMD and RTCD because these patients may not reliably trigger an IPAP/EPAP cycle because of respiratory muscle weakness or decreased respiratory system compliance. Patients with severely defective central control of ventilatory drive also almost always require a backup rate to prevent central apneas or hypoventilation. The timed mode is infrequently used for NPPV. However, there are individual patients who are more adequately treated with the timed mode than the ST mode. The timed mode using a set respiratory rate that is higher than the native rate may result in a more stable pattern of ventilation in some patients. Some

mask interfaces. This article focuses on NPPV using BPAP devices.

BPAP MODES FOR NPPV

NPPV using BPAP may be delivered in the spontaneous mode, in which the patient determines the time spent in IPAP (within the device IPAPtime

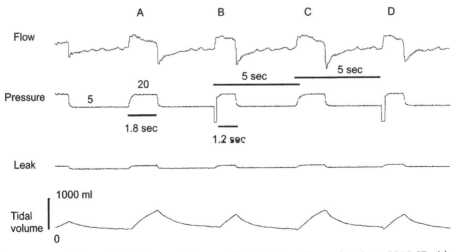

Fig. 1. Flow, pressure, leak, and tidal volume during an NPPV titration. The patient is on BPAP ST with a backup rate of 12 bpm. (A, C) Patient-initiated breaths. (B, D) Machine-cycled breaths. If the device does not cycle from EPAP to IPAP within a 5-second window, a machine breath (IPAPcycle) for the chosen inspiratory time (IPAPtime) occurs (B). The NPPV device supplies a negative pressure spike signifying a machine-triggered breath. Note the shorter inspiratory time in breath B compared with A. Although the peak flow rates are similar, the tidal volume differs between breaths A and B because of a different inspiratory time (IPAPtime). This illustrates the usefulness of recording tidal volume as well as flow.

patients may have adequate ventilation with lower PS and IPAP when using lower tidal volumes with a higher respiratory rate than their native respiratory rate.[47]

A NPPV delivery system consists of 3 main components: a NPPV device, a mask interface (nasal mask, nasal pillows mask, oronasal mask, or oral interface) held snug to the face by headgear, and a flexible hose that connects the device to the interface. NPPV devices used for titration with polysomnography (PSG) typically provide analog or digital outputs of flow, tidal volume, delivered pressure, and leak (total or unintentional, depending on the manufacturer). The outputs may be visualized by the sleep technologist using the software that controls the device or may be recorded along with other standard PSG information.

NPPV devices used for treatment can also store information such as adherence, leak, respiratory rate, percentage of patient-triggered breaths, and mean tidal volume. This information can be used by the clinician to make adjustments to treatment. A given set of NPPV settings may result in variable minute ventilation in the same patient in response to changes in respiratory system impedance, progression of muscle weakness, or alterations in central control as a result of medications or the underlying disease process. Therefore, adequate follow-up of the patient during NPPV therapy by a physician knowledgeable in the delivery of NPPV treatment is essential.

Indications for Initiation of NPPV

A consensus conference of the American College of Chest Physicians[48] outlined indications for initiation of NPPV (**Table 1**). Patients with nocturnal hypoventilation often complain of nocturnal dyspnea, morning headaches, disturbed sleep, or daytime sleepiness. Objective evidence supporting the need for nocturnal NPPV includes daytime hypoventilation (arterial P_{CO_2} >45 mm Hg) or nocturnal oximetry revealing an arterial oxygen saturation (Sp_{O_2}) $\leq$88% for 5 or more consecutive minutes. For patients with chronic progressive neuromuscular disorders a forced vital capacity (FVC) less than 50% of predicted, or maximum inspiratory pressure less than 60 cm H_2O are also considered indications for NPPV initiation.

Medicare has recently change the guidelines for BPAP reimbursement for NPPV treatment (local carrier determination 11,504). Such devices are termed respiratory assist devices (RADs) and include devices without a backup rate (E0470) and with a backup rate (E0471). The guidelines for reimbursement for RADs for patients with RTCD and NMD are unchanged (**Table 2**).[40] Devices with a backup rate are more expensive but the cost will be reimbursed if the clinician feels that a device with a backup rate is indicated. A formal sleep study is not needed to qualify these patients for RADs. However, patients will usually benefit from a sleep study, especially if there is a reason to suspect that obstructive sleep apnea (OSA) is present. A sawtooth pattern in the nocturnal oximetry tracings suggests that discrete events, such as obstructive apnea or hypopneas, are present.

In the case of OHS, if sufficient OSA is documented on a sleep study to qualify the patient for positive airway pressure (PAP) treatment, the cost of BPAP without a backup rate will be reimbursed if "A single level device (CPAP) has been tried and proven ineffective based on a therapeutic

| Table 1 | | |
Indications for NPPV treatment in restrictive thoracic chest wall disease and NMD		
RTCD	Symptoms of hypoventilation (morning headache, daytime somnolence) AND 1 of the following: Physiologic Criteria: • Pa_{CO_2} >45 mm Hg (daytime) • Nocturnal oximetry showing Sp_{O_2} $\leq$88% for 5 consecutive minutes or more	
NMD	Symptoms of hypoventilation (morning headache, daytime somnolence) AND 1 of the following: Physiologic Criteria: • Pa_{CO_2} >45 mm Hg (daytime) • Nocturnal oximetry showing Sp_{O_2} <88 % for 5 consecutive minutes or more • FVC<50% of predicted • Maximal inspiratory pressure <60 cm H_2O	

Data from American College of Chest Physicians. Clinical indications for noninvasive positive pressure ventilation in chronic respiratory failure due to restrictive lung disease, COPD, and nocturnal hypoventliation – a consensus conference report. Chest 1999;116:523, 524.

Table 2
Medicare guidelines for reimbursement for RADs

RTCD and NMD	Criterion A: There is documentation in the patient's medical record of an NMD (amyotrophic lateral sclerosis [ALS]) or severe thoracic cage abnormality AND Criterion B1 or B2 or B3 are met B1: $Paco_2$ ≥45 mm Hg while awake and breathing patient's prescribed Fio_2 B2: Sleep oximetry shows Sao_2 ≤88% for at least 5 min of nocturnal recording time while breathing prescribed Fio_2 (2 h minimum recording time) Criterion B3 (NMD only) maximal inspiratory pressure <60 cm H_2O or FVC <50% predicted AND Criterion C: COPD does not contribute significantly to the patient's pulmonary limitation If all criteria are met then E0470 or E0471 will be covered for the first 3 months of treatment

trial conducted in either a facility or in a home setting." If OHS patients qualify for BPAP under the OSA category, purchasers of BPAP with a backup rate will only be reimbursed at the lower-cost level of BPAP without a backup rate. If a backup rate is needed, OHS patients can now qualify under the new hypoventilation syndrome category (**Table 3**). In the International Classification of Sleep Disorders, 2nd edition,[49] OHS patients are included under the category "Sleep Related Hypoventilation/Hypoxemia due to Neuromuscular and Chest Wall Disorders."

Table 3
Medicare guidelines for hypoventilation syndrome

Hypoventilation syndrome (E0470 device)	Criterion A: arterial blood gas (ABG) $Paco_2$ ≥45 mm Hg while awake and breathing patient's prescribed Fio_2 AND Criterion B: Spirometry shows an FEV_1/FVC ≥70% and FEV_1 ≥50% of predicted AND criterion C or D Criterion C: an ABG Pco_2, done during sleep or immediately on awakening, and breathing the patient's prescribed Fio_2, show the beneficiary's Pco_2 worsened 7 mm Hg compared with original result in criterion A Criterion D: a facility-based PSG shows oxygen saturation <88% for 5 min of nocturnal recording time (minimal recording time of 2 h) that is not caused by obstructive upper airway events A EO470 will be covered for first 3 mo of treatment if criterion A, B, and C or D are met
Hypoventilation syndrome (E0471 device)	Criterion A: a covered E0470 device is being used AND Criterion B: Spirometry shows an FEV1/FVC >70% and FEV1 >50% of predicted AND criterion C or D Criterion C: an arterial blood gas Pco_2, done while AWAKE, and breathing the patient's prescribed Fio_2, show the beneficiary's Pco_2 worsened 7 mm Hg compared to the ABG result used to qualify the patient for the E0470 device (that is patient has worsened while using E0470) Criterion D: a facility-based PSG demonstrates oxygen saturation <88% for 5 minutes of nocturnal recording time (minimal recording time of 2 hours) that is not caused by obstructive upper airway events (AHI <5/h) WHILE USING an E0470 device A EO471 will be covered for first 3 months of treatment if criterion A, B and either C or D are met.

For patients with CRCD, the cost of NPPV treatment with a backup rate will be reimbursed if the patient qualifies under criteria for central apnea (**Table 4**). Previously, ruling out CPAP as an effective treatment was required but that requirement has been removed. If enough discrete central apneas (or central hypopneas) are not present, patients with CRCD may qualify under the hypoventilaton syndrome criteria (see **Table 3**).

Clinical indication for transitioning a patient with CRCD from tracheosotomy and volume ventilation to NPPV would require patient acceptance of NPPV, suitable social support, and evidence that NPPV was effective.

A high index of suspicion for hypoventilation is indicated in patients with disease processes known to be associated with hypoventilation. A clue that chronic hypoventilation might be present is an elevation in the CO_2 (HCO_3) on an electrolyte panel. In the absence of metabolic alkalosis, this is suggestive of renal compensation for chronic respiratory acidosis.[50] It is also reasonable to obtain pulmonary function tests, which may show a restrictive pattern with a reduced FVC in patients with OHS, RCTD, and NMD. The presence of orthopnea suggests diaphragmatic weakness. It has been suggested that a reduced supine FVC is useful at identifying diaphragmatic weakness.[51] Early in the course of disease, patients may exhibit hypoventilation only during sleep. Some of these patients may benefit from nocturnal NPPV. For example, in patients with severe chest wall restriction or progressive NMD, early intervention before the development of daytime hypoventilation may improve sleep quality or improve nocturnal symptoms of dyspnea. Although an FVC less than 50% of predicted has some value in identifying patients with nocturnal hypoventilation and desaturation, there are a considerable number of patients with an FVC greater than 50% of predicted who have significant nocturnal arterial oxygen desaturation (**Fig. 2**).[52] Therefore, patients with nocturnal symptoms and disease processes known to be associated with hypoventilation may benefit from screening nocturnal oximetry even if the daytime P_{CO_2} is normal.

Goals of NPPV Treatment

The goals of NPPV titration and treatment (**Box 2**) should be individualized. Different levels of NPPV support may be needed depending on the specific goals in an individual patient. Common treatment goals include (1) relief or improvement of nocturnal symptoms, (2) reduction in sleep fragmentation and improvement in sleep quality, (3) decrease in the work of breathing and providing respiratory muscle rest, and (4) normalization or improvement of gas exchange (nocturnal and diurnal). In patients with progressive neuromuscular dysfunction, the main goals may be palliation, especially if a short period of survival is anticipated. Improvement in quality of life and patient comfort may be the primary goals in this situation. Although most studies of NPPV have not evaluated objective changes in sleep quality at least two did show an improvement in sleep quality with NPPV treatment.[24,31] Although pulse oximetry provides some information about the adequacy of gas exchange during sleep, measurement of P_{CO_2} is the most precise method to determine the effects of NPPV support on hypoventilation. NPPV titration or treatment can be guided by transcutaneous P_{CO_2} (Pt_{CCO_2}) monitoring, end-tidal P_{CO_2} (PET_{CO_2}), or arterial blood gas (ABG) sampling.

If a goal of NPPV treatment is to decrease the work of breathing, monitoring the patient during sleep is the most precise way to adjust NPPV settings to achieve this goal. Monitoring of tidal volume, respiratory rate, and possibly respiratory muscle electromyogram (EMG) during sleep can determine whether NPPV treatment is adequate. Patients with respiratory muscle weakness or increased work of breathing often have a pattern

Table 4 Central apnea	
E0470 or E0471	Before initiating therapy, a complete facility-based attended PSG must be performed documenting the following criterion:
Central sleep apnea: (1) Apnea hypopnea index $\geq$5/h (2) Central apnea/hypopnea greater that 50% of the total apneas and hypopneas (3) Central apneas or hypopneas $\geq$5/h symptoms of excessive sleepiness or disturbed sleep	Criterion A: diagnosis of central sleep apnea AND Criterion B: significant improvement of the sleep-associated hypoventilation with the use of E0470 or E0471 device on settings that will be prescribed for initial use at home, while breathing the patient's usual prescribed F_{IO_2}

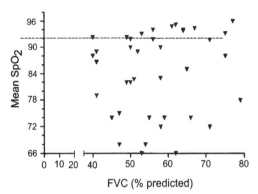

Fig. 2. Mean nocturnal Spo_2 by oximetry in patients with amyotrophic lateral sclerosis plotted against FVC as a percentage of predicted. An FVC less than 50% of predicted is a criterion for initiation of NPPV. However, a significant number of patients with higher FVC values still had significant nocturnal arterial oxygen desaturation. (*From* Morgan RK, McNally S, Alexander M, et al. Use of sniff nasal-inspiratory force to predict survival in amyotrophic lateral sclerosis. Am J Respir Crit Care Med 2005;171:269–74; with permission.)

of rapid shallow breathing (low tidal volume, high respiratory rate) and high levels of respiratory muscle EMG activity (including the accessory muscles of respiration) during sleep. Evidence that NPPV has reduced the work of breathing includes an increase in tidal volume and a reduction in respiratory rate.[53–57] An absence or reduction of inspiratory EMG activity of the muscle of respiration compared with baseline levels or those

---

Box 2
Goals and benefits of NPPV

Goals of NPPV treatment

- Relief of nocturnal dyspnea
- Reduction of sleep fragmentation and improvement in sleep quality
- Normalizing or improving nocturnal arterial Pco_2
- Respiratory muscle rest
- Elimination of obstructive apnea, hypopnea, and respiratory effort related arousals (RERAs)

Daytime benefits of NPPV (varies between CAH syndromes)

- Improved alertness
- Improvement in daytime Po_2 and Pco_2
- Improved pulmonary function (FVC)
- Improved respiratory muscle strength
- Improved quality of life
- Prevention of cor pulmonale

---

on lower amounts of NPPV support[55,56] (**Fig. 3**) would provide evidence of adequate NPPV support to achieve muscle rest.

Longer-term goals of NPPV treatment include prevention of cor pulmonale, a reduction in hospitalizations, delay or prevention of acute respiratory failure requiring intubation, and improved survival.

Benefits of NPPV

Studies of NPPV treatment in CAH syndromes have documented several benefits that vary with the disorder being treated. These include increased alertness (less daytime sleepiness), improvements in nocturnal or diurnal gas exchange, increases in muscle strength (some but not all studies), improved quality of life, and prevention of cor pulmonale.[1–45] RTCD and NMD studies have documented improvement in daytime Pco_2 and Po_2, and some studies in patients with RTCD found improvements in pulmonary function tests or muscle strength.[14,15] In OHS, NPPV resulted in reduced daytime Pco_2 and increased Po_2. Because of ethical considerations, randomized trials of NPPV versus supportive care regarding survival are problematic. In one study, 9 of 10 patients with NMD/RTCD in the control group of a randomized trial of NPPV deteriorated during 8 months of follow-up and had to be treated with NPPV.[19] In NMD, some studies have documented improved quality of life in patient groups such as those with motor neuron disease (amyotrophic lateral sclerosis [ALS]).[28,38] In a randomized controlled study of the effects of NPPV on survival and quality of life in ALS,[38] the subgroup of patients without moderate to severe bulbar dysfunction had improved survival.

Initiating NPPV

The goals of treatment and the side effects of NPPV treatment should be discussed in detail with the patient before the NPPV treatment. One approach is to initiate NPPV treatment based on a NPPV titration with PSG. Another approach would be initiation of NPPV treatment in an outpatient setting with low levels of BPAP. In either case, the patient should be carefully fitted with an appropriate mask with the goals of minimizing leak, maximizing comfort, and compensating for significant nasal obstruction. In the case of an NPPV titration, the patient should be acclimated to the NPPV equipment (ie, wearing the interface with the pressure at a low level) before turning lights off. Pressurizing a mask that seems to provide a reasonable fit may produce an unacceptable leak or require an uncomfortable degree of mask strap tightening. An appropriate intervention then

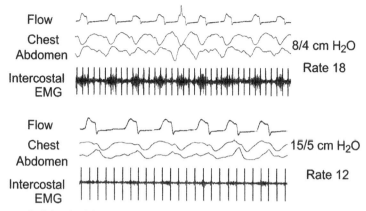

Fig. 3. Flow, chest and abdominal belt, and intercostals EMG tracings during NPPV titration. The BPAP was increased from 8/4 cm H_2O to 15/5 cm H_2O. The respiratory rate decreased from 18 to 12 bpm and the tidal volume increased. A higher level of PS was associated with higher tidal volume, lower respiratory rate, and reduced inspiratory muscle activity. Note also the paradoxic chest and abdomen movements before PS was increased. The narrow lines in the EMG are electrocardiograph artifact.

is possible before the start of the sleep study. In pediatric patients, behavioral modification techniques may be implemented to increase the tolerability and potential adherence to PAP therapy,[58–60] because children frequently have problems adjusting to PAP treatment.

NPPV TREATMENT INITIATED AFTER TITRATION WITH PSG

Attended NPPV titration with PSG has several advantages.[61] These include documentation of the effects of NPPV on sleep quality, obstructive apnea and hypopnea, ventilation, and nocturnal gas exchange. The NPPV device settings (EPAP, IPAP, backup rate, inspiratory time) can be manually adjusted to deliver adequate nocturnal ventilation and improve or normalize nocturnal P_{CO_2}. If necessary, supplemental oxygen can also be added. Mask interfaces can be changed or adjusted to maximize comfort and minimize leak. The PSG can document the effectiveness of NPPV settings in various body positions and sleep stages. It is common for NMD, RTCD, and OHS patients to have the most severe degree of hypoventilation during rapid eye movement (REM) sleep.[62] Therefore, it is important to document that NPPV settings selected for chronic treatment are effective in that situation.

Several studies documenting the effectiveness of NPPV in CAH syndromes used titration with PSG to determine the NPPV settings. These include studies in patients with NMD[29,31,33] and the OHS.[1,10,11] In most of the studies, the titration protocols were not presented in detail. However, the stated goals of titration usually were to

eliminate obstructive events and improve ventilation such that the Sa_{O_2} was more than 90% and the Ptc_{CO_2} was less than a set goal (eg, 45–50 mm Hg), if sufficient pressure to achieve these goals was tolerated.

Studies in patients with OHS[10] and NMD[63] have documented disturbances in sleep quality caused by patient-NPPV device asynchrony. Other studies noted that leak (particularly mouth leak)[64,65] also resulted in sleep disturbance. Such sleep disturbance would usually not be recognized without PSG. Fanfulla and colleagues[63] found that empiric NPPV settings that were effective and well tolerated during the day were associated with a substantial frequency of ineffective respiratory efforts and worsened sleep quality at night. Guo and colleagues[10] found that PSG detected periods of patient-NPPV device desynchronization (uncoupling of the onset of the patient's respiratory effort as detected by thoracoabdominal movement and the onset of an IPAP/EPAP pressure cycle), periodic breathing, or autotriggering in a group of OHS patients chronically treated with NPPV. Arousals from mouth leaks or patient-NPPV device desynchronization would not be apparent without monitoring with PSG during NPPV treatment.

NPPV TREATMENT INITIATED WITHOUT PSG

NPPV treatment can be initiated without PSG.[25,38,39] In some situations, such as patients with NMD with a low suspicion of having a component of OSA, NPPV can be empirically initiated at low pressure settings. Treatment pressures are then increased as tolerated over days to weeks, based on daytime P_{CO_2} measurements, nocturnal oximetry, subjective relief of symptoms, and, in some cases, nocturnal $Ptcco_2$ monitoring. Initiating NPPV in an outpatient setting at low levels of pressure may be indicated if the patient has severe difficulty tolerating NPPV or the major treatment goal is palliation. If the patient is suspected of having a component of OSA based on history, physical examination, or oximetry showing a sawtooth pattern, an NPPV titration with PSG would be more appropriate.

A common approach to initiating NPPV treatment without a titration is to start the patient on a low level of BPAP (8/4 cm H_2O) and a backup rate of 2 to 4 breaths per minute (bpm) less than the spontaneous breathing rate. The patient typically uses NPPV in the office or clinic under close supervision for a short period of time with adjustment of pressure settings, inspiratory time, and backup rate to maximize comfort. One could also use an NPPV machine controlled by a peripheral device or computer that could provide real-time information on tidal volume, rate, and leak during short NPPV trials in the outpatient setting. NPPV treatment is then initiated on the selected settings. Patients are seen at frequent intervals (1 week, 1 month, then 3 months) to make further adjustments. Some patients with NMD may be able to sleep with NPPV only a few hours per night at first until they adapt. Some clinicians use daytime P_{ETCO_2}, $Ptcco_2$, or ABG measurements to monitor treatment. Another approach would be to obtain an ABG immediately after periods of NPPV treatment to guide adjustment of NPPV device settings.

Several of the studies documenting the efficacy of NPPV treatment in CAH syndromes did not use PSG for NPPV titration. NPPV treatment was initiated in patients with RTCD,[13–17] NMD,[15,28,38] and OHS[3] without PSG for titration. Many of these studies admitted patients to the hospital for NPPV treatment initiation. In most settings today, hospital admission for NPPV titration alone would not be financially feasible or considered as medically necessary. Therefore, a practical approach would be starting NPPV in the office or clinic under close medical supervision with adjustment of NPPV settings to maximize patients' comfort.

NPPV IN DIFFERENT PATIENT GROUPS
OHS

The diagnostic criteria for the OHS include (1) daytime hypoventilation (2) obesity body mass index (BMI) greater than 30 kg/m^2, (3) absence of pulmonary disease that could explain hypoventilation. Most (80%–90%) patients with OHS have

OSA.[1–9] However, some have daytime hypoventilation that worsens during sleep in the absence of discrete obstructive events. Continuous positive airway pressure (CPAP) is often effective in preventing apnea, hypopnea, and snoring in individual OHS patients. Chronic CPAP treatment in OHS patients can also result in a reduction in daytime P_{CO_2} in some patients.[2] However, many OHS patients require high levels of CPAP and manifest residual arterial oxygen desaturation or continue to hypoventilate after upper airway patency is restored.[2,6] In such patients BPAP (NPPV) has been proven effective and, by augmenting ventilation, may prevent the need for supplemental oxygen.[2–10] A recent randomized trial[11] compared CPAP with BPAP for treatment of patients with OHS. Patients with significant residual desaturation (Spo_2 <80% for >10 minutes) on a level of CPAP that eliminated obstructive events, an acute increase in P_{CO_2} more than 10 mm Hg during REM sleep, or an increase in P_{CO_2} more than 10 mm Hg in the morning compared with the afternoon were excluded. An equivalent reduction in daytime P_{CO_2} was noted at 3 months in patients randomized to CPAP or BPAP. Adherence to the treatment modalities was also not significantly different. In the BPAP group, the mean IPAP and EPAP levels used were 16 and 10 cm H_2O respectively, and the spontaneous mode of BPAP was used. A few patients in both groups required supplemental oxygen in addition to PAP. The patients with the most severe OHS were excluded from this study and were treated with NPPV outside the study protocol. Patients with OHS may require high levels of EPAP to prevent obstructive apnea, and this tends to limit the available range of PS unless very high IPAP levels are used. In a study by Berger and colleagues[2] of the effect of NPPV in patients with OHS, EPAP values up to 14 cm H_2O and IPAP values up to 25 cm H_2O were needed. The mean IPAP and EPAP values were 18 and 8 cm H_2O, respectively.

NPPV treatment of patients with OHS is ideally initiated after a PSG titration. Because most patients have OSA, a titration is essential to select settings that will maintain upper airway patency. Patients often require the addition of supplemental oxygen, at least at the initiation of treatment. Other patients with OHS are started on NPPV treatment after admission to an intensive care unit for acute respiratory failure. BPAP settings are often chosen in the intensive care unit by direct observation with oximetry while the patients are sleeping. Once the patients are stable they may undergo a formal sleep study for diagnosis of OSA and optimization of NPPV settings. Many patients with OHS can be adequately treated without a backup rate. A recent study found that volume target ventilation was also effective in OHS patients.[43]

Restrictive Chest Wall Disorders

Several studies have documented that NPPV treatment can result in an improvement in quality of life and gas exchange in patients with RTCD. Most published studies concerning NPPV treatment in patients with RTCD [13,14] have not used an attended NPPV titration study to select levels of pressure. However, in one study[11] patients were admitted to the hospital for initiation of NPPV. Treatment NPPV settings were based on daytime ABG testing, nocturnal oximetry, or nocturnal $Ptcco_2$ monitoring. Because of a reduced thoracic compliance, patients with RTCD may require high levels of PS to deliver adequate tidal volumes. In one study, the mean IPAP and EPAP values were 21.1 and 3.1 cm H_2O, respectively, with a backup rate of 20 bpm.[14] The amount of improvement in the daytime Pco_2 correlated with the amount of PS. A study by Gonzalez and colleagues[13] used a mean backup rate of 15 bpm. Some RTCD patients may be more comfortably ventilated with a lower tidal volume and a higher respiratory rate.

Obstructive events can occur in patients with RTCD. For example, in one study by Gonzalez and colleagues[13] of patients with kyphoscoliosis the apnea hypopnea index averaged 13.9 events/h. Although concurrent OSA may be suspected in candidates for NPPV who report snoring and witnessed apnea, absence of these symptoms does not rule out significant obstructive events.

CRCD

Many patients with CRCD, such as those with congenital central hypoventilation, may have life-threatening events if not adequately ventilated during sleep. In these patients, documentation of the adequacy of NPPV treatment settings is essential before chronic NPPV treatment can be safely initiated. Patients with congenital central hypoventilation often require tracheostomy and volume ventilation from birth, at least during sleep. Those patients who do not require 24-hour ventilatory assistance may be transitioned to NPPV if they are motivated, found to be reliably adherent, and a sleep study documents efficacy of NPPV.[21–23] NPPV with a backup rate should be used in these patients because they may not reliably trigger IPAP/EPAP transitions because of abnormalities in ventilatory control.

The transition to NPPV often occurs when the patient attains an age sufficient to accept mask ventilation. However, selected patients have used NPPV from an early age. A potential complication of early use of mask ventilation is an association with the development of central facial hypoplasia.[66,67] This complication could be caused by the effects of chronic mask pressure. This problem is most likely to occur in patients needing mask ventilation during the day as well as during sleep.

NMD

There have been numerous studies of the effectiveness of NPPV in patients with NMD, although the benefits may vary depending on the specific disorder.[24–35,38] Attended NPPV titration with PSG in patients with NMD can provide rapid determination of an adequate level of support, intervention for OSA if present, and documentation of the effectiveness of the chosen NPPV settings in various sleep stages and body positions. Interventions for mask and leak problems can be made quickly. Several studies of NPPV in NMD patients did use NPPV titration with PSG.[19,29,31,33]

Some centers with considerable expertise in treating patients with NMD (eg, ALS) have structured programs for initiating NPPV on an outpatient basis during the daytime. NMD patients are often started on BPAP at low pressures after a period of daytime adaptation under direct supervision. If patients tolerate nocturnal NPPV with low pressures, the settings are increased over weeks to months based on symptoms or daytime arterial Pco_2 measurement (or estimates of arterial Pco_2 such as $Petco_2$). In one study of this approach in ALS patients,[25] symptom relief was provided in 4 of 18 patients with the low initial settings, whereas most other patients required 1 or 2 increases in pressure. Only 6/19 patients required PS of more than 10 cm H_2O. In patients with rapidly progressive NMD, the main goal of treatment is often palliation of symptoms and improvement in quality of life rather than normalization of nocturnal arterial Pco_2.

In a randomized controlled study of the effect of BPAP in the ST mode on survival and quality of life in ALS,[38] the average IPAP and EPAP settings were 15 and 6 cm H_2O respectively. In this study, only the subgroup of ALS patients without moderate to severe bulbar dysfunction had improved survival. However, all patients treated with NPPV had improvement in the quality of life. Patients with bulbar involvement may have more difficulty tolerating NPPV and mask ventilation. These patients may also have a greater risk of aspiration than those without upper airway dysfunction.[27]

NPPV TITRATION WITH PSG
NPPV Device and Monitoring

The NPPV device used for NPPV titration should ideally have the ability to function in the S, ST, and T modes. The ideal device should provide analog or digital outputs of flow, pressure, leak, and tidal volume that may be monitored during titration and recorded with other PSG data (see **Fig. 1**; **Table 5**). The flow and pressure signals are derived from accurate internal flow and pressure sensors. The airflow signal from the NPPV device is the recommended signal to detect apnea, hypopnea, and RERAs. The signal provides information concerning the magnitude and shape (contour) of airflow. A flattened inspiratory shape is evidence of airflow limitation and is usually associated with high upper airway resistance. Snoring is usually detected by a microphone or by piezoelectric transducers attached to the neck or chest. A vibratory pattern in mask pressure may also be used to detect snoring. The airflow signal from NPPV devices is usually too filtered or undersampled to detect snoring.

Most NPPV devices also provide a signal that gives a breath-by-breath estimate of tidal volume for display in the software or on the peripheral device remotely controlling the unit. The tidal volume is derived from integration of the device's flow. The tidal volume signal should be recorded if possible. Although airflow provides some information concerning ventilation, the tidal volume depends on airflow and inspiratory time (see **Fig. 1**). The product of the estimated tidal volume and respiratory rate provides an estimate of the minute ventilation. It is also useful to record the pressure signal from the NPPV device outlet or mask using an external pressure transducer or the signal generated from the NPPV device based on the internal pressure sensor. Recording of delivered pressure is helpful to the technologist and physician reviewing the sleep recording. The pressure signal clearly shows the IPAP/EPAP cycle and is especially helpful in determining the pattern of response of the NPPV device in situations in which the backup rate is frequently activated. Some NPPV devices output a brief signal (intentional artifact) before each machine-triggered breath (see **Fig. 1**). Another method to identify machine-triggered breaths is to observe that they often have a different inspiratory time than spontaneous breaths.

Respiratory Muscle EMG

Recording respiratory muscle EMG activity with bipolar surface electrodes and techniques similar to those used for recording the anterior tibialis EMG may be helpful during NPPV titration in

Table 5		
Monitoring during NPPV titration		
Recommended Parameter to be Monitored During NPPV Titration	**Recommended Method**	**Use**
Airflow	NPPV device output (accurate internal flow sensor)	Detection of apnea, hypopnea, and RERAs
Tidal volume	NPPV device output (from integration of flow signal)	Estimate of tidal volume
Snoring	Piezoelectric sensor or microphone	Detection of snoring
Pressure	External pressure transducer or NPPV device signal (internal pressure sensor)	Documentation of amount and pattern of pressure delivery
Respiratory muscle EMG	bipolar monitoring use surface electrodes over the diaphragm or intercostal muscles	Absence or reduction in respiratory muscle EMG suggests adequate respiratory muscle rest has been achieved
Chest and abdominal movement	Respiratory inductance plethysmography	Differentiating central and obstructive events, detection of paradox
P_{ETCO_2}	Side stream via nasal cannula in nares under the mask	Breath-by-breath estimate of arterial P_{CO_2}
Transcutaneous P_{CO_2} (Pt_{CCO_2})	Transcutaneous sensor	Estimate of trends in arterial P_{CO_2}

patients with NMD or an increased effort of breathing. Adequate NPPV support for muscle rest is associated with the absence or decrease in inspiratory EMG activity of the respiratory muscles during sleep. Surface diaphragm EMG recording uses 2 electrodes about 2 cm apart horizontally in the seventh and eighth intercostal spaces in the right anterior axillary line.[56,57] The right side of the body is used to reduce artifacts on the electrocardiogram. Other sites include the sternocleidomastoid (an accessory muscle of respiration) and the right parasternal area (second and third intercostal spaces in the midaxillary line). In normal individuals, the accessory muscles are usually quiet during sleep, except during periods following arousal. Inspiratory EMG activity is noted in the intercostal muscles and the diaphragm during non-REM (NREM) sleep. During REM sleep the intercostal activity is inhibited but diaphragmatic activity persists (although frequently diminished during bursts of eye movements). In contrast, in patients with respiratory muscle weakness or increased work of breathing, the EMG of accessory muscles often shows inspiratory activity during NREM sleep. During the NPPV titration, a reduction in the EMG activity of respiratory muscles (accessory, intercostals, diaphragm) may be a useful indicator that sufficient PS is being administered to allow muscle rest (see **Fig. 3**).

Measurement of P_{CO_2} During NPPV Titration and Treatment

ABG testing at a given level of NPPV support (commonly immediately after awakening) is the most accurate method for determining the effects of NPPV on the arterial P_{CO_2}. However, this measurement is invasive and requires special expertise. In addition, rapid access to a laboratory where the sample can be processed may be problematic for sleep centers located outside a hospital. In pediatric patients, sampling of a capillary blood gas (arterialized blood) is often used as an alternative to ABG testing. Another limitation of ABG monitoring is that serial testing during sleep is impractical.

Other methods for estimating arterial P_{CO_2} during NPPV titration include measurement of Ptc_{CO_2} and $P_{ET}CO_2$. Ptc_{CO_2} monitoring provides a continuous reading and maybe useful for NPPV titration when the device is calibrated and the readings are within 10 mm Hg of the concurrent P_{CO_2} value obtained by ABG (or capillary blood gas) testing during stable breathing. Because of a slow response time, changes in Ptc_{CO_2} generally are delayed following changes in the arterial P_{CO_2}. Storre and colleagues[68] compared 250 paired

samples of ABG and $PtcCO_2$ measurements in a group of 8 subjects undergoing NPPV for acute or chronic hypoventilation caused by COPD. They found that the Ptc_{CO_2} provided a reasonable estimate of ABGs, with the best results obtained by comparing a given arterial P_{CO_2} value with a Ptc_{CO_2} result 2 minutes later. In an earlier study, Sanders and colleagues[69] did not find Ptc_{CO_2} to be a valid indicator of the arterial P_{CO_2} during sleep. Pavia and colleagues[70] performed Ptc_{CO_2} monitoring during NPPV and found evidence of nocturnal hypoventilation (Ptc_{CO_2} >50 mm Hg) in 21 patients of a group of 50 with normal daytime P_{CO_2} (capillary blood gas) who had no nocturnal desaturation on oximetry. The information supplied by Ptc_{CO_2} may be useful if the accuracy can be verified. Ideally, the Ptc_{CO_2} device is calibrated before monitoring and the results are validated by ABG sampling at the start of or during the study. Caution is advised in making clinical decisions based on Ptc_{CO_2} monitoring alone, especially if the results do not correlate with other findings.

Capnography is the measurement of exhaled CO_2 (**Fig. 4**). The $P_{ET}CO_2$ provides an estimate of the arterial P_{CO_2}. There is always a gradient between the arterial P_{CO_2} and $P_{ET}CO_2$. In normal individuals, the gradient (arterial P_{CO_2} to $P_{ET}CO_2$) is around 4 to 6 mm Hg but can exceed 10 mm Hg if lung disease is present. In addition, to be accurate the signal should show an alveolar plateau. Sampling of gas at the nares rather than at the mask is required for optimal measurement of $P_{ET}CO_2$ during NPPV titration. The $P_{ET}CO_2$ should ideally be validated by concurrent P_{CO_2} measurement using arterial or capillary blood gas testing during stable breathing. Sanders and colleagues[69] found poor agreement between $P_{ET}CO_2$ and ABG testing in adult patients during diagnostic PSG. However, gas was sampled from a mask covering the nose and mouth rather than the nares. In contrast, Kirk and colleagues[71] found reasonable agreement between $P_{ET}CO_2$ and Ptc_{CO_2} during pediatric PSG. In the commonly used sidestream capnography method, exhaled gas is suctioned via a nasal cannula to an external CO_2 sensor. The major challenge for $P_{ET}CO_2$ monitoring during NPPV titration is dilution of the exhaled sample by flow from the NPPV device (especially if gas is sampled at the mask). One approach is to have the patient wear a sampling nasal cannula under the NPPV mask interface. Using this approach, gas is sampled as it is exhaled from the nares rather than suctioned from the mask. A similar method was used by Parreira and colleagues[47] during their study of BPAP in normal subjects. A disadvantage of this approach is that

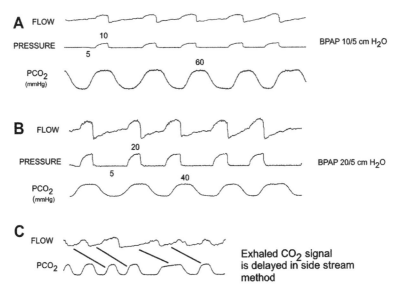

Fig. 4. Flow, pressure, and PETCO$_2$ during NPPV titration. (*A*) BPAP is 10/5 cm H$_2$O and the PETCO$_2$ is 60 mm Hg. (*B*) the BPAP is 20/5 cm H$_2$O and tidal volume is higher and PETCO$_2$ much lower (40 mm Hg). The PETCO$_2$ signal is delayed following each exhalation as the side-stream method was used (*C*). A nasal cannula under the mask was used to sample the exhaled gas. Note the curved shape of the pressure pulses resulting from a long rise time.

the presence of the cannula passing under the mask seal could cause excessive leak.

NPPV Mask Interfaces and Humidification for NPPV Titration and Treatment

A comfortable and well-fitting mask interface is essential for adequate NPPV titration and treatment. A variety of different types of PAP interfaces (ie, nasal masks, nasal pillows, full-face mask) and accessories (chinstraps, heated humidifier) should be available.[72,73] Nasal masks or nasal pillows mask are often better tolerated, especially in patients with claustrophobia. Patients with substantial mouth leak or nasal congestion may require the use of a full-face mask. Some patients may prefer an oral interface. Pediatric (in addition to small adult) interfaces should be available for titration in patients less than 12 years old. Pediatric patients benefit from introduction to potential interfaces and acclimatization before the night of the NPPV titration. Introduction of the interfaces should be developmentally appropriate for the child's age.

Heated humidification should be available for patients undergoing NPPV titration. The addition of humidification is indicated if the patient complains of significant oral or nasal dryness (unless humidification is not tolerated by the patient). It is consistent with clinical guidelines for the manual titration of CPAP and BPAP in patients with OSA.[73] The American Academy of Sleep Medicine (AASM) Standards of Practice for CPAP and BPAP treatment also states "the

addition of heated humidification is indicated to improve PAP use."[72] Two controlled studies were not able to document an improvement in patient acceptance of CPAP treatment with the prophylactic use of heated humidity.[74,75] However, the level of CPAP was low (around 10 cm H$_2$O) and the nasal symptoms were mild in one study. NPPV treatment frequently uses high pressures and is associated with high intentional and unintentional leak. A bench study documented that NPPV devices deliver air at a reduced relative humidity compared with ambient air and that increasing IPAP lowered the delivered relative humidity.[76] Initiation of humidification at the start of the study may be useful in selected patients with significant nasal congestion or a history of severe mucosal dryness during sleep, in particularly in dry locales, or during the winter in cold climates. At the minimum, heated humidity should be available for patients who develop severe nasal congestion or dryness during the night.

NPPV Titration Protocol

There is no widely accepted protocol for NPPV titration in the sleep center. The AASM Board of Directors appointed an NPPV Titration Task Force to develop consensus guidelines. The guidelines were still being finalized at the time this article was written. The titration suggestions discussed later reflect some of the preliminary thoughts of the task force as well as industry protocols. The reader is encouraged to read the AASM NPPV titration guidelines when they are finalized and disseminated. The initial IPAP/EPAP levels are typically 8/4 cm H_2O. During the titration the minimum PS usually varies between 4 cm H_2O and 20 cm H_2O. In the AASM Clinical Guidelines for titration of CPAP and BPAP in patients with OSA, the recommended minimum IPAP-EPAP difference was 4 cm H_2O and the maximum was 10 cm H_2O.[73] However, in the case of OSA, the major objective is to maintain airway patency. Budweiser and colleagues[14] used a mean PS of 18 cm H_2O in a study of patients with RTCD. Patients with low respiratory system compliance may require a high level of PS to augment ventilation during sleep. The maximum available IPAP varies between devices (20–30 cm H_2O). Most NPPV devices used for PSG have a maximum IPAP of 30 cm H_2O. The maximum recommended IPAP for the titration of BPAP in OSA was 30 cm H_2O in adults and 20 cm H_2O in children.[73] During titration, PS is usually increased in 1- to 2-cm H_2O increments. A maximum incremental change of 2 cm H_2O is recommended to avoid overtitration.

Adjustment of IPAP and EPAP to eliminate obstructive events

IPAP and EPAP should be adjusted to eliminate obstructive apneas, hypopneas, RERAs, and snoring following the AASM Clinical Guidelines for the Manual Titration of PAP in Patients with OSA.[73] These guidelines (summarized in **Table 6**) provide a protocol for increasing the IPAP and EPAP to eliminate obstructive apneas, hypopneas, RERAs, and snoring. For obstructive apnea, IPAP and EPAP are increased by 1 or more cm H_2O (eg, a change from 8/4 to 9/5 for obstructive apnea). For other events, the IPAP is increased by 1 cm H_2O or more, no more rapidly than every 5 minutes. If stable breathing (minimal obstructive

events) is obtained for 30 minutes or more, a downward titration of pressure could be tried.

Adjustment of PS during NPPV titration

A protocol for adjusting PS is listed in **Table 7**. The PS is increased every 5 to 10 minutes if the tidal volume is less than an acceptable goal. An acceptable tidal volume goal for most patients ranges from 6 to 8 mL/kg using ideal body weight. An optimal tidal volume may vary with the disorder being treated and the respiratory rate. Tidal volumes of 6 to 8 mL/kg at typical respiratory rates usually deliver normal minute ventilation. If lung disease is present, a higher minute ventilation is needed to deliver adequate alveolar ventilation because of an increase in physiologic dead space. In normal individuals, the dead space is approximately equal to 2 cm^3/kg. The recommended tidal volume target for VT-BPAP is 8 mL/kg using ideal body weight.[43,45] Slightly lower tidal volumes with higher respiratory rates may be better tolerated in individual patients (particularly in RTCD).

The PS is increased if the arterial P_{CO_2} or surrogates (P_{ETCO_2}, P_{tcCO_2}) remain 10 mm H_2O more than the goal at the current settings for 10 minutes or more. An acceptable goal for P_{CO_2} is usually a value less than or equal to the awake P_{CO_2}. Changing PS based on the P_{ETCO_2} or P_{tcCO_2} assumes that these measurements have been documented to accurately reflect the arterial P_{CO_2} in a given patient. In normal subjects, there is a small increase in arterial P_{CO_2} during sleep of about 5 to 10 mm Hg. However, because most patients being treated with NPPV have daytime hypoventilation, an ideal goal of treatment would consist of preventing a further increase in the arterial P_{CO_2} during sleep. The daytime awake P_{CO_2} may decrease with chronic nocturnal NPPV treatment in a substantial number of patients with

Table 6 Changes in IPAP and EPAP for obstructive events		
	Event Triggers	
	Adults/Children >12 y	**Children <12 y**
Increase IPAP and EPAP by $\geq$1 cm H_2O Increase no more rapidly than every 5 min	$\geq$2 obstructive apneas	$\geq$1 obstructive apneas
Increase IPAP $\geq$1 cm H_2O Increase no more rapidly than every 5 min	$\geq$3 hypopneas $\geq$5 RERAs $\geq$3 min of loud unambiguous snoring	$\geq$1 hypopneas $\geq$3 RERAs $\geq$1 min of loud unambiguous snoring

Adapted from Kushida CA, Chediak A, Berry RB, et al. Clinical guidelines for the manual titration of positive airway pressure in patients with obstructive sleep apnea. J Clin Sleep Med 2008;4:163,164.

Table 7
Adjustment of pressure support (PS) during NPPV titration

Pressure Change	Trigger	Duration Between Changes	Goal
IPAP/EPAP increased	Eliminate apnea, hypopnea, RERA (see **Table 6**)	$\geq$5 min	Prevent apnea, hypopnea, RERAs, snoring
PS increased 1–2 cm H_2O	Low tidal volume (<6–8 cm^3/kg ideal body weight)	$\geq$5 min	Adequate tidal volume
PS increased 1–2 cm H_2O	P_{CO_2} >10 mm Hg more than goal	$\geq$10 min	Adequate ventilation and P_{CO_2}
PS increased 1–2 cm H_2O	Respiratory muscle rest not achieved	$\geq$10 min	Adequate respiratory muscle rest Reduction of respiratory rate with higher tidal volumes or reduction in inspiratory respiratory EMG activity
PS increase 1–2 cm H_2O	Sa_{O_2} <90% with tidal volume <8 cm^3 kg (assumes discrete apnea, hypopnea, RERAS not present)	$\geq$5 min	Adequate oxygenation

CAH. Thus, the level of nocturnal P_{CO_2} on NPPV treatment may eventually be lower than the initial goal. However, some patients may not initially tolerate a level of PS adequate to meet the chosen P_{CO_2} goal. Daytime and nocturnal P_{CO_2} may decrease over time with chronic NPPV treatment.

If a goal of NPPV is to provide respiratory muscle rest, PS may be increased if respiratory muscle rest has not been achieved by NPPV treatment at the current settings for 10 minutes or more. Adequate respiratory muscle rest during NPPV is associated with resolution or improvement in tachypnea or excessive inspiratory effort as measured by phasic EMG activity of inspiratory muscles (see **Fig. 3**).

If the Sa_{O_2} remains less than 90% for 5 minutes and the tidal volume is less than ideal (<8 mL/kg), an increase in the PS may be tried. The rationale behind this recommendation is that an increase in PS may increase tidal volume and reduce or eliminate residual hypoventilation, thereby improving oxygenation. If not successful, the addition of supplemental oxygen may be needed. If discrete obstructive apneas or hypopneas are present, the clinical guidelines for PAP titration in OSA patients should be followed.[73] Although criteria for chronic oxygen therapy often use an Sa_{O_2} of less than 88% as an indication for supplemental oxygen, the slightly higher goal of 90% allows for a margin of error because the tidal volume associated with a level of PS could vary with the clinical condition of the patient.

Use of ST and Timed Modes During Titration

Indications for the use of the ST mode (backup rate) are listed in **Box 3**. Most clinicians would use the ST mode in all patients with central hypoventilation or significantly impaired respiratory

Box 3
Indications for use of the ST mode (backup rate)

- All patients with disorders of central ventilatory control or impaired ventilatory drive
- Patients with NMD
- Patients with episodically low respiratory efforts (REM sleep) and tidal volume caused by muscle weakness or high work of breathing
- Frequent central apneas are present at baseline or during NPPV titration/treatment
- Inappropriately low respiratory rate
- Respiratory muscle rest not achieved with maximum PS (or maximum tolerated PS)
- Adequate ventilation is not achieved with maximum PS (or maximum tolerated PS)

drive. The ST mode (backup rate) should be used if frequent and significant central apneas are present at baseline or during the NPPV titration, if the respiratory rate is inappropriately low, or if the patient fails to reliably cycle the NPPV device between EPAP and IPAP because of muscle weakness. Many physicians routinely use the ST mode in all patients with NMD and RTCD. Because muscle strength may vary over time in patients with NMD, most clinicians would use a backup rate for chronic treatment in these patients even if not required during the NPPV titration. If adequate ventilation or adequate muscle rest is not achieved by the maximum PS or maximally tolerated PS, then a backup rate may be used. For example, patients with RTCD may be treated with lower tidal volumes and more rapid respiratory rates. Prior studies have used the ST mode in NMD,[28,33,38] and RTCD.[13,14,16] Some studies have also used a backup rate in patients with OHS.[7,10] If NPPV using the ST mode is not successful, the timed mode with a fixed respiratory rate may be tried. This mode may be tried if the patient cannot adequately trigger IPAP/EPAP cycles or there is difficulty in patient-NPPV synchrony. Choice of the backup rate (ST mode) or respiratory rate (timed mode) and inspiratory time (IPAPtime) are discussed later.

Choosing and Adjusting the Backup Rate (ST Mode) or Respiratory Rate (Timed Mode)

The initial backup rate for the ST mode should be equal to or less than the patient's spontaneous sleeping respiratory rate (≥ 10 bpm) (**Box 4**). If the sleeping respiratory rate is not known, the spontaneous awake respiratory rate may be used. Some industry protocols[77] and sleep centers start with a backup rate 2 to 4 bpm less than the spontaneous backup rate. The initial setting for the respiratory rate in the timed mode should be equal to or slightly less than the patient's spontaneous sleeping respiratory rate or the current backup rate if switching from the ST to timed mode.

In a study of patients with NMD, Katz and colleagues[33] used a backup rate 10% less than the patient's resting breathing rate. One industry protocol suggests starting at a minimum rate of 8 to 10 bpm or 2 bpm less than the patient's resting rate.[74–77] Gonzalez and colleagues[13] used a backup rate of 15 bpm in a group of patients with RTCD. Mellies and colleagues[31] used backup rates ranging from 14 to 24 (mean 19.6) bpm in a group of children with NMDs. Tuggey and colleagues[16] used a mean backup rate of 15 bpm in a study of NPPV and patients with RTCD,

---

Box 4
Choosing and adjusting the backup rate and IPAP time

Choosing and adjusting the backup rate

- Initial rate 1 to 2 bpm less than spontaneous respiratory rate (≥ 10 bpm)
- Increased in 1 to 2 bpm increments until goal achieved
- Decreased backup rate if patient reports discomfort or if NPPV device triggered and patient-triggered breaths are frequently superimposed (stacking of breaths).

Choosing the IPAP time (inspiratory time)

- Usually 1.2 to 1.6 seconds (depending or respiratory rate and desired %IPAPtime)
- Based on respiratory rate, choose inspiratory time so that %IPAPtime is 30% to 40%
- %IPAPtime 30% useful for obstructive lung disease (allows more expiratory time)
- %IPAPtime of 40% useful for chest wall disease (allows adequate inspiratory time)

---

whereas another study[14] used a backup rate of 20 bpm in a similar population.

The backup rate (ST mode) or specified respiratory rate (timed mode) should be increased in increments of 1 to 2 bpm, usually no more frequently than every 10 minutes, if the desired goal of the backup rate (or fixed respiratory rate) is not attained with lower rates. The backup rate (ST mode) or respiratory rate (timed mode) should be decreased if the patient reports discomfort that is believed to be related to a high respiratory rate or if NPPV device–triggered and patient-triggered breaths are frequently superimposed (stacking of breaths).

Choosing the Inspiratory Time (IPAPtime) in the ST and Timed Modes

When NPPV devices are used in the ST mode, the backup rate and the duration of IPAP (inspiratory time or IPAPtime) for machine-triggered breaths must be specified (although the devices do have default values) (see **Box 4**). In the timed mode, the respiratory rate and the IPAPtime time are specified by the physician for all breaths. The inspiratory time on BPAP is similar to IPAPtime, although inspiratory flow may cease before IPAP cycles to EPAP.

The IPAPtime for machine-triggered breaths in the ST mode, or all breaths in the timed mode, is chosen based on the respiratory rate and the need to provide an adequate tidal volume and an appropriate inspiratory time to expiratory time ratio

(I/E ratio). Another method of expressing the I/E ratio is the %IPAP time, which is the IPAP time as a percentage of the cycle time (**Table 8**). The cycle time equals 60/respiratory rate and is also equal to IPAPtime + EPAPtime. The recommended %IPAPtime is usually between 30% and 40%. A lower %IPAP time and I/E ratio is desirable in patients with obstructive airway disease to allow a sufficient expiratory time because expiratory airflow is reduced in these patients. A greater %IPAP time (greater I/E ratio) is preferred in patients with restrictive lung disease to allow for a longer inspiratory time. As the respiratory rate becomes faster, the inspiratory time must be decreased to maintain an adequate I/E ratio.

The default inspiratory time on NPPV devices is commonly 1.2 seconds. At a respiratory rate of 15 bpm, the IPAPtimes corresponding to %IPAP-times of 30% or 40% are 1.2 and 1.6 seconds. The IPAPtime in the ST or timed modes should be adjusted to maximize ventilation, patient/NPPV synchrony, and patient comfort.

Adjustments for Patient Comfort and Synchrony with the NPPV Device

Several interventions can be made for patient comfort during NPPV titration or treatment (**Box 5**). During an NPPV titration or treatment, if the patient awakens and complains that the IPAP, EPAP, or both are too high, the appropriate pressure(s) should be decreased to a lower pressure(s), chosen so that the patient reports a degree of comfort adequate to allow return to sleep (titration) or tolerate NPPV (treatment).

NPPV devices have some adjustments that can be made during titration or chronic treatment to improve patient comfort. The rise time (time duration for pressure to change from EPAP to set IPAP) should be increased or decreased for patient comfort. Typical rise times vary from 100 to 600 milliseconds. Patients with obstructive airway disease often prefer shorter rise times (100– 400 milliseconds) and patients with restrictive disease

(NMD, RTCD) often prefer longer rise times (300–600 milliseconds). A rise time of approximately 200 milliseconds is usually the default on NPPV devices. Adjustment of the rise time may improve tolerance to NPPV in certain patients.

NPPV devices transition from IPAP to EPAP during a patient-triggered breath when flow falls to less than a set value. In patients with a stiff chest wall (decreased compliance), flow rates may decrease as the lung volume increases. An early decrease in the absolute flow rates may prematurely trigger the transition to EPAP. Certain devices provide a minimum IPAPtime (IPAPtime-min) to ensure that IPAP lasts long enough to allow delivery of an adequate tidal volume. In situations of high leak (continued flow) or muscle weakness, the IPAP to EPAP transition may be unduly delayed. A default maximum IPAP duration of 3 seconds exists on some devices, whereas in other devices a maximal IPAP time (IPAPtime-max) may be chosen.

VT-BPAP

VT-BPAP, a mode of NPPV that automatically adjusts the IPAP within the pressure range of IPAPmin to IPAPmax (set by the clinician) to deliver the targeted tidal volume.[43–45] VT-BPAP may used in the spontaneous, ST, and timed modes. VT-BPAP has the potential advantage of automatically varying the PS to deliver a targeted tidal volume. For example, if respiratory muscle strength declined and the tidal volume decreased, the device would deliver higher PS to return the delivered tidal volume to the targeted amount. Few studies on VT-BPAP have been published. To date, only one VT-BPAP device is available in the United States (Average Volume Assured Pressure Support [AVAPS], Philips-Respironics).

When VT-BPAP is used, the purpose of a titration is to select a level of EPAP that eliminates obstructive events (obstructive apnea and hypopnea) and document that the device does deliver

| Table 8 |||||
| IPAPtime (inspiratory time) at different respiratory rates (RR) and %IPAPtime |||||
%IPAPtime	RR	Cycle Time (s)	Inspiratory Time = IPAPtime (s)
30	12	5	1.5
	15	4	1.2
	20	3	0.9
40	12	5	2.0
	15	4	1.6
	20	3	1.2

Cycle time = 60/respiratory rate in bpm. %IPAPtime = IPAPtime × 100/cycle time. EPAP time = cycle time − IPAP time.

<table>
<tr><td>

Box 5
Adjusting NPPV setting for patient comfort

- Adjust rise time (time from start of IPAP cycle to when set IPAP is reached)

  Rise time 100 to 600 milliseconds (default usually 200 milliseconds)

  Shorter rise time (100–400 milliseconds) often preferred with obstructive lung disease or when patient complains of too much air

  Longer rise time (300–600 milliseconds) often preferred by patients with restriction chest wall disease or when patient complains of not enough air

- Adjust minimum IPAPtime (IPAPtime-min), if available

  Increase IPAPtime-min if IPAP cycles off too early (chest wall disease)

- Adjust maximum allowed IPAP time (IPAP-time-max), if available

  Decrease IPAPtime-max if IPAP cycles off too late because of high leak or muscle weakness

</td><td>

Box 6
Addition of supplemental oxygen to NPPV during titration or treatment

Indications

- Add supplemental O_2 during the NPPV treatment when the patient's awake supine Sao_2 while breathing room air is less than 88%
- Add supplemental O_2 when the PS and respiratory rate have been optimized but the Sao_2 remains less than 90% for 5 to 10 minutes or more
- Weaning off O_2 supplementation by using a higher PS or respiratory rate (if the patient tolerates these increases) can be attempted

Adjusting supplemental oxygen flow

- The minimum starting O_2 flow rate is usually 1 L/min
- The O_2 flow rate is typically increased in increments of 1 L/min about every 5 minutes, until Sao_2 is more than 90%

</td></tr>
</table>

adequate tidal volumes. According to the manufacture's recommendations, a target volume of 8 cm^3/kg (based on ideal body weight) is selected. Initial settings are EPAP = 4 cm H_2O, IPAPmin = EPAP + 4 cm H_2O, and IPAPmax = 25 to 30 cm H_2O. If volume-targeted PS is used in the ST or timed modes, the backup rate and inspiratory time may be chosen based on the recommendations discussed earlier.

Studies comparing VT-BPAP with BPAP (ST) have shown slightly lower Pco_2 and higher ventilation on VT-BPAP.[43,44] The sleep quality was similar[43,44] or worse[45] on VT-BPAP. The role of VT-BPAP in the NPPV treatment of patients with CAH remains to be determined.

Addition of Supplemental Oxygen

Individual patients may continue to have desaturation on the maximum NPPV settings (or on the maximal tolerated settings). In this case, supplemental oxygen can be added during an NPPV titration or to NPPV treatment based on nocturnal oximetry performed on an outpatient's current settings. Suggested indications for the addition of supplemental oxygen during NPPV titration are listed in **Box 6**. These are similar to the AASM guidelines for administration of supplemental oxygen in patients undergoing CPAP or BPAP titration.[73] Supplemental oxygen should be added during the NPPV titration when the patient's

supplemental oxygen is needed to maintain an adequate awake supine Sao_2 during stable breathing. Supplemental O_2 is also added when PS and respiratory rate have been optimized but the Sao_2 remains less than 90% for 5 minutes or more. The supplemental oxygen flow rate is typically increased in increments of 1 L/min about every 5 minutes, until Sao_2 is more than 90%. The use of 90% as the criterion to add supplemental oxygen is made with the understanding that pulse oximetry can overestimate the actual arterial oxyhemoglobin saturation in some circumstances.

Dependence of the Effective Oxygen Concentration on Flow Rate

The effective fractional concentration of oxygen (Fio_2) that the patient breaths during NPPV treatment depends on the flow rate of the supplemental oxygen and the machine flow. The machine flow increases as pressure increases because of higher controlled leak (nonrebreathing orifices) and higher unintentional leak (mask or mouth leak). The increase in machine flow decreases the effective Fio_2 at a given flow of supplemental oxygen.[78–81] The Fio_2 does not seem to vary with the amount of PS or the respiratory rate. Therefore an increase in pressure can decrease the effective Fio_2. The optimal location at which supplemental oxygen should be connected to the NPPV circuit has been studied by several investigators and the results are somewhat conflicting likely due to different locations of oxygen concentration (Fio_2) measurement. Most studies recommend attachment of the supplemental oxygen tubing to the junction between the NPPV device and the pressure tubing leading to the mask. This results in a more stable oxygen concentration.

Mask and Other Interventions for Leak

The total leak is equal to the sum of the intentional leak (required to prevent rebreathing) and unintentional leak (mask or mouth leak depending on whether a nasal or full-face mask is being used). The intentional leak depends on the type of mask (type of leak port/device) and increases with higher pressure. Intentional leak can be appreciable with most interfaces at high pressure. Therefore, it is difficult to identify a maximum value for an acceptable leak. In general, an unacceptable leak could be defined as one that is much higher than might be expected for a given mask interface and pressure. The leak value provided by some NPPV devices during titration is an estimate of total leak and, in others, an estimate of unintentional leak (mask interface can be specified in NPPV device setup). The trend in leak is often more informative than an absolute value. For example, if the leak suddenly increases using a nasal mask without a change in pressure or body position, one should suspect mouth leak. NPPV devices used for treatment also often provide leak information that can be reviewed during patient visits or with uploads of data from memory cards or modems. During the NPPV titration or treatment mask refit, adjustment, or change in mask type, should be performed whenever any significant unintentional leak is observed or the patient complains of mask discomfort.

Mouth leak is a significant problem in patients on NPPV treatment and may cause arousals even if the NPPV device is able to maintain the desired IPAP and EPAP.[64,65] Teschler and colleagues[65] studied a group of patients being treated with nasal BPAP who complained of symptomatic mouth leak. Taping the mouth substantially reduced arousals and increased the amount of REM sleep. Substantial mouth leak is often associated with complaints of oral dryness that may persist despite the use of heated humidification. Interventions for mouth leak include chin straps or a full-face mask. Some mouth leak may be inevitable, especially if high pressures are used.

Follow-up of Patients on NPPV Treatment

Close follow-up after initiation of NPPV by appropriately trained health care providers under the supervision of an experienced physician is indicated to establish effective use patterns (ideally using objective adherence data), remediate

problems including NPPV side effects and interface issues, and ensure that the equipment is maintained in good repair and disposable equipment is changed on a regular schedule as clinically indicated. As in PAP treatment of OSA, adherence to NPPV for CAH is essential for success.

Minimal information is available concerning adherence to NPPV treatment except for patients with the OHS.

Because BPAP at fixed settings does not deliver a set tidal volume, pressure settings determined during an NPPV titration may not remain adequate if patient characteristics such as muscle strength change during chronic treatment. In addition, concurrent medical problems or medications might affect the effectiveness of treatment. Patients on chronic NPPV treatment should be assessed with measures of oxygenation and ventilation (ABG, end-tidal CO_2, $Ptcco_2$) on a regular follow-up basis or if signs of clinical deterioration are present. Some patients may benefit from a repeat NPPV titration.

In patients with progressive NMD, the time patients spent on NPPV may increase until NPPV is used during the day and night. End-of-life decisions ideally should be discussed before acute respiratory failure occurs. The clinical condition of patients may change (weight gain, reduction in muscle strength, progression of the underlying cause of CAH) with the result that current NPPV treatment may no longer be adequate. The assessment of oxygenation and ventilation in such cases is typically performed during quiet breathing while awake and at rest. Overnight oximetry can be performed on an outpatient basis.

REFERENCES

1. Perez de Llano LA, Golpe R, Montserrat OP, et al. Short-term and long-term effects of nasal intermittent positive pressure ventilation in patients with obesity hypoventilation syndrome. Chest 2005;128: 587–94.
2. Berger KI, Ayappa I, Chatr-Amontri B, et al. Obesity hypoventilation syndrome as a spectrum of respiratory disturbances during sleep. Chest 2001;120: 1231–8.
3. Pérez de Llano LA, Golpe R, Piquer MO, et al. Clinical heterogeneity among patients with obesity hypoventilation syndrome: therapeutic implications. Respiration 2008;75:34–9.
4. Rapoport DM, Sorkin B, Garay SM, et al. Reversal of the "Pickwickian syndrome" by long-term use of nocturnal nasal-airway pressure. N Engl J Med 1982;307:931–3.

5. Masa JF, Bartolome RC, Riesco JA, et al. The Obesity Hypoventilation Syndrome can be treated with noninvasive mechanical ventilation. Chest 2001;119:1102–7.

6. Banerjee D, Yee BJ, Piper AJ, et al. Obesity Hypoventilation Syndrome: hypoxemia during continuous positive airway pressure. Chest 2007;131:1678–84.

7. Budweiser S, Riedl SG, Jörres RA, et al. Mortality and prognostic factors in patients with obesity-hypoventilation syndrome undergoing noninvasive ventilation. J Intern Med 2007;261:375–83.

8. de Lucas-Ramos P, de Miguel-Diez J, Santacruz-Siminiani A, et al. Benefits at 1 year of nocturnal intermittent positive pressure ventilation in patients with obesity hypoventilation syndrome. Respir Med 2004;98:961–7.

9. Redolfi S, Corda L, La Piana G, et al. Long-term non-invasive ventilation increases chemosensitivity and leptin in obesity-hypoventilation syndrome. Respir Med 2007;101:1191–5 Curr Opin Pulm Med. 2007; 13: 490–6.

10. Guo YF, Sforza E, Janssens JP. Respiratory patterns during sleep in obesity-hypoventilation patients treated with nocturnal pressure support: a preliminary report. Chest 2007;131:1090–9.

11. Piper AJ, Wang D, Yee BJ, et al. Randomized trial of CPAP vs bilevel support in the treatment of obesity hypoventilation syndrome without severe nocturnal desaturation. Thorax 2008;63:395–401.

12. Ellis ER, Grunstein RR, Chan S, et al. Noninvasive ventilatory support during sleep improves respiratory failure in kyphoscoliosis. Chest 1988;94:811–5.

13. Gonzalez C, Ferris G, Diaz J, et al. Kyphoscoliotic ventilatory insufficiency: effects of long-term intermittent positive-pressure ventilation. Chest 2003; 124:857–62.

14. Budweiser S, Heinemann F, Fischer W, et al. Impact of ventilation parameters and duration of ventilator use on non-invasive home ventilation in restrictive thoracic disorders. Respiration 2006;73:488–94.

15. Piper AJ, Sullivan CE. Effects of long-term nocturnal ventilation on spontaneous breathing during sleep in neuromuscular and chest wall disorders. Eur Respir J 1996;9:1515–22.

16. Tuggey JM, Elliott MW. Randomized crossover study of pressure and volume non-invasive ventilation in chest wall deformity. Thorax 2005;60:859–64.

17. Simonds AK, Elliott MW. Outcome of domiciliary nasal intermittent positive pressure ventilation in restrictive and obstructive disorders. Thorax 1995; 50:604–9.

18. Leger R, Bedicam JM, Cornetta A, et al. Nasal intermittent positive pressure ventilation: long term follow-up in patients with severe chronic respiratory insufficiency. Chest 1994;105:100–5.

19. Ward S, Chatwin M, Heather S, et al. Randomised controlled trial of non-invasive ventilation (NIV) for nocturnal hypoventilation in neuromuscular and chest wall disease patients with daytime normocapnia. Thorax 2005;60:1019–24.

20. Masa JF, Celli BR, Riesco JA, et al. Noninvasive positive pressure ventilation and not oxygen may prevent overt ventilatory failure in patients with chest wall disease. Chest 1997;112:207–13.

21. Tibballs J, Henning RD. Noninvasive ventilatory strategies in the management of a newborn infant and three children with congenital central hypoventilation syndrome. Pediatr Pulmonol 2003;36:544–8.

22. Ramesh P, Boit P, Samuels M. Mask ventilation in the early management of congenital central hypoventilation syndrome. Arch Dis Child Fetal Neonatal Ed 2008;93:F400–3.

23. Nielson DW, Black PG. Mask ventilation in congenital central alveolar hypoventilation syndrome. Pediatr Pulmonol 1990;9:44–5.

24. Ellis ER, Bye PT, Bruderer JW, et al. Treatment of respiratory failure during sleep in patients with neuromuscular disease. Positive-pressure ventilation through a nose mask. Am Rev Respir Dis 1987;135:148–52.

25. Gruis KL, Brown DL, Lisabeth LD, et al. Longitudinal assessment of noninvasive positive pressure ventilation adjustments in ALS patients. J Neurol Sci 2006; 247:59–63.

26. Toussaint M, Chatwin M, Soudon P. Mechanical ventilation in Duchenne patients with chronic respiratory insufficiency: clinical implications of 20 years published experience. Chron Respir Dis 2007;4:167–77.

27. Benditt JO. Respiratory complications of amyotrophic lateral sclerosis. Semin Respir Crit Care Med 2002;23:239–47.

28. Bourke SC, Bullock RE, Williams TL, et al. Noninvasive ventilation in ALS: indications and effect on quality of life. Neurology 2003;61:171–7.

29. Guilleminault C, Philip P, Robinson A. Sleep and neuromuscular disease: bilevel positive airway pressure by nasal mask as a treatment for sleep disordered breathing in patients with neuromuscular disease. J Neurol Neurosurg Psychiatry 1998;65:225–32.

30. Lechtzin N, Weiner CM, Clawson MC, et al. Use of noninvasive ventilation in patients with amyotrophic lateral sclerosis. Amyotroph Lateral Scler Other Motor Neuron Disord 2004;5:9–15.

31. Mellies U, Ragette R, Dohna Schwake C, et al. Long-term noninvasive ventilation in children and adolescents with neuromuscular disorders. Eur Respir J 2003;22:631–6.

32. Vianello A, Bevilacqua M, Salvador V, et al. Long-term nasal intermittent positive pressure ventilation in advanced Duchenne's muscular dystrophy. Chest 1994;105:445–8.

33. Katz S, Selvadurai H, Keilty K, et al. Outcome of noninvasive positive pressure ventilation in paediatric neuromuscular disease. Arch Dis Child 2004;89:121–4.

34. Jackson CE, Lovitt S, Gowda N, et al. Factors correlated with NPPV use in ALS. Amyotroph Lateral Scler 2006;7:80–5.

35. Berlowitz DJ, Detering K, Schachter L. A retrospective analysis of sleep quality and survival with domiciliary ventilatory support in motor neuron disease. Amyotroph Lateral Scler 2006;7:100–6.

36. Bach JR, Alba AS. Management of chronic alveolar hypoventilation by nasal ventilation. Chest 1990;97:52–7.

37. Alves RS, Resende MB, Skomro RP, et al. Sleep and neuromuscular disorders in children. Sleep Med Rev 2009;13:133–48.

38. Bourke SC, Tomlinson M, Williams TL, et al. Effects of non-invasive ventilation on survival and quality of life in patients with amyotrophic lateral sclerosis: a randomized controlled trial. Lancet Neurol 2006;5:140–7.

39. Perrin C, Unterborn JN, Ambrosio CD, et al. Pulmonary complications of chronic neuromuscular diseases and their management. Muscle Nerve 2004;29:5–27.

40. Ozsancak A, D'Ambrosio C, Hill NS. Nocturnal noninvasive ventilation. Chest 2008;133:1275–86.

41. Casey KR, Cantillo KO, Brown LK. Sleep-related hypoventilation/hypoxemic syndromes. Chest 2007;1318:1936–48.

42. Robert D, Argaud L. Non-invasive positive ventilation in the treatment of sleep-related breathing disorders. Sleep Med 2007;8:441–52.

43. Storre JH, Seuthe B, Fiechter R, et al. Average volume-assured pressure support in obesity hypoventilation: a randomized crossover trial. Chest 2006;130:815–21.

44. Ambrogio C, Lowman X, Kuo M, et al. Sleep and noninvasive ventilation in patients with chronic respiratory failure. Intensive Care Med 2009;35:306–13.

45. Janssens JP, Metzger M, Sforza E. Impact of volume targeting on efficacy of bi-level non-invasive ventilation and sleep in obesity hypoventilation syndrome. Respir Med 2009;103:165–72.

46. Sanders MH, Kern N. Obstructive sleep apnea treated by independently adjusted inspiratory and expiratory positive airway pressures via nasal mask. Physiologic and clinical implications. Chest 1990;98:317–24.

47. Parreira VF, Delguste P, Jounieaux V, et al. Effectiveness of controlled and spontaneous modes in nasal two-level positive pressure ventilation in awake and asleep normal subjects. Chest 1997;112:1267–77.

48. American College of Chest Physicians. Clinical indications for noninvasive positive pressure ventilation in chronic respiratory failure due to restrictive lung disease, COPD, and nocturnal hypoventilation – a consensus conference report. Chest 1999;116:521–34.

49. Iber C, Chesson A, Ancoli-Israel S, et al. The scoring of sleep and associated events rules, terminology, and technical specifications. 1st edition. Westchester (IL): American Academy of Sleep Medicine; 2007.

50. Berry RB, Sriram PS. Evaluation of hypoventilation. Semin Respir Crit Care Med 2009;30:303–14.

51. Lechtzin N, Wiener CM, Shade DM, et al. Spirometry in the supine position improves the detection of diaphragmatic weakness in patients with amyotrophic lateral sclerosis. Chest 2001;121:436–42.

52. Morgan RK, McNally S, Alexander M, et al. Use of sniff nasal-inspiratory force to predict survival in amyotrophic lateral sclerosis. Am J Respir Crit Care Med 2005;171:269–74.

53. Fanfulla F, Delmastro M, Berardinell A, et al. Effects of different ventilator settings on sleep and inspiratory effort in patients with neuromuscular disease. Am J Respir Crit Care Med 2005; 172:619–24.

54. Tuggey JM, Elliott MW. Titration of non-invasive positive ventilation in chronic respiratory failure. Respir Med 2006;100:1262–9.

55. Pankow W, Hijjeh N, Schullter F, et al. Influence of noninvasive positive pressure ventilation on inspiratory muscle activity in obese subjects. Eur Respir J 1997;10:2847–52.

56. Carrey Z, Gottfried SB, Levy RD. Ventilatory muscle support in respiratory failure with nasal positive pressure ventilation. Chest 1990;97:150–8.

57. White JES, Drinnan MJ, Smithson AJ, et al. Respiratory muscle activity and oxygenation during sleep in patients with muscle weakness. Eur Respir J 1995;8: 808–14.

58. Rains JC. Treatment of obstructive sleep apnea in pediatric patients. Behavioral intervention for compliance with nasal continuous positive airway pressure. Clin Pediatr (Phila) 1995;34:535–41.

59. Kirk VG, O'Donnell AR. Continuous positive airway pressure for children: a discussion on how to maximize compliance. Sleep Med Rev 2006;10:119–27.

60. Slifer KJ, Kruglak D, Benore E, et al. Behavioral training for increasing preschool children's adherence with positive airway pressure: a preliminary study. Behav Sleep Med 2007;5:147–75.

61. Lofaso F, Quera-Salva MA. Polysomnography for the management of progressive neuromuscular disorders. Eur Respir J 2001;19:989–90.

62. Weinberger J, Klefbeck, Borg J, et al. Polysomnography in chronic neuromuscular disease. Respiration 2003;62:349–54.

63. Fanfulla F, Taurino AE, Lupo ND, et al. Effect of sleep on patient/ventilator asynchrony in patients undergoing chronic non-invasive mechanical ventilation. Respir Med 2007;101:1702–7.

64. Meyer TJ, Pressman MR, Benditt J, et al. Air leaking through the mouth during nocturnal nasal ventilation: effect on sleep quality. Sleep 1997;20:561–9.

65. Teschler H, Stampa J, Ragette R, et al. Effect of mouth leak on effectiveness of nasal bilevel ventilatory assistance and sleep architecture. Eur Respir J 1999;14:1251–7.

66. Fauroux B, Lavis JF, Nicot F, et al. Facial side effects during noninvasive positive pressure ventilation in children. Intensive Care Med 2005;31:965–9.

67. Villa MP, Pagani J, Ambrosio R, et al. Mid-face hypoplasia after long-term nasal ventilation. Am J Respir Crit Care Med 2002;166:1142–3.

68. Storre JH, Steurer B, Kabitz HJ, et al. Transcutaneous Pco_2 monitoring during initiation of noninvasive ventilation. Chest 2007;132:1810–6.

69. Sanders MH, Kern NB, Costantino JP, et al. Accuracy of end-tidal and transcutaneous Pco_2 monitoring during sleep. Chest 1994;106:472–83.

70. Paiva R, Krivec U, Aubertin G, et al. Carbon dioxide monitoring during noninvasive respiratory support in children. Intensive Care Med 2009;35:1068–74.

71. Kirk VG, Batuyong ED, Bohn SG. Transcutaneous carbon dioxide monitoring and capnography during pediatric polysomnography. Sleep 2006; 29:1601–8.

72. Kushida CA, Littner MR, Hirshkowitz M, et al. Practice parameters for the use of continuous and bilevel positive airway pressure devices to treat adult patients with sleep-related breathing disorders. Sleep 2006;29:375–80.

73. Kushida CA, Chediak A, Berry RB, et al. Positive Airway Pressure Titration Task Force. American Academy of Sleep Medicine. Clinical guidelines for the manual titration of positive airway pressure in patients with obstructive sleep apnea. J Clin Sleep Med 2008;4:157–71.

74. Duong M, Jayram L, Camfferman D, et al. Use of heated humidification during nasal CPAP titration in obstructive sleep apnea syndrome. Eur Respir J 2005;26:679–85.

75. Wiest GH, Harsch IA, Fuchs FS, et al. Initiation of CPAP therapy for OSA: does prophylactic humidification during CPAP titration improve initial patient acceptance and comfort? Respiration 2002;69: 406–12.

76. Holland AE, Denehy L, Buchan CA, et al. Efficacy of a heated passover humidifier during noninvasive ventilation: a bench study. Respir Care 2007;52: 38–44.

77. Titration Protocol Philips-Respironics. 2007.

78. Thys F, Liistro G, Dozin O, et al. Determinants of Fio_2 with oxygen supplementation during noninvasive two-level positive pressure ventilation. Eur Respir J 2002;19:653–7.

79. Yoder EA, Klann K, Strohl KP. Inspired oxygen concentrations during positive pressure therapy. Sleep Breath 2004;8:1–5.

80. Schwartz AR, Kacmarek RM, Hess DR. Factors affecting oxygen delivery with bilevel positive airway pressure. Respir Care 2004;49:270–5.

81. Miyoshi E, Fujino Y, Uchiyama A, et al. Effects of gas leak on triggering function, humidification, and inspiratory oxygen fraction during noninvasive positive airway pressure ventilation. Chest 2005; 128:3691–8.

Index

Note: Page numbers of article titles are in **boldface** type.

sleep.theclinics.com

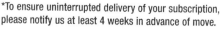

Printed and bound by CPI Group (UK) Ltd, Croydon, CR0 4YY

03/10/2024

01040357-0019